AF575019

Neurobrucellosis

Mehmet Turgut • Fuad Sami Haddad
Oreste de Divitiis
Editors

Neurobrucellosis

Clinical, Diagnostic and Therapeutic Features

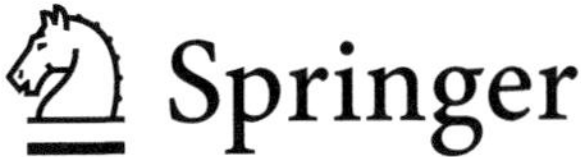

Editors
Mehmet Turgut
Department of Neurosurgery
Adnan Menderes University
School of Medicine
Aydin
Turkey

Fuad Sami Haddad[†]
Department of Surgery
American University of Beirut
Beirut
Lebanon

Oreste de Divitiis
Department of Neurosciences
Reproduction and Odontostomatological
Sciences
School of Medicine and Surgery
University of Naples Federico II
Naples
Italy

ISBN 978-3-319-24637-6 ISBN 978-3-319-24639-0 (eBook)
DOI 10.1007/978-3-319-24639-0

Library of Congress Control Number: 2015958921

Springer Cham Heidelberg New York Dordrecht London

Printed on acid-free paper

Springer International Publishing AG Switzerland is part of Springer Science+Business Media (www.springer.com)

This book is dedicated to the memory of Professor Fuad Sami Haddad, MD, FRCS (C), FACS, whose untimely death has saddened his colleagues and the scientific community. Professor Haddad, an eminent neurosurgeon in the Middle East, founded the Lebanese Society of Neurology, Neurosurgery and Psychiatry, the Middle East Neurosurgical Society, and the Arab Society of Neurological Sciences. He was an internationally recognized teacher of neurosurgery and a leader in Lebanon during the last half century. He was highly energetic and academically productive. He published his experience in highly respected journals and books. We found ourselves fortunate to work with him on our book, which is his latest scientific activity. Unfortunately, he passed away just before the publication of this book, which celebrates his outstanding contribution to science and humanity. Now it is clear to us that the written and published documents can be accepted as a reliable indicator of our accomplishments on earth.

Foreword

It is more than a hundred years since Themistocles Zammit showed that brucellosis could be transmitted to humans by milk from goats and that a simple test could show which goats were infected. Simple public health measures could reduce the risk of disease although these were difficult to apply in practice. Education of the public was difficult, and diagnosis of the disease has also been a problem for doctors as the symptoms are very difficult to separate from other diseases.

Even on the small islands of Malta, it has been a long struggle to eliminate the disease and to ensure that all goats are healthy. Humans are resistant to change and will subvert health measures when money is involved. Unnoticed outbreaks of the disease have occurred even when competent medical care was available. While it is possible to repeat that victory on other islands and communities, it is a dream which has been sadly disrupted by recent wars and conflicts around the Mediterranean. Refugees, displacement of hundreds of thousands into tented camps, and mass hunger and disease can mean that brucellosis is easily spread. Although infection is common among those who work with goats and their products, epidemics are also likely among whole populations.

Brucellosis is also common among wildlife animals in many countries and can be transmitted to unwary humans. This disease is widespread and will not be easily contained. It is difficult to diagnose and treat, so this new book about complications of the disease is most welcome.

Leeds, UK H.V. Wyatt

Preface

Brucellosis is still widely spread around the world especially in the Mediterranean basin, where it was first described, as well as in Central and South America. It has received a great deal of interest among the different scientific centers and a great deal has been written about it. However, brucellosis of the nervous system did not receive a similar wide interest in the current literature. This subject needs an in-depth study, reviewing all the aspects of the involvement of the central as well as the peripheral nervous systems. A book encompassing a review of the symptomatic as well as the therapeutic aspects of neurobrucellosis could fulfill an existing gap in the bibliography on the management of brucellosis of the nervous system.

In this multiauthored book, we shall try to cover the entire subject in depth, including the cranial, spinal, and peripheral systems, describing the presentations of this disease in these various areas as well as its treatment. With these ideas in mind, we tried at best to select authorities on the subject from different countries to obtain a global picture of the condition. The opinions of these authors are theirs and we cannot be accountable for their ideas or findings, although we share most of their opinions. We hope that this concise treatise may be helpful to the medical community and researchers in this field at large.

The book is divided into 21 chapters written by 44 specialists from the different countries of the Mediterranean basin, Europe, Asia, and Africa. It highlights the diagnosis, the course of the disease, and the management and prognosis in different parts of the nervous system, updating the literature on the prevention of complications of neurobrucellosis and also by including the authors' personal thoughts. The editors hope this book will be useful to neurosurgeons, neurologists, pediatric neurologists, radiologists, and residents.

Neurobrucellosis: Clinical, Diagnostic, and Therapeutic Features would not have been possible without the enthusiastic response from the contributors who shared their expertise. We sincerely thank them all. We would also like to express our appreciation to Springer personnel and specifically Claus-Dieter Bachem, Irmela Bohn, Sylvana Freyberg, and Antonia von Saint-Paul for their patience and experienced advice in the production of this book. Finally, we also thank our wives and children for their support and devotion.

Aydın, Turkey — Mehmet Turgut, MD, PhD
Beirut, Lebanon — Fuad Sami Haddad, MD, FACS, FRCS, ABNS
Naples, Italy — Oreste de Divitiis, MD

Contents

About the Editors

Mehmet Turgut, MD, PhD, graduated from the Ege University School of Medicine, İzmir, Turkey, in 1984 and later specialized in neurosurgery at the Hacettepe University Hospital, Ankara, Turkey. In 2004, he received a PhD degree from the Department of Embryology and Histology, Ege University Health Sciences Institute, İzmir, Turkey. He is currently Associate Professor in the Department of Neurosurgery, Adnan Menderes University School of Medicine, Aydın, Turkey. His fields of expertise and research interests are broad and include infectious diseases of the central nervous system, developmental neuroscience, pediatric neurosurgery, and peripheral nerve surgery. He spent time studying abroad during his early research career with grants from the DAAD (German Academic Exchange) and European Society for Stereotactic and Functional Neurosurgery (ESSFN). Dr. Turgut is an editorial board member for 20 international journals, including the *Journal of Neurological Surgery Part A*: *Central European Neurosurgery*, *Journal of Spine*, *Journal of Pediatric Neurology*, *Journal of Spine & Neurosurgery*, and *Journal of Neurosciences in Rural Practice*, and a reviewer for a wide range of international journals and research programs. He is the lead or coauthor of about 200 scientific publications as articles in international journals as well as many book chapters and other publications.

Fuad Sami Haddad† BA, MD, FRCS (C), FACS, graduated from the School of Medical Sciences at the American University in Beirut, Lebanon, in 1948, and trained in neurosurgery under Wilder Penfield at the Montreal Neurological Institute. When he returned to Beirut, towards the end of 1955, he was one of the first, if not the first, fully trained neurosurgeons in the Middle East. He returned to his alma mater where he reached the position of Clinical Professor of Neurosurgery and Chairman of the Department of Surgery. He held the position of Visiting Professor of Neurosurgery at many universities in the USA among others, the University of Chicago, the University of Iowa, the Cleveland Clinics, the University of New York, and the University of Arkansas. He was the founder of the Lebanese Society of Neurology, Neurosurgery, and Psychiatry, the Middle East Neurosurgical Society, the Lebanese Society for the Welfare of the Physically Disabled, Le Club International de Neurochirurgie, the Lebanon Chapter of the American College of Surgery, the Arab Society of Neurological Sciences, the World Association of Lebanese Neurosurgeons, and the Lebanese Society of

Surgical Neurologists. He held the position of Editor in Chief of the Lebanese Medical Journal. He is at present retired from medical practice. He has written many scientific articles (over 160) and several books and edited others.

Oreste de Divitiis, MD, graduated from the Federico II University School of Medicine in Naples, Italy, in 1992 and subsequently specialized in neurosurgery at the La Statale University School of Medicine in Milan, Italy. Since 2005, he has been Associate Professor in the Division of Neurosurgery, Federico II University, School of Medicine, in Naples, Italy, where he holds the position of Chief of the Oncological Microneurosurgical Department. In 2008, he spent time abroad, including at the Institute of Anatomy of the University of Vienna and the International Neuroscience Institute of Hannover, Germany. His fields of expertise and research interests are broad and include oncological neurosurgery, spinal neurosurgery, infectious diseases of the central nervous system, and peripheral nerve surgery. Dr. de Divitiis is an editorial board member of international journals including *World Neurosurgery* and *Indian Neurology* and is a reviewer for a wide range of international journals and research programs. He is the lead or coauthor of numerous publications in international journals as well as many book chapters and other publications.

Contributors

Farhad Abbasi, MD Department of Infectious Diseases, Bushehr University of Medical Sciences, Bushehr, Iran

Sadaf Anwar, MBBCh, PGDCC Department of Cardiology, National Heart Institute New Delhi, New Delhi, India

George F. Araj, PhD, D(ABMM), FAAM Department of Pathology and Laboratory Medicine, American University of Beirut Medical Center, Beirut, Lebanon

Rouf Asimi, MD, DM Department of Neurology, SKIMS Kashmir, Kashmir, India

Gull Mohammad Bhat, MD, DM Department of Medical Oncology, SKIMS Kashmir, Kashmir, India

Recep Brohi, MD Department of Neurosurgery, State Hospital, Ankara, Turkey

Chiara Caggiano, MD Department of Neurosciences and Reproductive and Odontostomatological Sciences, School of Medicine and Surgery, Università degli Studi di Napoli Federico II, Naples, Italy

Ana Cerván, MD Department of Orthopedic Surgery and Traumatology, Hospital Universitario Costa del Sol., University of Malaga, Marbella (Málaga), Spain

Michelangelo de Angelis, MD Department of Neurosciences and Reproductive and Odontostomatological Sciences, School of Medicine and Surgery, University of Naples Federico II, Naples, Italy

Oreste de Divitiis, MD Department of Neurosciences, Reproduction and Odontostomatological Sciences, School of Medicine and Surgery, University of Naples Federico II, Naples, Italy

Pelin Demir, MD Department of Radiology, Numune Training and Research Hospital, Ankara, Turkey

Andrea Elefante, MD Department of Advanced Biomedical Sciences, School of Medicine and Surgery, University of Naples Federico II, Naples, Italy

Department of Advanced Biomedical Sciences, "Federico II" University, Naples, Italy

Fatih Erdi, MD Department of Neurosurgery, Necmettin Erbakan University, Meram Faculty of Medicine, Konya, Turkey

Ersen Ertekin, MD, PhD Department of Radiology, Adnan Menderes University School of Medicine, Aydın, Turkey

Francesco Faella, MD, PhD I Division of Infectious Diseases, Department of Infectious Diseases, "D. Cotugno" Hospital, AORN "Dei Colli", Naples, Italy

Enrique Guerado, MD, PhD, MSc Department of Orthopedic Surgery and Traumatology, Hospital Universitario Costa del Sol., University of Malaga, Marbella (Málaga), Spain

Güliz Uyar Güleç, MD Department of Infectious Diseases, Adnan Menderes University School of Medicine, Aydın, Turkey

Fuad Sami Haddad, MD, FACS, FRCS, ABNS Department of Surgery, American University of Beirut, Beirut, Lebanon

Miguel Hirschfeld, MD Department of Orthopedic Surgery and Traumatology, Hospital Universitario Costa del Sol., University of Malaga, Marbella (Málaga), Spain

Roula Hourani, MD Department of Diagnostic Radiology, American University of Beirut Medical Center, Beirut, Lebanon

Basharat Mujtaba Jan, MS Department of Neurosurgery, SKIMS Kashmir, Kashmir, India

Erdal Kalkan, MD Department of Neurosurgery, Necmettin Erbakan University, Meram Faculty of Medicine, Konya, Turkey

Saliha Kanık-Yüksek, MD Department of Pediatric Infectious Disease, Ankara Hematology Oncology Children's Training and Research Hospital, Ankara, Turkey

Bülent Kaya, MD Department of Neurosurgery, Necmettin Erbakan University, Meram Faculty of Medicine, Konya, Turkey

Dheeraj Khurana, MD Department of Neurology, Postgraduate Institute of Medical Education and Research, Chandigarh, India

Soolmaz Korooni, MD Department of Internal Medicine, Bushehr University of Medical Sciences, Bushehr, Iran

Ebru Kursun, MD Department of Infectious Diseases and Clinical Microbiology, Baskent University School of Medicine, Ankara, Turkey

Huwayda Murad, MD Department of Diagnostic Radiology, American University of Beirut Medical Center, Beirut, Lebanon

Hamid Reza Naderi, MD Department of Infectious Diseases, Mashhad University of Medical Sciences, Mashhad, Iran

Marzieh Nojomi, MD, MPH Department of Community Medicine, Iran University of Medical Sciences, Tehran, Iran

Roopa Rajan, MD Department of Neurology, Postgraduate Institute of Medical Education and Research, Chandigarh, India

Mitra Ranjbar, MD Department of Infectious Diseases, Iran University of Medical Sciences, Tehran, Iran

Miguel Rodriguez, MD Department of Orthopedic Surgery and Traumatology, Hospital Universitario Costa del Sol., University of Malaga, Marbella (Málaga), Spain

Stylianos Roupakias, MD Department of Pediatric Surgery, University of Patras, Patras, Greece

Arif Hussain Sarmast, MS Department of Neurosurgery, SKIMS Kashmir, Kashmir, India

Hakim Irfan Showkat, MBBCh, MD, DNB Department of Cardiology, National Heart Institute New Delhi, New Delhi, India

Xenophon Sinopidis, MD, PhD Department of Pediatric Surgery, University of Patras, Patras, Greece

Teresa Somma, MD Department of Neurosciences and Reproductive and Odontostomatological Sciences, School of Medicine and Surgery, Università degli Studi di Napoli Federico II, Naples, Italy

Abbas Tafakhori, MD Department of Neurology, Imam Khomeini Hospital, Tehran University of Medical Sciences, Tehran, Iran

Enrico Tedeschi, MD Department of Advanced Biomedical Sciences, School of Medicine and Surgery, Università degli Studi di Napoli Federico II, Naples, Italy

Naime Altınkaya Tokmak, MD Department of Radiology, Baskent University School of Medicine, Ankara, Turkey

Ahmet Tuncay Turgut, MD Department of Radiology, Hacettepe University School of Medicine, Ankara, Turkey

Mehmet Turgut, MD, PhD Department of Neurosurgery, Adnan Menderes University School of Medicine, Aydın, Turkey

Venugopalan Y. Vishnu, MD Department of Neurology, Postgraduate Institute of Medical Education and Research, Chandigarh, India

Part I

General Considerations

Historical Preview

1

Fuad Sami Haddad†

Contents

Abstract

A review of the historical landmarks of neurobrucellosis is given starting in 1861 with Allen Marston and going up to the present days mentioning the landmark through that period. It includes the contributions of Allen Marston, David Bruce, Mathews Hughes, Bernhard Bang, Almroth Wright, Themistocles Zammit and Caruana Scicluna.

Keywords

Brucella • Brucellosis • Bang's disease • Mediterranean gastric remittent fever

Abbreviations

CNS Central nervous system

1.1 Introduction

Brucellosis is a zoonotic infection caused by an intracellular bacterium of the genus *Brucella* [7, 9, 11]. It is transmitted to humans through the ingestion of infected milk or its raw products as well as by direct contact with infected animals. First historical reports of this disease have been described between the end of the nineteenth and the beginning of the twentieth century. Surgeon-General

† Author was deceased at the time of publication.

F.S. Haddad, MD, FACS, FRCS, ABNS
Department of Surgery, American University of Beirut, Beirut, Lebanon
e-mail: fshaddad@aub.edu.lb

M. Turgut et al. (eds.), *Neurobrucellosis: Clinical, Diagnostic and Therapeutic Features*,
DOI 10.1007/978-3-319-24639-0_1

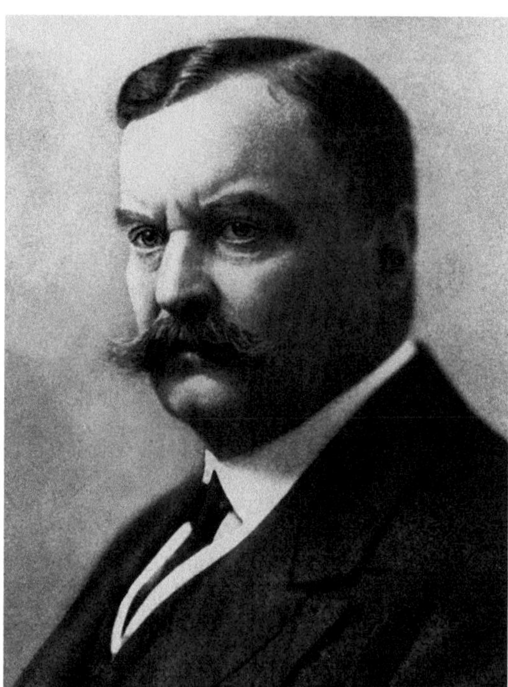

Fig. 1.1 Photograph of Major General Sir David Bruce (From https://en.wikipedia.org/wiki/David_Bruce_(microbiologist))

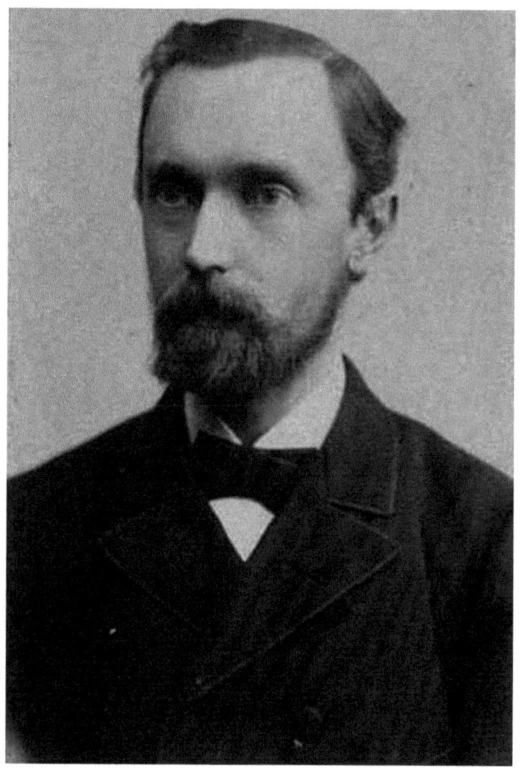

Fig. 1.2 Photograph of Bernard Lauritz Frederik Bang (From https://commons.wikimedia.org/wiki/File:Bernhard_Bang_2.jpg))

Jefferey Allen Marston (1832–1911), in 1861, shortly after leaving Malta, contracted a fever which prevailed in that island and he described it in great the first time, hence the eponym of this condition Malta fever [10]; he called this condition "Mediterranean gastric remittent fever". In 1887, General Sir David Bruce (1855–1931) was the first to isolate the organism from the spleen of a cadaver who had died from this disease (Fig. 1.1) [4]. A year later, he named it *Micrococcus melitensis* [5]. This genus was later renamed by Karl Meyer, a veterinary scientist at the Hooper Foundation in San Francisco, "*Brucella*", in honour of Dr. Bruce [6].

Surgeon-Captain Mathews Louis Hughes (1867–1899), in 1897, isolated the organism from the meninges of a patient who had died as a consequence of this infection. This same year, Bernhard Lauritz Frederik Bang (1848–1932) isolated the organism, now known as *Brucella abortus* (Fig. 1.2) [3]. This is why brucellosis is also known as Bang's disease. That same year, Sir Almroth Edward Wright (1861–1947) developed a specific agglutination diagnostic test named after him. In 1905, Themistocles Zammit (1864–1935) found Malta fever to be transmitted to humans through goat's milk [16]. In 1986, George F Araj (1947–) developed a *Brucella-specific* enzyme-linked immunosorbent assay test for the rapid and accurate diagnosis of brucellosis involving the peripheral or central nervous system (CNS) [1].

1.2 History of Brucellosis

This is the well-known part of the history of brucellosis. Nevertheless, the other side of the coin is described by Edwards and Jawad (2006) [8] in a comment on an article by Dr. H Vivian Wyatt [15] in the *Journal of the Royal Society of Medicine* of October 2005, where they say, "First, Dr. Carruana-Secluna (the proper spelling is 'Scicluna', editor's note) who accompanied Zammit to Chadwick

Lakes, carried out a great deal of work for Sir David Bruce-he prepared the agar plates and the culture media and cultured the causative organism from the spleen samples of fatal cases. He never received proper recognition for his work and Sir David Bruce did not allow him to be co-author on any of his publications. Secondly, Surgeon Captain Matthew Louis Hughes assisted Bruce in his studies and first named the disease 'undulant fever'. He also named the organism Micrococcus melitensis, although he was wrong about the source of infection, believing it to be resident in the soil and inhaled by humans." Hughes was killed in the Boer war at the age of 32.

Sir David's wife, Lady Bruce née Mary Elizabeth Steele, was a trained microbiologist and helped her husband's research, drawing the fine illustrations to his papers.

Towards the middle of last century, the commonest species that infected humans in the States was *B. abortus*. The infection with this species is a self-limited condition. *B. melitensis* was less frequent. Other species, like *B. suis*, are rare in humans. At present, most human infections are related to *B. melitensis* [12]. A case of marine mammal neurobrucellosis has been reported in a laboratory technician working on this strain [14]. This disease is on the decrease around the world, but it is still an important affliction in Central and South America and especially in the Mediterranean basin. It is characterized by fever which is usually recurrent in nature, hence its eponym "recurrent undulant fever". It is a protean condition and may affect a large number of the body organs. The CNS is one of its important localization, thus neurobrucellosis has become, along with cardiac brucellosis, an important clinical group. Neurobrucellosis is estimated, by some, at 10 % of the total numbers of *Brucella* cases [7, 13]; others estimate it at 8 % [2] and some at less than 5 % [8] and still others as low as 1.7 % [6].

1.3 Neurobrucellosis

Under the heading of neurobrucellosis, we shall include not only the CNS but also its coverings, as well as its appendages; hence, it shall include the scalp and the skull as well as the vertebrae, the dura mater with its epidural and subdural spaces. In the brain and spinal cord, it may involve their substance in the form of encephalitis and myelitis. It may grow masses and abscesses within the brain or the spinal cord. It may affect the vascular system of both brain and spinal cord. Afterwards, it may affect the patient's psyche and behaviour.

Neurobrucellosis in all these locations as well as their diagnosis and treatment shall be discussed in the book by specialists, each in his or her respective field.

Conclusion

In conclusion, it is fair to say that the history of neurobrucellosis has been described in many a varied way and that different persons claimed different rights. We have tried to simplify this history and give, what we thought, was a fair account of this history.

References

1. Araj GF, Lulu AR, Saadeh MA, Mousa AM, Strannegard IL, Shakir RA (1986) Rapid diagnosis of central nervous system brucellosis by ELISA. J Neuroimmunol 12:173–182
2. Asadipooya K, Dehghanian A, Omrani GHR, Abbasi F (2011) Short course treatment in neurobrucellosis: a study in Iran. Neurol India 59:101–103
3. Bang B (1897) The aetiology of porcine infection warping (in German). Verwerfens Ztschr f Tiermed 1:241
4. Bruce D (1887) Note on the discovery of a microorganism in Malta fever. Practitioner 39:161–170
5. Bruce D (1888) The micrococcus of Malta Fever. Practitioner 40:241–249
6. Colmenero JD, Reguera JM, Martos F, Sanchez-De-Mora D, Delgado M, Causse M, Martin-Farfan A, Juarez C (1996) Complications associated with Brucella melitensis infection: a study of 530 cases. Medicine (Baltimore) 75:195–211
7. Demiroğlu YZ, Turunç T, Karaca S, Arlıer Z, Alışkan H, Colakoğlu S, Arslan H (2011) Neurological involvement in brucellosis; clinical classification, treatment and results. Mikrobiyol Bul 45:401–410
8. Edwards C, Jawad ASM (2006) History of brucellosis. J R Soc Med 99:54
9. Haji-Abdolbagi M, Rasooli-Nejad M, Yaghoubzadeh M, LoutiShahrokh B (2001) Epidemiological, clinical, diagnostic, and therapeutic survey in 505 cases with brucellosis. J Tehran Facul Med 4:34–46

10. Marston JA (1861) Report on Fever (Malta), medical report for 1861. Army Medical Department, London, pp 486–521
11. Spink WW (1952) Some biologic and clinical problems related to intracellular parasitism in brucellosis. N Engl J Med 247:603–610
12. Spink WW (1953) Observations on brucellosis due to Brucella melitensis. Bull World Health Organ 9:385–398
13. Spink WW (1956) The nature of brucellosis. University of Minnesota Press, Minneapolis
14. Sohn AH, Probert WS, Glaser CA, Gupta N, Bollen AW, Wong JD, Grace EM, McDonald WC (2003) Human neurobrucellosis with intracerebral granuloma caused by a marine mammal Brucella spp. Emerg Infect Dis 9:485–488
15. Wyatt HV (2005) How Themistocles Zammit found Malta Fever (brucellosis) to be transmitted by the milk of goats. J R Soc Med 98:451–454
16. Wyatt HV (2009) Brucellosis and Maltese goats in the Mediterranean. J Maltese Hist 1:1–15

2 Human Brucellosis and Its Complications

George F. Araj

Contents

Abstract

Brucellosis has been an important zoonotic disease globally. Since *Brucella* can infect and survive without inducing a massive inflammatory response, this bacteria was labeled as "stealth pathogen." Its protean and diverse clinical presentation can mimic other infectious and noninfectious diseases, posing challenges to physicians in reaching a diagnosis, and merited the label "disease of mistakes." The complications of brucellosis are common and can involve a wide range of body organs and localization, neurobrucellosis being among the most serious ones. Awareness about the disease and the use of appropriate *Brucella*-specific tests can expedite the accurate diagnosis.

Keywords

Clinical features • Complications • Diagnosis • Human brucellosis

Abbreviations

BCV *Brucella*-containing vacuoles
CSF Cerebrospinal fluid

G.F. Araj, PhD, D(ABMM), FAAM
Department of Pathology and Laboratory Medicine, American University of Beirut Medical Center, PO Box 11-0236, Beirut 1107-2020, Lebanon
e-mail: garaj@aub.edu.lb

M. Turgut et al. (eds.), *Neurobrucellosis: Clinical, Diagnostic and Therapeutic Features*, DOI 10.1007/978-3-319-24639-0_2

2.1 Introduction

The medical literature is flooded with numerous studies from different parts of the world, especially those endemic with brucellosis, addressing the clinical and complication aspects of this most widespread zoonotic disease. Among a considerable number of papers published on this topic, there is a shortlist that we can consider as landmark in this field [8, 10–15, 25–28, 30, 37, 40]. On a more specific aspect dealing with neurobrucellosis, a couple of studies on this critical complication have been well noted in the literature [18, 35].

Though the clinical and complication aspects have not changed, brucellosis remains a significant zoonotic disease that is emerging or reemerging in many parts of the world. In addition, the inclusion of *Brucella* spp. in the potential biological weapon lists of most authorities has renewed interest in this these pathogens [17]. However, the improved knowledge and awareness, as well as the introduction of newer technology and tests, have helped detect and reveal more of such episodes in a short time [1, 3].

Whatever is presented in this chapter essentially refers to the above noted studies.

2.2 Disease Synonyms and *Brucella* Species

Brucellosis has been known with many synonyms mainly pertaining to the geographic locations where the disease occurred, e.g., Malta fever, Gibraltar fever, Mediterranean fever, and Cyprus fever [21].

Brucella spp. are common zoonoses among domestic animals and wildlife and have been recovered from marine mammals. Though over 10 *Brucella* spp. have been recognized, only four have been well recognized to cause human infections, and, together with their preferred/predominant host, they are *B. melitensis* (mostly in goats, sheep, and camels), *B. abortus* (mostly in cattle), *B. suis* (mostly in swine), and *B. canis* (in dogs). *Brucella* spp. recovered from marine animals were reported to cause human infections [21].

2.3 Virulence and Pathogenicity

The descriptive characteristics of *Brucella* spp. include small gram-negative coccobacilli, live intracellularly, and are facultative in aeration. In endemic area, the infection is mostly acquired by ingestion of fresh unpasteurized milk or its products, while in the nonendemic areas, it is mainly occupational due to accidents at clinical or research laboratories and contacts with infected laboratory animals.

The incubation period may be long but the symptoms can appear in a short time (within 1–4 weeks). Once the organisms enter the body by various routes, they are encountered by the polymorphonuclear and mononuclear phagocytes. The intracellular location contributes to their virulence and pathogenesis, as they preferentially replicate within phagocytic cells. *Brucella* uses several mechanisms to avoid being killed and establish a survival niche within macrophages. To help evade the immune system and facilitate propagation, and persistence within macrophages and other cells, the pathogen forms *Brucella-containing* vacuoles (BCV) and inhibits the phagosome-lysosome. Subsequently, they are transported through regional lymph nodes into the circulatory system to seed and involve a wide range of body organs or systems, with tropism for the reticuloendothelial system, resulting in different clinical phases of disease [22].

Though receiving close attention, the exact nature of the immune response and protective antigens/factors involved in this disease are still being investigated, and the pathogenic mechanisms of reinfection remain unknown. Recently, the production of cytokines, chemokines, and matrix metalloproteinases has been associated with induced osteoclastogenesis in *Brucella* arthritis and osteomyelitis, and the outer membrane protein 19 lipoprotein, together with tumor necrosis factor-alpha, was reported to be associated with astrocyte apoptosis in neurobrucellosis [9].

Since *Brucella* can infect and survive without inducing a massive inflammatory response, this bacteria was labeled as "stealth pathogen" [22, 29].

2.4 Epidemiology and Transmission

Though present worldwide, *Brucella* spp. endemicity is well noted in many regions such as the Arabian Peninsula, Middle East, eastern Mediterranean basin, Latin America, Southern Europe, Central Asia, and the Indian subcontinent [16].

Globally, around 500,000 cases are reported annually. Because of nonspecific presentation of its signs and symptom features, it is estimated that for each reported case, 25 cases are not reported [41].

In many countries, brucellosis remains continuing or reemerging causing significant economic losses, not only from cost associated with clinical treatment and lost productivity in human infections but also by economic costs associated with reproductive losses in livestock [31].

Animals are generally asymptomatic carriers of these bacteria, and the major symptoms appear during infectious abortion of the animal fetus and placenta. In humans, its epidemiology differs between areas of endemicity and nonendemicity in terms of age, sex, season, and risk factors. In regions of endemicity, the disease occurs among the general population, with the levels of infection being almost equal among adults and children of both sexes and mostly due to ingestion of unpasteurized dairy products (e.g., soft cheese, ice cream) from goat, sheep, cow, and camel [26, 34].

In nonendemic areas, infection is seen predominantly among adult males, acquired occupationally by handling or manipulating infected animals or cultures of the pathogen and by transmission through direct skin contact (e.g., accidental inoculation through skin cuts and abrasions) and through inhalation of infected aerosols or aerosols inoculated into the eye, mouth, and nose. These infections occur mostly among dairy industry professionals, veterinarians, abattoir workers, and clinical and research microbiology staff. Most cases of laboratory-acquired disease result from mishandling and misidentification of the organism [38].

2.5 Clinical Categories: Features and Complications of Human Brucellosis

Infection of humans with *Brucella* spp. ranges from asymptomatic to full-blown clinical features. Among the latter, different criteria has been suggested to define clinical categories of human brucellosis. For example, in 1956, Spink [37] based them on the duration of symptoms: acute (presentation ≤2 months), subacute (2–12 months), and chronic (≥12 months). Subsequently, others based them primarily on extent of clinical manifestations (e.g., subclinical, localized, chronic, and active, with or without localized disease, including bacteremic and serological classifications) [13, 27, 41]. It is interesting to note that the variation in the incident rates of clinical presentation and complications reported among different published studies can be attributed to the lack of consensus/uniform categorization definition used.

Brucella has a very low infectious dose ($\leq 10^2$ organisms) and a variable incubation period. The disease onset is insidious and can present with a diverse range of over 30 nonspecific clinical signs and symptoms mainly fever, weakness, malaise, headache, sweats, joint manifestations, myalgia,, fatigue, cough, loss of appetite, weight loss, hepatomegaly, and splenomegaly. All these can be present but at variable rates in the acute, subacute, or chronic clinical categories [11, 26].

2.6 Complications

Brucellosis complications can involve different body sites with common localization. The routine hematology and biochemical profiles are usually within normal limits. Some elevation in liver function tests and erythrocyte sedimentation rate can be noted [11, 15, 19, 26, 28, 32, 40].

Complications of human brucellosis remains medically problematic and challenging [11, 26, 32]. They present in diverse features and can occur at variable rates in the acute, subacute, or chronic clinical categories [26]. The variability in the reported rates among different studies could be attributed to the variable delay in the diagnosis of brucellosis [3, 26].

The most involved sites of *Brucella* complications include the joints and bone, genitals of males and females, neurological, cardiac, pulmonary, and renal. Mortality is very low (<1 %) and is almost exclusively due to cardiac complications [12, 13, 26–28, 39].

2.6.1 Osteoarticular Complications

Osteoarticular complications occur mostly as arthritis (10–70 %) and rarely as osteomyelitis (<1 %). The joints most frequently involved are, in descending order, sacroiliac, knee, hip, vertebra, ankle, and multiple other joints. Generally, *Brucella* arthritis can be misdiagnosed as rheumatoid arthritis, rheumatic fever, tuberculosis, and systemic lupus erythematosus [12, 26].

2.6.2 Neurobrucellosis

Neurobrucellosis (detected in 3–5 % of patients with brucellosis) can affect both adults and children with diverse presentations, including fever, headache, meningeal signs, coma, or paresis. Depression, psychosis, and mental fatigue are not uncommon complaints [18, 24, 35]. Manifestations of neurobrucellosis include meningitis, meningoencephalitis, brain or epidural abscess, and demyelinating disorders [23].

Cerebrospinal (CSF) analysis, of both adults and children, is nonspecific and can overlap with other central nervous system diseases, such as mycobacterial, viral, syphilitic, tuberculous, or fungal infections, or with noninfectious diseases, such as psychiatric problems, multiple sclerosis, and cancer [35]. The yield of *Brucella* culture from CSF is low (5–30 %). Therefore, the use of *Brucella* serology tests, especially indirect Coombs', Brucellacapt, or enzyme-linked immunosorbent assay, on CSF specimens is essential to diagnose neurobrucellosis [2–6, 35]. With appropriate treatment, the prognosis is usually good for acute presentations and varies in the setting of chronic disease.

2.6.3 Genital Complications

Genital complications in males (6–8 % of cases) are mostly orchitis or epididymo-orchitis [11, 26]. Other rare complications reported for females include cervicitis, salpingitis, tubo-ovarian abscess, and ovarian dermoid cyst.

2.6.4 Relapse

Relapse is considered one of the most important features of brucellosis and its complications. The exact factors associated with relapse remain to be determined but some were noted to include positive blood culture, ineffective therapy, and ≤10 days' duration of symptoms before initiation of treatment [7, 11, 36].

2.7 Prevention

Vaccines have been successful in the control of livestock infections, which can subsequently reduce infections in humans. Most veterinary vaccines focus on live, attenuated strains, namely, strains S 19 and RB51 of *B. abortus* for cows, strain Rev-1 of *B. melitensis* for sheep and goats, and strain 2 of *B. suis* for swine. However, the developed vaccine for humans still suffers from limited efficacy and serious medical reactions [33]. Heating of dairy products and related foods has also been effective in preventing disease transmission. The most cost-effective approach to control and prevent brucellosis relies on raising public awareness about the disease and having the human and animal health sectors consolidate their efforts and cooperation in this regard [20].

Conclusion

The diversified clinical presentations and complications of brucellosis especially neurobrucellosis necessitate awareness to consider this disease in the differential diagnosis. Requesting the appropriate and *Brucella* relevant tests on blood and CSF would help provide the specific diagnosis.

References

1. Al Dahouk S, Sprague LD, Neubauer H (2013) New developments in the diagnostic procedures for zoonotic brucellosis in humans. Rev Sci Tech 32:177–188
2. Araj GF (1997) Enzyme linked immunosorbent assay, not agglutination test is the test of choice for the diagnosis of neurobrucellosis (letter). Clin Infect Dis 25:942
3. Araj GF (2010) Update on laboratory diagnosis of human brucellosis. Int J Antimicrob Agents 36(suppl 1): S12–S17
4. Araj GF, Lulu AR, Khateeb MI, Saadah MA, Shakir RA (1988) ELISA versus routine tests in the diagnosis of patients with systemic and neurobrucellosis. Acta Pathol Microbiol Scand 96:171–176
5. Araj GF, Lulu AR, Mustafa MY, Khateeb MI (1986) Evaluation of ELISA in the diagnosis of acute and chronic brucellosis in human beings. J Hyg (London) 97:457–469
6. Araj GF, Lulu AR, Saadah MA, Mousa AM, Strannegard I-L, Shakir RA (1986) Rapid diagnosis of central nervous system brucellosis by ELISA. J Neuroimmunol 12:173–182
7. Ariza J, Corredoira J, Pallares R, Vilarich PF, Rufi G, Pujol M, Gudiol F (1995) Characteristics of and risk factors for relapse of brucellosis in humans. Clin Infect Dis 20:1241–1249
8. Aygen B, Doĝanay M, Sümerkan B, Yildiz O, Kayabaş U (2002) Clinical manifestations, complications and treatment of brucellosis: a retrospective evaluation of 480 patients. Med Mal Infect 32:485–493
9. Baldi PC, Giambartolomei GH (2013) Immunopathology of Brucella infection. Recent Pat Antiinfect Drug Discov 8:18–26
10. Barroso Garcia P, Rodriguez-Contreras Pelayo R, Gil Extremera B, Maldonado Martin A, GuilarroHeratas G, Martin Salguero A, Baron Carreno T (2002) Study of 1595 brucellosis cases in the Almeria province (1972–1998) based on epidemiological data from disease reporting. Rev Clin Esp 202:577–582
11. Buzgan T, Karahocagil MK, Irmak H, Baran AI, Karsen H, Evirgen O, Akdeniz H (2010) Clinical manifestations and complications in 1028 cases of brucellosis: a retrospective evaluation and review of the literature. Int J Infect Dis 14:e469–e478
12. Colmenero JD, Reguera JM, Martos F, Sanchez-De-Mora D, Delgado M, Causse M, Martin-Farafan A, Juarez C (1996) Complications associated with Brucella melitensis infection: a study of 530 cases. Medicine (Baltimore) 75:195–211
13. Corbel MJ (1997) Brucellosis: an overview. Emerg Infect Dis 3:213–221
14. Dalrymple-Champneys W (1960) Clinical features, Brucella infection and undulant fever in man. Oxford University Press, London
15. Dean A, Crump L, Greter H, Hattendorf J, Schelling E, Zinsstag J (2012) Clinical manifestations of human brucellosis: a systematic review and meta-analysis. PLoS Negl Trop Dis 6, e1929. doi:10.1371/journal.pntd.0001929
16. Dean A, Crump L, Greter H, Schelling E, Zinsstag J (2012) Global burden of human brucellosis: a systematic review of disease frequency. PLoS Negl Trop Dis 6, e1865. doi:10.1371/journal.pntd.0001865
17. Doganay G, Doganay M (2013) Brucella as a potential agent of bioterrorism. Recent Pat Antiinfect Drug Discov 8:27–33
18. Erdem H, Ulu-Kilic A, Kilic S, Karahocagil M, Shehata G, Eren-Tulek N, Yetkin F, Celen MK, Ceran N, Gul H, Mert G, Tekin-Koruk S, Dizbay M, Inal A, Nayman-Alpat S, Bosilkovski M, Inan D, Saltoglu N, Abdel-Baky L, Adeva-Bartolome MT, Ceylan B, Sacar S, Turhan V, Yılmaz E, Elaldi N, Kocak-Tufan Z, Uğurlu K, Dokuzoğuz B, Yılmaz H, Gundes S, Guner R, Ozgunes N, Ulcay A, Unal S, Dayan S, Gorenek L, Karakas A, Tasova Y, Usluer G, Bayindir Y, Kurtaran B, Sipahi O, Leblebicioglu H (2011) Efficacy and tolerability of antibiotic combinations in neurobrucellosis: results of the Istanbul Study. Antimicrob Agents Chemother 56:1523–1528
19. Franco MP, Mulder M, Gilman RH, Smits HL (2007) Human brucellosis. Lancet Infect Dis 7:775–786
20. Godfroid J, AlDahouk S, Pappas G, Roth F, Matope G, Mama J, Marcotty T, Pfeiffer D, Skjerve E (2013) A "One Health" surveillance and control of brucellosis in developing countries: moving away from improvisation. Comp Immunol Microbiol Infect Dis 36:241–248
21. Godfroid J, Cloeckaert A, Liautard JP, Kohler S, Fretin D, Walravens K, Garin-Bastuji B, Letesson JJ (2005) From the discovery of the Malta fever's agent to the discovery of a marine mammal reservoir, brucellosis has continuously been a re-emerging zoonosis. Vet Res 36:313–326
22. Gorvel J-P (2014) "If you bring an alarm, we will destroy it", said Brucella to the host cell. Virulence 5:460–462
23. Gul HC, Erdem H, Bek S (2009) Overview of neurobrucellosis: a pooled analysis of 187 cases. Int J Infect Dis 13:e339–e343
24. Guven T, Ugurlu K, Ergonul O, Celikbas AK, Gok SE, Comoglu S, Baykam N, Dokuzoguz B (2013) Neurobrucellosis: clinical and diagnostic features. Clin Infect Dis 56:1407–1412
25. HasanjaniRoushan MR, Mohrez M, SmailnejadGangi SM, SolemaniAmiri MJ, Hajiahmadi M (2004) Epidemiological features and clinical manifestations in 469 adult patients with brucellosis in Babol, Northern Iran. Epidemiol Infect 132:1109–1114
26. Lulu AR, Araj GF, Khateeb MI, Mustafa MY, Yusuf AR, Fenech FF (1988) Human brucellosis in Kuwait: a prospective study of 400 cases. Q J Med 66:39–54
27. Madkour MM (1989) Brucellosis. Butterworths, London
28. Mantur BG, Amarnath SK, Shinde RS (2007) Review of clinical and laboratory features of human brucellosis. Indian J Med Microbiol 25:188–202

29. Martirosyan A, Moreno E, Gorvel JP (2011) An evolutionary strategy for a stealthy intracellular Brucella pathogen. Immunol Rev 240:211–234
30. Memish Z, Mah MW, Al Mahmoud S, Al Shaalan M, Khan MY (2000) Brucella bacteraemia: clinical and laboratory observations in 160 patients. J Infect 40:59–63
31. Olsen SC, Palmer MV (2014) Advancement of knowledge of Brucella over the past 50 years. Vet Pathol 51:1076–1089
32. Pappas G, Akritidis N, Bosilkovski M, Tsianos E (2005) Brucellosis. N Engl J Med 352:2325–2336
33. Perkins SB, Smither SJ, Atkins HS (2010) Towards a Brucella vaccine for humans. FEMS Microbiol Rev 34:379–394
34. Rubach MP, Halliday JE, Cleaveland S, Crump JA (2013) Brucellosis in low-income and middle-income countries. Curr Opin Infect Dis 26:404–412
35. Shakir RA, Al-Din ASN, Araj GF, Lulu AR, Mousa AR, Saadah MA (1987) Clinical categories of neurobrucellosis: a report on 19 cases. Brain 110:213–223
36. Solera J, Martinez-Alfaro E, Espinosa A, Castillejos ML, Geijo P, Rodriguez-Zapata M (1998) Multivariate model for predicting relapse in human brucellosis. J Infect 36:85–92
37. Spink WW (1956) The nature of brucellosis. University of Minnesota Press, Minneapolis
38. Traxler RM, Guerra MA, Morrow MG, Haupt T, Morrison J, Saah JR, Smith CG, Williams C, Fleischuauer AT, Lee PA, Stanek D, Trevino-Garrison I, Franklin P, Oakes P, Hand S, Shadomy SV, Blaney DD, Lehman MW, Benoit TJ, Stoddard RA, Tiller RV, De BK, Bower W, Smith TL (2013) Review of brucellosis cases from laboratory exposures in the United States in 2008 to 2011 and improved strategies for disease prevention. J Clin Microbiol 51:3132–3136
39. Young EJ (2010) Brucella species. In: Mandell GL, Bennet JE, Dolin R (eds) Principles and practice of infectious diseases. Churchill Livingstone, Philadelphia, pp 2921–2925
40. Young EJ (1983) Human brucellosis. Rev Infect Dis 5:821–842
41. Young EJ (1995) An overview of human brucellosis. Clin Infect Dis 21:283–290

Part II

Cranial and Intracranial Brucellosis

Scalp and Cranium Neurobrucellosis

3

Ersen Ertekin, Mehmet Turgut, Ahmet Tuncay Turgut, and Fuad Sami Haddad†

Contents

Abstract

Brucellosis is a worldwide zoonotic disease of domestic and wild animals. The infection is transmitted to humans by direct contact with the tissues of infected animals, ingestion of food and drinks with risk, and inhalation of infectious aerosols. Brucellosis can involve any organ or system in the body. Osteoarticular brucellosis is the most frequent complication of brucellosis. Sacroiliitis, spondylitis, peripheral arthritis, and osteomyelitis of the long bones are the most frequent sites of skeletal brucellosis. Cranial bone involvement in brucellosis is considered to be extremely rare and cutaneous manifestations of brucellosis are also uncommon. Scalp involvement is also extremely rare in brucellosis. The findings of both skeletal and cutaneous brucellosis are nonspecific. For differential diagnosis, a thorough history including job, journey to endemic areas, and ingestion of contaminated food or water, clinical evaluation, laboratory tests including serology or polymerase chain reaction assay combined with culture, and radiologic tests should be evaluated.

Keywords

Brucellosis • Cranium • Scalp

† Author was deceased at the time of publication.

E. Ertekin, MD, PhD (✉)
Department of Radiology, Adnan Menderes University School of Medicine, Aydın, Turkey
e-mail: drersen@hotmail.com

M. Turgut, MD, PhD
Department of Neurosurgery, Adnan Menderes University School of Medicine, Aydın, Turkey
e-mail: drmturgut@yahoo.com

A.T. Turgut, MD
Department of Radiology, Hacettepe University School of Medicine, Ankara, Turkey
e-mail: ahmettuncayturgut@yahoo.com

F.S. Haddad, MD, FACS, FRCS, ABNS
Department of Surgery, American University of Beirut, Beirut, Lebanon
e-mail: fshaddad@aub.edu.lb

M. Turgut et al. (eds.), *Neurobrucellosis: Clinical, Diagnostic and Therapeutic Features*,
DOI 10.1007/978-3-319-24639-0_3

Abbreviations

CT Computed tomography
MRI Magnetic resonance imaging
PCR Polymerase chain reaction
PET-CT Positron emission tomography-computed tomography

3.1 Introduction

Brucellosis is a worldwide zoonotic disease of domestic and wild animals, caused by members of the genus *Brucella*. In animals, brucellosis is a chronic and persistent infection during the life. Infection is transmitted to humans by direct contact with infected animal tissues, consumption of contaminated food or beverage, and inhalation of infectious aerosols [10, 22, 54].

There are a total of four species of *Brucella* that recognized in humans and each has several biovars: *Brucella melitensis* (sheep, goats, and camels), *B. abortus* (cattle), *B. suis* (pigs), and *B. canis* (dogs) [22, 54].

After entering the human body from epithelial cell of skin, conjunctiva, or mucosal cells, *Brucella* organisms induce a nonspecific cellular response. Brucellae survive and multiply within the phagocytic cells of the host [10, 54]. Brucellae in phagocytes are transferred from regional lymph nodes into the blood circulation and seed throughout all organs of the body, especially to the reticuloendothelial system including bone marrow, spleen, and liver. Leukocytes, epithelioid cells, and lymphocytes form granulomas in tissues and organs [9].

Brucellosis is one of the most important causes of unknown fever and febrile neutropenia in endemic areas [3, 26, 29]. In humans, incubation period is about 1–3 weeks, but it may take up to several months. The most frequent presenting symptoms are fever, arthralgia, fatigue, sweating, and lower back pain seen in up to 75–100 % of cases. Fever, splenomegaly, hepatomegaly, and lymphadenopathy are the most common clinical findings [5, 12, 23].

Human brucellosis can be classified as subclinic, acute, subacute, and chronic [16]. The localized form of brucellosis is referred to when a specific organ involvement is detected [1, 14]. Reappearance of the symptoms and clinical findings with or without positive culture is defined as recurrence of brucellosis [52].

3.2 Brucellosis of Scalp

3.2.1 Cutaneous Brucellosis in General

Cutaneous manifestations of brucellosis are uncommon and reported in 2–10 % of brucellosis cases [10, 22]. Skin lesions occur less frequently in the acute phase of brucellosis compared with the subacute and chronic phases. It may depend on the incomplete formation of pathophysiological mechanisms [2]. In some studies, cutaneous lesions occur more frequently in woman. This could be explained with cellular and humoral immune responses in women that are more intense [2, 31].

3.2.2 Brucellosis of Scalp

Although the cutaneous brucellosis is usually seen in the upper and lower limbs and trunk of the body, cutaneous lesions can rarely be seen in the scalp, especially the contact urticaria lesions.

3.2.2.1 Mode of Transmission to Scalp

Pathogenic microorganisms can affect the skin by direct invasion or hematogenously. But some cutaneous lesions occur as a hypersensitivity reaction.

3.2.2.2 Course

This process may appear in any stage of the disease but occur most frequently in subacute or chronic phases of the disease. Response to the antibiotic treatment is well in cutaneous brucellosis. The lesions may disappear spontaneously without treatment within 2 weeks, leaving no trace of the papules.

3.2.2.3 Signs and Symptoms

Most frequent cutaneous findings are maculopapular eruptions and erythematous lesions. The other skin lesions of brucellosis are papulonodular eruptions, psoriasiform lesions, contact dermatitis, rashes, purpura and petechiae, cutaneous or subcutaneous abscess, vasculitis, superficial thrombophlebitis, etc. [2, 32].

3.2.2.4 Pathology

Pathogenesis of cutaneous lesions is hypersensitivity reactions, direct inoculation, depositing immune complexes, or invasion by the *Brucella* organism.

Contact urticaria, called as "erythema brucellum," is an erythematous eruption occurring as occupational disease especially in veterinarians. In early stages, before the contact urticaria begins, a hypersensitivity reaction may induce pruritus and erythema within a few hours after exposure. Erythematous lesions occur usually in upper extremities, rarely in face and neck, and they improve within 2–3 weeks [31, 32, 50]. Chronic ulcerations and cutaneous and subcutaneous abscesses also occur most frequently as an occupational disease.

Disseminated erythematous papulonodular lesions usually occur in lower extremities. Focal granulomatous lesions in the dermis occur due to hematogenous spread of bacteria and perivascular infiltration of histiocytes and leukocytes [6].

Erythema nodosum-like lesions occur as a result of hypersensitivity reaction or hematogenous spread of bacteria, but pathogenesis of maculopapular eruption is unknown yet. Although some cases of allergic, leukocytoclastic, necrotizing, or granulomatous vasculitis have been reported, relationship of these lesions with brucellosis is not fully understood [31, 32].

3.2.2.5 Diagnosis

Due to the lack of specificity of the skin lesions, a thorough history including the occupation, consumption of risk foods and beverages, and travel to endemic areas is necessary for the differential diagnosis. Also, clinical evaluation, laboratory tests including serology, or polymerase chain reaction (PCR) assay combined with culture helps diagnosis. The lack of alternative reason for these lesions and their disappearance with anti-brucellar therapy can contribute to the diagnosis [31].

The most significant finding for diagnosis is positive culture [22, 54]. Blood and bone marrow are the most suitable specimens [28, 41]. Also in some cases, brucellae could be cultured from subcutaneous papules and abscesses.

The most used serological test for Brucella is serum agglutination tests that measures *B. abortus* antigen. The other serological tests are Coombs' antiglobulin test, enzyme-linked immunosorbent assay, the fluorescence polarization assay, complement fixation test, PCR, etc. [22, 38, 49, 53].

Negative laboratory tests do not exclude the diagnosis. Positive laboratory test does not always refer to active infection, because Brucella antibodies can persist after the treatment up to 2 years in 5–7 % of cases [22, 43, 54].

Laboratory tests including erythrocyte sedimentation rate, complete blood count, and C-reactive protein are not specific for the diagnosis.

3.2.2.6 Treatment

Systemic antibiotic treatments are used for scalp brucellosis. There is no evidence of focal treatment methods in the literature. A new and effective treatment is Zithromax whose active ingredient is azithromycin. The advised dose is two tablets, 250 mg each, on the first day, followed by one tablet daily for 4 days.

3.3 Calvarial Brucellosis

3.3.1 Osseous Brucellosis in General

Osseous involvement is the most common complication and ranges from 10 to 85 % [17, 20, 47]. The osseous involvement is important because of its high prevalence and its association with functional sequelae. The prevalence and pattern of osseous involvement depend on the infecting *Brucella* species, the duration of disease, and patient's age [20].

Sacroiliitis, spondylitis, peripheral arthritis, and osteomyelitis of the long bones are the most frequent sites of skeletal brucellosis. The other, rare sites of skeletal brucellosis are calcaneus, phalanges, sternum, carpal and tarsal bones, ribs, clavicle, and pelvic bones [15, 20, 47].

3.3.2 Skull Brucellosis

Although the osseous involvement is the most common complication of the brucellosis, calvarial involvement is considered to be extremely rare [47]. Few cases of cranial bone involvement have been reported in brucellosis [30, 39, 47].

3.3.2.1 Mode of Transmission

Pathogenic microorganisms transmitted to the calvarium by direct invasion or hematogenously.

3.3.2.2 Course

The infection reaches the skull through its marrow and, for some unknown reasons, does not spread in this tissue but remains at the site of infection, involving the outer and inner tables. The process may be so invasive as to destroy both tables and produce a rugged edge whole in the skull. This process is not self-limited and in extreme cases may destroy galea, scalp, and dura and the brain may appear on the surface.

3.3.2.3 Signs and Symptoms

If the scalp is intact, there is usually a lump underneath it which is mildly tender neither movable nor fluctuating.

3.3.2.4 Pathology

The destruction in osteoarticular brucellosis may be owing to direct invasion of *Brucella* or a result of ongoing inflammatory response. *Brucella* spp. can infect the osteoblasts and live within them. The infected osteoblasts secrete cytokines and chemokines as pro-inflammatory and metalloproteases that may induce the osteoarticular brucellosis. Additionally, *Brucella* spp. induce osteoclasts activation and cause bone resorption [45].

3.3.2.5 Diagnosis

A thorough history, clinical evaluation, laboratory tests, culture, and radiologic tests help the diagnosis. The most significant finding for diagnosis is positive culture [22, 54]. Positive culture rates range from 15 to 90 %. Blood and bone marrow are the most suitable specimens [28, 41].

The most frequently used imaging modalities for the diagnosis of skeletal involvement in brucellosis are plain radiographs. The plain radiographic findings suggestive of osteomyelitis are periosteal new bone formation (periosteal reaction), periosteal elevation which can indicate periosteal abscess, and lytic lesions or sclerosis indicating subacute or chronic disease (Fig. 3.1) [47]. Nevertheless, a normal plain radiogram, especially in early days (7 days of symptoms onset), does not exclude the disease [13, 36].

Magnetic resonance imaging (MRI) has a high sensitivity, specificity, and accurate rates for identification of bone, periosteal, and soft tissue involvements [11]. MRI is useful for identifying early bone marrow changes, osteomyelitis, and subperiosteal or soft tissue collections such as abscesses. On MRI, active inflammation shows decreased signal on T1-weighted images and increased signal in T2-weighted images and fat-

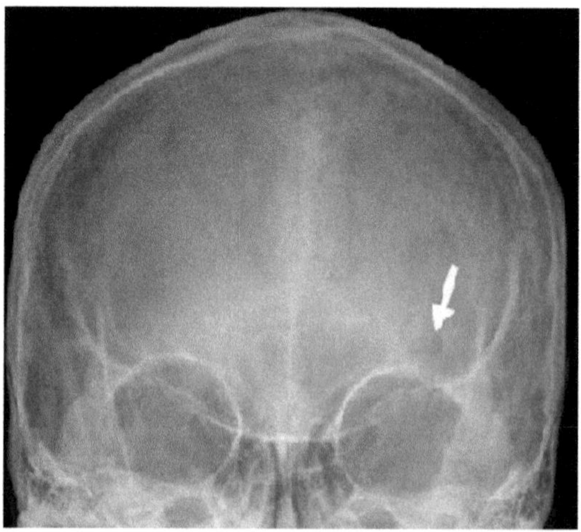

Fig. 3.1 Plain radiograph demonstrating a radiolucent osteolytic lesion in the left supraorbital region in the same patient (*white arrow*) (From Sohn et al. [47], with permission)

suppression sequences (Fig. 3.2), [47]. In T1-weighted images, high signal intensity between the abscess and sclerotic bone marrow, called "penumbra sign," is characteristic of osteomyelitis. The use of contrast agents is generally not necessary for MRI [11].

Scintigraphy is useful when the infection cannot be localized or multifocality is suspected [13]. The three-phase bone scan is usually performed; it consists of a nuclear angiogram (2–5 s after injection), a blood pool phase (5–10 min after injection), and a delayed phase (2–4 h after injection). In the first two phases, increased uptake can be caused by any inflammation that increased the blood flow. However, the increased uptake in the third (delayed) phase reflects the osteoblastic activity. Tc-99 m methylene diphosphonate and Ga 67 citrate are sensitive agents for detecting bone involvement, but they have a low specificity (Fig. 3.3) [47]. A higher specificity has been shown with Tc-99 m polyclonal human immunoglobulin, Tc-99 interleukin-8, In-111 granulocytes, radiolabeling leukocytes, and monoclonal Fab fragments [21, 25, 44].

Computed tomography (CT) indications for osteomyelitis are lack of availability of MRI or contraindications to MRI, the arrangement of the surgical intervention to debridement of sequestra, and identification of bone damage in chronic osteomyelitis. CT findings of osteomyelitis are increased bone marrow density, periosteal new bone formation, and periosteal purulence.

Ultrasonography usually does not help for the diagnosis of osteomyelitis. It can be used for detection of fluid collections and improve the percutaneous drainage procedures.

Ioannou et al. [24] demonstrated that positron emission tomography-computed tomography (PET-CT) scan may provide useful information in osteoarticular brucellosis. Fluorodeoxyglucose uptakes of infected tissues increased as standard uptake value max values. Sensitivity and specificity of the PET-CT is ranging 94–100 % and 87–100 %, respectively. However, this study has been limited to a small number of patient, and therefore, further studies are necessary to clarify these results. PET-CT is better than the other modalities to

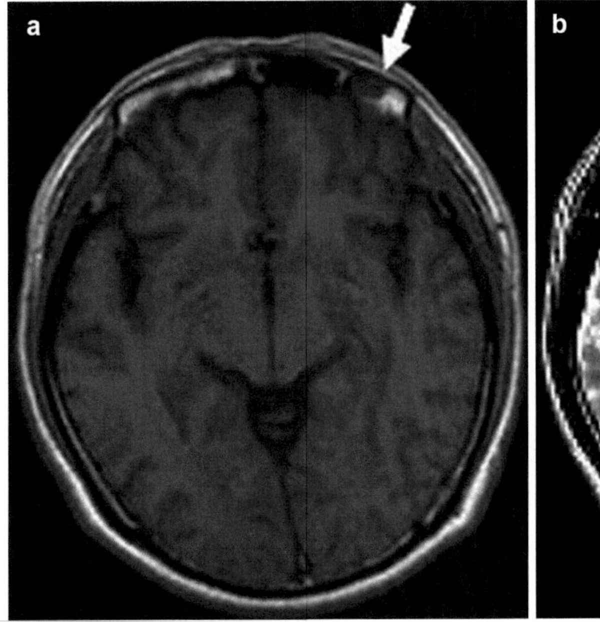

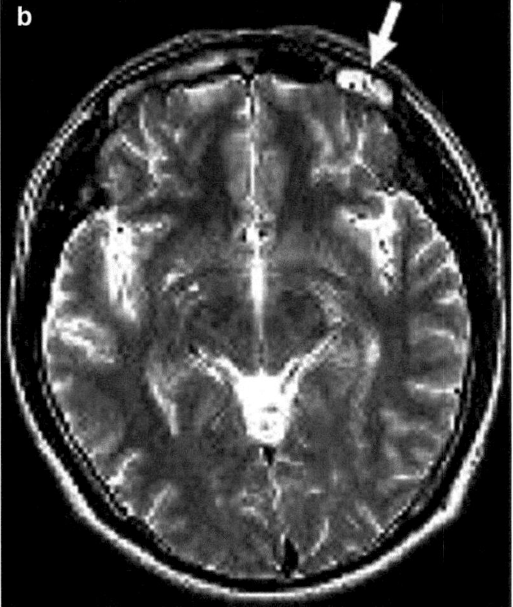

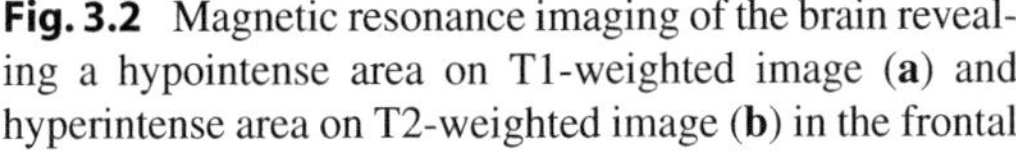

Fig. 3.2 Magnetic resonance imaging of the brain revealing a hypointense area on T1-weighted image (**a**) and hyperintense area on T2-weighted image (**b**) in the frontal bone, with a pathological diagnosis of brucellar granulomatous lesion (*white arrows*) (From Sohn et al. [47], with permission)

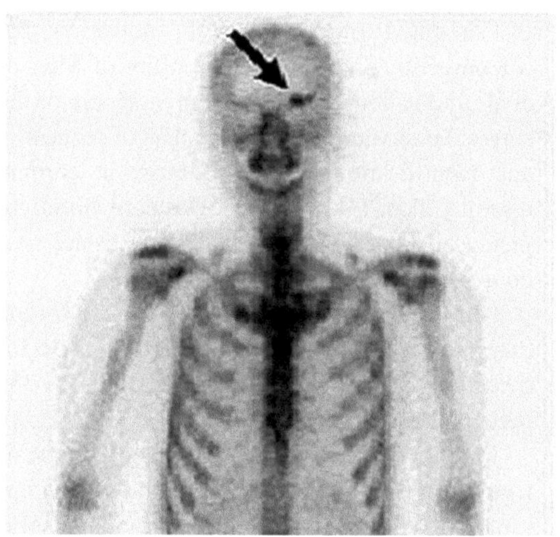
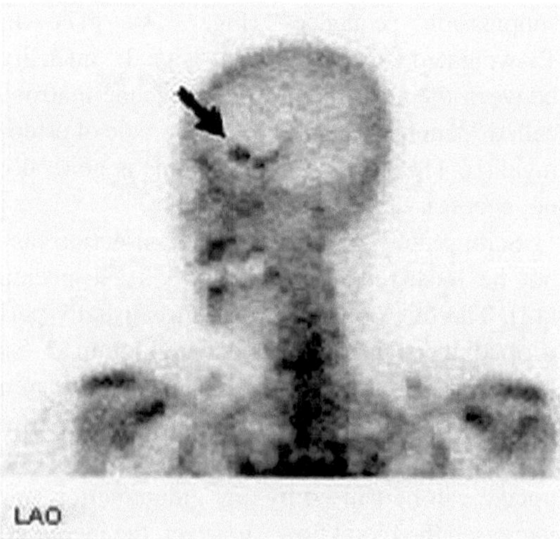

Fig. 3.3 Tc-99 m MDP bone scintigraphy showing a focal increased tracer uptake in the left supraorbital region in a patient with symptoms of fever and myalgia for 2 weeks (*black arrows*) (From Sohn et al. [47], with permission)

show the spread of infection and multifocal lesions in a multisystemic brucellosis disease.

3.3.2.6 Treatment

Treatment is used to shorten the duration of symptoms and to prevent complications and recurrence of the disease. Doxycycline, rifampin, trimethoprim-sulfamethoxazole, ceftriaxone, streptomycin, and ciprofloxacin have been proved very effective in many studies [6, 7, 18, 51]. Monotherapies or a combination of two or three drugs is currently used. Therapeutic failure was more common when monotherapy is used. Duration of the therapy depends on the condition of the patient, presence of complications, and time from onset of symptoms to beginning of the treatment. A minimum of 6 weeks of combined antibiotic treatment has a lower frequency of relapse.

3.4 Prevention and Prognosis

Brucellosis is not usually transmitted from human to human. Nevertheless, rarely, transmission of the *Brucella* by bone marrow transplantation, blood transfusion, sexual intercourse, ingestion of breast milk, and through the placenta has been reported [1, 19, 34, 37, 42].

Humans can be prevented from brucellosis by eradication of infection in animals by vaccination and other veterinary control methods. There is no brucellosis vaccine for humans yet [14, 33, 35]. In endemic regions, pasteurization of products such as milk, butter, cheese, etc., is an effective security precaution for the prevention of the diseases. Unpasteurized products at the dairy and undercooked meat or other animal products should not be ingested. Precautions should be taken for occupational disease such as hygiene and protective clothing or equipment [4, 10, 22, 40, 54].

Reappearance of the symptoms and clinical findings with or without positive culture is defined as recurrence of brucellosis [52]. The relapse rate varies from about 5 to 45 % depending on the treatment protocol used [8, 46, 52]. It often occurs 6 months after termination of the treatment and is often associated with poor compliance to therapy. Relapse tends to be milder than the primary disease [27, 46, 48].

Conclusion

- Scalp and cranial bone involvement is considered to be extremely rare.
- The most frequent findings are immobile, non-fluctuating lump for cranial osteomyelitis and erythema brucellum, maculopap-

ular eruptions, erythema nodosum-like lesions for scalp involvement.

- Due to the lack of specific skin and osseous lesions, a thorough history, clinical evaluation, serological tests, and culture are needed for diagnosis
- Plain radiography, MRI, and bone scintigraphy are the most frequently used imaging methods for cranial brucellosis
- Combined antibiotic therapy protocols for at least 6 weeks have therapeutic success. Surgery may be needed when abscesses are present.

References

1. Akçakuş M, Esel D, Cetin N, Kisaarslan AP, Kurtoglu S (2005) Brucella melitensis in blood cultures of two newborns due to exchange transfusion. Turk J Pediatr 47:272–274
2. Akcali C, Savas L, Baba M, Turunc T, Seckin D (2007) Cutaneous manifestations in brucellosis: a prospective study. Adv Ther 24:706–711
3. Ali-Eldin FA, Abdelhakam SM, Ali-Eldin ZA (2011) Clinical spectrum of fever of unknown origin among adult Egyptian patients admitted to Ain Shams University Hospitals: a hospital based study. J Egypt Soc Parasitol 41:379–386
4. Al-Shaar L, Chaaya M, Ghosn N, Mahfoud Z (2014) Brucellosis outbreak in Chouf district of Lebanon in 2009: a case control study. East Mediterr Health J 20:250–256
5. Andriopoulos P, Tsironi M, Deftereos S, Aessopos A, Assimakopoulos G (2007) Acute brucellosis: presentation, diagnosis, and treatment of 144 cases. Int J Infect Dis 11:52–57
6. Ariza J, Servitje O, Pallares R, Fernandez VP, Rufi G, Peyri J, Gudiol F (1989) Characteristic cutaneous lesions in patients with brucellosis. Arch Dermatol 125:380–383
7. Asadipoova K, Dehghanian A, Omrani GH, Abbasi F (2011) Short-course treatment in neurobrucellosis: a study in Iran. Neurol India 59:101–103
8. Aygen B, Doganay M, Sumerkan B, Yildiz O, Kayabas U (2002) Clinical manifestations, complications and treatment of brucellosis: a retrospective evaluation of 480 patients. Med Mal Infect 32:485–493
9. Baldi PC, Giambartolomei GH (2013) Pathogenesis and pathobiology of zoonotic brucellosis in humans. Rev Sci Tech 32:117–125
10. Beeching NJ, Madkour MM (2014) Brucellosis. In: Farrar J, Hotez P, Junghanss T, Kang G, Lalloo D, White NJ (eds) Manson's tropical diseases, 23rd edn. Elsevier Saunders, Philadelphia, pp 371–378
11. Browne LP, Mason EO, Kaplan SL, Cassady CI, Krishnamurthy R, Guillerman RP (2008) Optimal imaging strategy for community-acquired Staphylococcus aureus musculoskeletal infections in children. Pediatr Radiol 38:841–847
12. Buzgan T, Karahocagil MK, Irmak H, Baran AI, Karsen H, Evirgen O, Akdeniz H (2010) Clinical manifestations and complications in 1028 cases of brucellosis: a retrospective evaluation and review of the literature. Int J Infect Dis 14:469–478
13. Capitanio MA, Kirkpatrick JA (1970) Early roentgen observations in acute osteomyelitis. Am J Roentgenol Radium Ther Nucl Med 108:488–496
14. Chand P, Chhabra R, Naqrq J (2015) Vaccination of adult animals with a reduced dose of Brucella abortus S19 vaccine to control brucellosis on dairy farms in endemic areas of India. Trop Anim Health Prod 47:29–35
15. Colmenero JD, Reguera JM, Fernandez-Nebro A, Cabrera-Franquelo F (1991) Osteoarticular complications of brucellosis. Ann Rheum Dis 50:23–26
16. Doganay M, Algen B (2003) Human brucellosis: an overview. Int J Infect Dis 7:173–182
17. Ekici MA, Ozbek Z, Gökoğlu A, Menkü A (2012) Surgical management of cervical spinal epidural abscess caused by Brucella melitensis: report of two cases and review of the literature. J Korean Neurosurg Soc 51:383–387
18. El Miedany YM, El Gaafary M, Baddour M, Ahmed I (2003) Human brucellosis: do we need to revise our therapeutical policy? J Rheumatol 30:2666–2672
19. Ertem M, Kurekci AE, Aysev D, Unal E, Ikinciogulları A (2000) Brucellosis transmitted by bone marrow transplantation. Bone Marrow Transplant 26:225–226
20. Fowler TP, Keener J, Buckwalter JA (2004) Brucella osteomyelitis of the proximal tibia: a case report. Iowa Orthop J 24:30–32
21. Grats S, Rennen HJJM, Boerman OC, Oyen WJG, Burma P, Corstens FHM (2001) ^{99m}Tc-Interleukin-8 for imaging acute osteomyelitis. J Nucl Med 42:1257–1264
22. Gul HC, Erdem H (2015) Brucellosis (Brucella species). In: Bennett J, Dolin R, Blaser MJ (eds) Mandell, Douglas, and Bennett's principles and practice of infectious diseases, 8th edn. Elsevier Saunders, Philadelphia, pp 2584–9e3
23. Güven T, Ugurlu K, Ergonul O, Celikbas AK, Gok SE, Comoglu S, Baykam N, Dokuzoguz B (2013) Neurobrucellosis: clinical and diagnostic features. Clin Infect Dis 56:1407–1412
24. Ioannou S, Chatziioannou S, Pneumaticos SG, Zormpala A, Sipsas NV (2013) Fluorine-18 fluoro-2-deoxy-D-glucose positron emission tomography/computed tomography scan contributes to the diagnosis and management of brucellar spondylodiskitis. BMC Infect Dis 13:73
25. Kadanali A, Varoglu E, Kerek M, Tasyaran MA (2005) Tc-99 m polyclonal human immunoglobulin scintigraphy in brucellosis. Clin Microbiol Infect 11:480–485
26. Li JJ, Sheng ZK, Tu S, Bi S, Shen XM, Sheng JF (2012) Acute brucellosis with myelodysplastic syn-

drome presenting as pancytopenia and fever of unknown origin. Med Princ Pract 21:183–185
27. Lulu AR, Araj GF, Khateeb MI, Mustafa MY, Yusuf AR, Fenech FF (1988) Human brucellosis in Kuwait: a prospective study of 400 cases. Q J Med 66:39–54
28. Maio E, Begeman L, Bisselink Y, van Tulden P, Wiersma L, Hiemstra S, Ruuls R, Grone A, Roest HI, Willemsen P, van der Giessen J (2014) Identification and typing of brucella spp. in stranded harbour porpoises (Phocoena phocoena) on the Dutch coast. Vet Microbiol 173:118–124
29. Manson-Bahr P, Willoughby H (1929) A critical study of undulant fever: from a series of six cases in the Hospital for Tropical Diseases, London. Br Med J 1:633–635
30. Marandian MH, Soltanabadi A, Sabouri-Deliamy M, Yalda A, Shoukouhi JJ (1986) Cranial osteitis in two 7- and 8-years old brothers with associated chronic cerebral brucellosis in one brother. Ann Radiol (Paris) 29:545–548
31. Metin A, Akdeniz H, Buzgan T, Delice I (2001) Cutaneous findings encountered in brucellosis and review of the literatures. Int J Dermatol 40:434–438
32. Millionis H, Christou L, Elisaf M (2000) Cutaneous manifestations in brucellosis: case report and review of the literatures. Infection 28:124–126
33. Moreno E (2014) Retrospective and prospective perspectives on zoonotic brucellosis. Front Microbiol 5:213
34. Mosayebi Z, Movahedian AH, Ghayomi A, Kazemi B (2005) Congenital brucellosis in a preterm neonate. Indian Pediatr 42:599–601
35. Osman AE, Hassan AN, Ali AE, Abdoel TH, Smits HL (2015) Brucella melitensis Biovar 1 and Brucella abortus S19 vaccine strain infections in milkers working at cattle farms in the Khartoum Area, Sudan. PLoS One 10, e0123374
36. Overturf GD (2011) Bacterial infections of the bone and joints. In: Remington JS, Klein JO, Wilson CB et al (eds) Infectious diseases of the fetus and newborn, 7th edn. Elsevier Saunders, Philadelphia, p 296
37. Palanduz A, Palanduz S, Guler K, Guler N (2000) Brucellosis in a mother and her young infant: probable transmission by breast milk. Int J Infect Dis 4:55–56
38. Patra KP, Saito M, Atluri VL, Rolan HG, Young B, Kerrinnes T, Smits H, Ricaldi JN, Goluzzo E, Gilman RH, Tsolis RM, Vinets JM (2014) A protein-conjugate approach to develop a monoclonal antibody-based antigen detection test for the diagnosis of human brucellosis. PLoS Negl Trop Dis 8, e2926
39. Piampiano P, McLeary M, Young LW, Janner D (2000) Brucellosis: unusual presentations in two adolescent bpys. Pediatr Radiol 30:355–357
40. Ragan V, Vroegindewey G, Babcock S (2013) International standards for brucellosis prevention and management. Rev Sci Tech 32:189–198
41. Rai A, Gautam V, Gupta PK, Sethi S, Rana S, Ray P (2014) Rapid detection of Brucella by an automated blood culture system at a tertiary care hospital of north India. Indian J Med Res 139:776–778
42. Reine NJ (2004) Infection and blood transfusion: a guide to donor screening. Clin Tech Small Anim Pract 19:568–574
43. Rolan HG, Xavier MN, Santos RL, Tsolis RM (2009) Natural antibody contributes to host defense against an attenuated Brucella abortus virB mutant. Infect Immun 77:3004–3013
44. Schauwecker DS, Park HM, Mock BH, Burt RW, Kernick CB, Ruoff AC III, Sinn HJ, Wellman HN (1984) Evaluation of complicating osteomyelitis with Tc-99 m MDP, In-111 granulocytes, and Ga-67 citrate. J Nucl Med 25:849–853
45. Scian R, Barrionuevo P, Fossati CA, Giambartolomei GH, Delpino MV (2012) Brucella abortus invasion of osteoblasts inhibits bone formation. Infect Immun 80:2333–2345
46. Shaalan MA, Memish ZA, Mahmoud SA, Alomari A, Khan MY, Almuneef M, Alalola S (2002) Brucellosis in children: clinical observations in 115 cases. Int J Infect Dis 6:182–186
47. Sohn MH, Lim ST, Jeong YJ, Kim DW, Jeong HJ, Lee CS (2010) Unusual case of occult Brucella osteomyelitis in the skull detected by bone scintigraphy. Nucl Med Mol Imaging 44:161–163
48. Tanir G, Tufekci SB, Tuygun N (2009) Presentation, complications, and treatment outcome of brucellosis in Turkish children. Pediatr Int 51:114–119
49. Thepsuriyanont P, Intrapuk A, Chanket P, Tunyong W, Kalambaheti T (2014) ELISA for brucellosis detection based on three Brucella recombinant proteins. Southeast Asian J Trop Med Public Health 45:130–141
50. Trunell TN, Waisman M, Trunnell TL (1985) Contact dermatitis caused by Brucella. Cutis 35:379–381
51. Ulu-Kilic A, Karakas A, Erdem H, Turker T, Inal AS, Ak O, Turan H, Kazak E, Inan A, Duygu F, Demiraslan H, Kader C, Sener A, Dayan S, Deveci O, Tekin R, Saltoglu N, Aydın M, Horasan ES, Gul HC, Ceylan B, Kadanalı A, Karabay O, Karagoz G, Kayabas U, Turhan V, Engin D, Gulsun S, Elaldı N, Alabay S (2014) Update on treatment options for spinal brucellosis. Clin Microbiol Infect 20:O75–O82
52. Ulu-Kılıc A, Metan G, Alp E (2013) Clinical presentations and diagnosis of brucellosis. Recent Pat Antiinfect Drug Discov 8:34–41
53. Wang Y, Wang Z, Zhang Y, Bai L, Zhao Y, Liu C, Ma A, Yu H (2014) Polymerase chain reaction-based assays for the diagnosis of human brucellosis. Ann Clin Microbiol Antimicrob 13:31
54. Young E (2014) Brucellosis. In: Cherry JD, Harrison GJ, Kaplan SL, Steinbach WL, Hotez PJ (eds) Feigin and Cherry's textbook of pediatric infectious diseases, 7th edn. Elsevier Saunders, Philadelphia, pp 1611–1615

Epidural and Subdural Brucellar Empyema

4

Abbas Tafakhori, Ahmet Tuncay Turgut, Saliha Kanık-Yüksek, and Mehmet Turgut

Contents

A. Tafakhori, MD (✉)
Department of Neurology, Imam Khomeini Hospital, Tehran University of Medical Sciences, Tehran, Iran
e-mail: a_tafakhori@tums.ac.ir

A.T. Turgut, MD
Department of Radiology, Hacettepe University School of Medicine, Ankara, Turkey
e-mail: ahmettuncayturgut@yahoo.com

S. Kanık-Yüksek, MD
Department of Pediatric Infectious Disease, Ankara Hematology Oncology Children's Training and Research Hospital, Ankara, Turkey
e-mail: salihakanik@gmail.com

M. Turgut, MD, PhD
Department of Neurosurgery, Adnan Menderes University School of Medicine, Aydın, Turkey
e-mail: drmturgut@yahoo.com

Abstract

Neurobrucellosis is a rare but important complication of brucellosis with a rate of about 3–5 %. Intracranial epidural and subdural empyemas are less common and present with nonspecific signs and symptoms including several days of fever, headache, altered mental status and confusion, seizures, and focal neurological deficits. Neuroimaging is very crucial in the diagnosis. Surgical and medical treatments are the cornerstone of therapy. The purposes of this chapter are to emphasize the brucellar epidural and subdural empyemas to keep these neurobrucellosis forms in mind and to review the diagnostic and treatment modalities.

Keywords

Complication • Epidural empyema • Neurobrucellosis • Subdural empyema • Treatment

Abbreviations

2-ME 2-Mercaptoethanol
CSF Cerebrospinal fluid

M. Turgut et al. (eds.), *Neurobrucellosis: Clinical, Diagnostic and Therapeutic Features*,
DOI 10.1007/978-3-319-24639-0_4

CT Computed tomography
MRI Magnetic resonance imaging
PCR Polymerase chain reaction

4.1 Introduction

Neurobrucellosis is a focal and partly rare complication of brucellosis that has been detected in approximately 3–5 % of the patients with brucellosis [5, 15, 24, 31, 34] although reported different ratios in different studies [6, 17, 25]. In a systematic review of clinical manifestation of brucellosis that was published in 2012, authors concluded that 4 % of brucellosis patients can evolve neurobrucellosis in their course of disease [9].

In a review of 31 cases of neurobrucellosis [17], frequencies of presenting signs were detected as meningoencephalitis (45 %), meningitis (39 %), polyradiculopathy (8 %), brain abscess (3 %), and epidural abscess (3 %). Other studies support such findings in neurobrucellosis [29]. Epidural and subdural empyemas of the brain due to *Brucella*, the subject of this chapter, are exceedingly rare [23, 37]. Brucellar epidural abscess, which has been reported in less than 1.5 % of cases with neurobrucellosis, is usually associated with spondylitis [26, 34]. Interestingly, the routes of infection of the epidural and subdural abscesses are completely different: direct extension, lymphatics, and bloodstream. The rarity of this issue makes the diagnosis very difficult. Epidural and subdural brucellar empyemas can involve the intracranial and spinal structures [40, 41]; the latter is discussed in Chap. 15.

4.2 Signs and Symptoms

Despite having an onset of weeks to months, neurobrucellosis is generally defined for at least 4 weeks [39]. However, the reported latency period between the onset of clinical brucellosis and the onset of cerebral symptoms in intracranial abscess is approximately 2 months [16, 30]. Headache is a prominent early symptom of neurobrucellosis [36]. The complaints such as hypoesthesia, hemiparesis, paraplegia, dysarthria, confusion, convulsion, and coma have been also reported [15, 17] and can be the only presenting symptoms. [1] Epidural and subdural empyemas usually present with nonspecific signs and symptoms including several days of fever, headache, altered mental status and confusion, seizures, and focal neurological deficits (hemiparesis, facial paresis, etc.), as in the other cases of brain abscess [26, 27].

In children, signs of increased cranial pressure such as vomiting, depressed responsiveness, and headache can be detected, especially in intracranial subdural empyemas. In infants, enlarged head circumference, bulging fontanel, and persistent fever may also be observed. In intracranial epidural empyemas of children, nonspecific symptoms and signs of intracranial suppurative processes may be observed [21]. Spinal epidural abscess presents as localized or generalized back or flank pain. Additionally, focal neurological deficits (sensory or motor) can develop. Spinal subdural abscess presents similar to epidural abscess [8]. Neurobrucellosis-related brain abscesses located in the epidural or subdural spaces appear to be a subtle disease and require attention, especially in patients with unexplained neurological symptoms.

4.3 Neurological Examination

Examination reveals few focal findings, but signs of meningeal irritation such as neck stiffness are common [39]. Papilledema, ophthalmoplegia, hemiparesis, hyperreflexia, and Babinski sign must be evaluated. The clinical manifestation of subdural and epidural empyemas may be similar, but the course of subdural empyema is more severe [11, 27]. In neurological examination of intracranial subdural empyemas, bulging fontanel, depressed responsiveness, meningismus, increased head circumference, papilledema, hemiparesis, or hemiplegia can be determined in children and infants [11]. Mental status changes, focal neurological deficits, papilledema, or meningeal signs may be detected in intracranial epidural abscess [21].

4.4 Neuroimaging

Imaging abnormalities of neurobrucellosis are various and may mimic other infectious or inflammatory processes [2]. Neuroimaging plays a critical role in the diagnosis of epidural and subdural empyemas. Computed tomography (CT) scan is an inexpensive modality, and empyema can be seen as an extra-axial mass in CT scan [2, 14, 21]. Often empyema appears as an extra-axial mass in low density in non-contrast CT scan, and enhancement with contrast agent can differentiate empyema from other collections like effusions or hematomas [8, 15].

In magnetic resonance imaging (MRI), empyema presents as a low or isointense extra-axial mass in T1-weighted and high-signal lesions in T2-weighted imaging. It enhances on gadolinium use; contrast enhancement is present in a heterogeneous manner [14, 15, 21]. Frequently, a leptomeningeal involvement and arachnoiditis are a dominant feature [15, 28].

4.5 Laboratory Tests

The diagnosis of neurobrucellosis is based on seroagglutination methods and cultures of blood and cerebrospinal fluid (CSF), but they have relatively low sensitivity [42]. The gold standard of diagnosis of brucellosis is isolation of the organism from an affected tissue such as blood, brain, or bone marrow (Fig. 4.1) [6, 12]. Nevertheless, its yield remains suboptimal (40–70 %) and expensive. The duration of illness is important for a positive culture, especially the first 2 weeks of the illness [4, 6]. There are also alternative serological tests such as slide agglutination test, serum agglutination test, microagglutination test, indirect Coombs (antihuman globulin) test, enzyme-linked immunosorbent assay, indirect fluorescent antibody test, or immunochromatographic lateral flow assay, and one of these may be preferred in the absence of a positive culture [4]. Using a standard agglutination test, the most commonly used and most standardized test, for patients presenting with symptoms suggestive of brucellosis should be considered, and a titer of 1:≥160 may be interpreted as a positive *Brucella* serology test [6, 42].

Laboratory confirmation of neurobrucellosis should be made by the presence of any 1 of the following criteria: (1) isolation of microorganism from CSF; (2) presence of anti-*Brucella* antibodies in CSF; (3) detection of lymphocytosis, increased protein, and decreased glucose levels of the CSF; and (4) findings associated with neurobrucellosis in CT or MRI [4]. Lumbar puncture

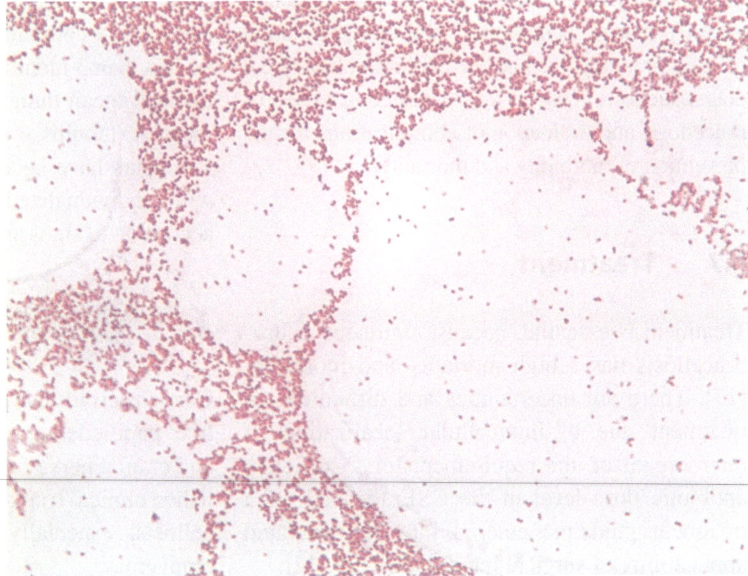

Fig. 4.1 *Brucella* organisms on gram stain of colonies from blood culture of a patient with brucellosis, × 1000 (Courtesy of G.F. Araj, M.D.)

can be a dangerous procedure in intracranial space-occupying lesions such as subdural or epidural empyemas and should not be performed [27]. Serological tests of CSF can be negative in empyemas, and mild nonspecific inflammatory changes in CSF may be detected only [4]. Furthermore, the culture of surgical specimens may reveal a localized infection caused by *Brucella* species [42]. Polymerase chain reaction (PCR) method is being studied for diagnosis of brucellosis as a promising test due to its sensitivity and specificity and can be a diagnostic modality of choice in brucellosis [19, 20]. PCR is not a routine test, but can be helpful after 10 days of infection, and it can be performed in any tissue [22].

4.6 Differential Diagnosis

Intracranial space-occupying lesions such as hematomas, effusions, calcification or metastatic dural involvement, and other infectious and inflammatory conditions such as tuberculosis, *Leptospira* species, *Borrelia burgdorferi*, syphilis, poliomyelitis, and fungal infections should be considered in differential diagnosis of epidural and subdural empyemas. In particular, the differential diagnosis should be that of the epidural and subdural spaces brucellosis. Contrast enhancement may help to distinguish infectious lesions [15, 27]. Neurobrucellosis may mimic many different central and peripheral nervous system pathologies, and a combination of neuroimaging techniques and microbiological diagnostic tests is useful for the detection of neurobrucellosis and evaluation of complications for the prevention of morbidity and mortality.

4.7 Treatment

Treatment is essential, because untreated neurobrucellosis has a high mortality and morbidity [15]. There are uncertainties and difficulties in treatment due to intracellular localization of microorganism, the requirement for a sufficient antibiotic dose level in the CSF, the lack of a treatment guideline entered into practice, and applicability of surgical intervention [25, 42].

4.7.1 Surgical Treatment

Presence of the neurological symptoms and deficits determines the indication of surgical intervention. A combination of surgical and medical therapy is appropriate in patients with neurological deficit [32, 33, 38]. Follow-up only with medical therapy may be an appropriate approach in some cases without neurological deficit [38]. Intracranial epidural and subdural empyemas must be evacuated surgically, and positive culture of the specimens can establish the diagnosis [29, 30].

4.7.2 Antibiotic Therapy

There is no consensus in the literature regarding optimal antimicrobial regimen and appropriate duration of treatment of neurobrucellosis [25, 42]. The medical treatment regimens must include the antibiotics that have penetration feature to the hematoencephalic barrier and sufficient concentrations in the CSF and maintain intracellular activity [3]. Dual-triple combination therapies are recommended including rifampin, tetracyclines, trimethoprim-sulfamethoxazole, ceftriaxone, and aminoglycosides [6, 7, 13, 22]. Single-agent regimens are contraindicated in the treatment of brucellosis [7, 13]. Although there is no certainty about the duration of treatment, the regimens including a combination therapy are advised for no less than 3 months [3, 6, 13]. While the recommended mean duration of neurobrucellosis treatment is 6 months, elongated treatment durations to 1–2 years have been reported in various studies, with individualized treatment in many cases according to signs and symptoms [6, 10].

4.7.3 Corticosteroid Treatment

Corticosteroids can be helpful in some conditions like papilledema, myelopathy, polyneuropathy, and cranial nerve palsies [27]. There is not established clinical trial about steroid use in neurobrucellosis, especially in epidural and subdural empyemas.

4.7.4 Antiepileptic Therapy

In acute stage, if the seizure attacks are frequent, a potent antiepileptic drug such as phenytoin (with landing dose) should be initiated to control the attacks [22]. Also levetiracetam, lamotrigine, or sodium valproate may be suitable alternative options for this purpose [21]. Rifampin can diminish the level of valproic acid, and this should be considered in therapeutic use of valproate. Rifampin also can increase metabolism of lamotrigine and diminish the level of drug in serum. After the termination of the seizure episodes, antiepileptics can be stopped within a short period [25, 29].

4.8 Follow-Up

Follow-up of patients with clinical symptoms and serial neuroimaging is necessary for monitoring of relapse and complications [17]. Relapse or reinfection occurs in 3–9 % of treated patients, and serial follow-ups are recommended [29, 35]. The 2-mercaptoethanol (2-ME) agglutination test measures IgG antibodies and is a good biomarker for relapsed brucellosis. High IgG levels in 2-ME test indicate relapse [35].

Conclusion

- Brucellar epidural and subdural empyemas are less common than the other forms of neurobrucellosis and present with nonspecific signs and symptoms.
- Brucellar epidural and subdural empyemas should be kept in mind in patients presenting with related symptoms, and required microbiological and neuroimaging tests should be performed in suspected cases.
- Treatment should be scheduled as soon as possible to decrease the mortality and morbidity.
- Presence of the neurological symptoms and deficits determines the indication of surgery.
- Follow-up of patients is necessary for monitoring of relapse and complications of neurobrucellosis.

References

1. Al Deeb SM, Yaqub BA, Sharif HS, Phadke JG (1989) Neurobrucellosis: clinical characteristics, diagnosis, and outcome. Neurology 39:498–501
2. Al-Sous MW, Bohlega S, Al-Kawi MZ, Alwatban J, McLean DR (2004) Neurobrucellosis: clinical and neuroimaging correlation. AJNR Am J Neuroradiol 25:395–401
3. American Academy of Pediatrics (2009) Brucellosis. In: Pickering LK, Baker CJ, Kimberlin DW, Long SS (eds) Red book: 2009 report of the Committee of Infectious Diseases, 28th edn. American Academy of Pediatrics, Elk Grove Village, pp 237–239
4. Araj GF (2010) Update on laboratory diagnosis of human brucellosis. Int J Antimicrob Agents 36:12–17
5. Bruce D (1887) Note on the discovery of a micro-organism in Malta fever. Practitioner 39:161–170
6. Ceran N, Turkoglu R, Erdem I, Inan A, Engin D, Tireli H, Goktas P (2011) Neurobrucellosis: clinical, diagnostic, therapeutic features and outcome: unusual clinical presentations in an endemic region. Braz J Infect Dis 15:52–59
7. Corbel MJ, Beeching NJ (2012) Brucellosis. In: Braunwald BE, Fauci AS, Kasper DL, Hauser SL (eds) Harrison's principles of internal medicine, 18th edn. McGraw Hill, New York, pp 1295–1296
8. Danner RL, Hartman AJ (1987) Update of spinal epidural abscess: 35 cases and review of the literature. Rev Infect Dis 9:265–274
9. Dean AS, Crump L, Greter H, Hattendorf J, Schelling E, Zinsstag J (2012) Clinical manifestations of human brucellosis: a systematic review and meta-analysis. PLoS Negl Trop Dis 6, e1929
10. Demiroğlu YZ, Turunç T, Karaca S, Arlıer Z, Alışkan H, Colakoğlu S, Arslan H (2011) Neurological involvement in brucellosis; clinical classification, treatment and results. Mikrobiyol Bul 45:401–410
11. Dill SR, Cobbs CG, McDonald CK (1995) Subdural empyema: analysis of 32 cases and review. Clin Infect Dis 20:372–386
12. Doganay M, Aygen B (2003) Human brucellosis: an overview. Int J Infect Dis 7:173–182
13. Erdem H, Ulu-Kilic A, Kilic S, Karahocagil M, Shehata G, Eren-Tulek N, Yetkin F, Celen MK, Ceran N, Gul HC, Mert G, Tekin-Koruk S, Dizbay M, Inal AS, Nayman-Alpat S, Bosilkovski M, Inan D, Saltoglu N, Abdel-Baky L, Adeva-Bartolome MT, Ceylan B, Sacar S, Turhan V, Yilmaz E, Elaldi N, Kocak-Tufan Z, Ugurlu K, Dokuzoguz B, Yilmaz H, Gundes S, Guner R, Ozgunes N, Ulcay A, Unal S, Dayan S, Gorenek L, Karakas A, Tasova Y, Usluer G, Bayindir Y, Kurtaran B, Sipahi OR, Leblebicioglu H (2012) Efficacy and tolerability of antibiotic combinations in neurobrucellosis: results of the Istanbul study. Antimicrob Agents Chemother 56:1523–1528
14. Erdem M, Namiduru M, Karaoglan I, Kecik VB, Aydin A, Tanriverdi M (2012) Unusual presentation

of neurobrucellosis: a solitary intracranial mass lesion mimicking a cerebral tumor: a case of encephalitis caused by Brucella melitensis. J Infect Chemother 18:767–770
15. Gul HC, Erdem H, Gorenek L, Ozdag MF, Kalpakci Y, Avci IY, Besirbellioglu BA, Eyigun CP (2008) Management of neurobrucellosis: an assessment of 11 cases. Intern Med 47:995–1001
16. Guvenc H, Kocabay K, Okten A, Bertas S (1989) Brucellosis in a child complicated with multiple brain abscesses. Scand J Infect Dis 21:33–36
17. Haji-Abdolbagi M, Rasooli-Nejad M, Jafari S, Hasibi M, Soudbakhsh A (2008) Clinical and laboratory findings in neurobrucellosis: review of 31 cases. Arch Iran Med 11:21–25
18. Köse Ş, Senger SS, Çavdar G, Yavaş S (2011) Case report on the development of a brucellosis-related epidural abscess. J Infect Dev Ctries 5:403–405
19. Mantur BG, Amarnath SK, Shinde RS (2007) Review of clinical and laboratory features of human brucellosis. Indian J Med Microbiol 25:188–202
20. Mantur BG, Biradar MS, Bidri RC, Mulimani MS, Veerappa Kariholu P, Patil SB, Mangalgi SS (2006) Protean clinical manifestations and diagnostic challenges of human brucellosis in adults: 16 years' experience in an endemic area. J Med Microbiol 55: 897–903
21. McIntyre PB, Lavercombe PS, Kemp RJ, McCormack JG (1991) Subdural and epidural empyema: diagnostic and therapeutic problems. Med J Aust 154: 653–657
22. McLean DR, Russell N, Khan MY (1992) Neurobrucellosis: clinical and therapeutic features. Clin Infect Dis 15:582–590
23. Papaioannides D, Giotis C, Korantzopoulos P, Akritidis N (2003) Brucellar spinal epidural abscess. Am Fam Physician 67:2071–2072
24. Pappas G, Akritidis N, Bosilkovski M, Tsianos E (2005) Brucellosis. N Engl J Med 352:2325–2336
25. Pappas G, Akritidis N, Christou L (2007) Treatment of neurobrucellosis: what is known and what remains to be answered. Expert Rev Anti Infect Ther 5: 983–990
26. Perez-Calvo J, Matamala C, Sanjoaquin I, Rodriguez-Benavente A, Ruiz-Laiglesia F, Bueno-Gomez J (1994) Epidural abscess due to acute Brucella melitensis infection. Arch Intern Med 154:1410–1411
27. Pradilla G, Ardila GP, Hsu W, Rigamonti D (2009) Epidural abscesses of the CNS. Lancet Neurol 8: 292–300
28. Rajan R, Khurana D, Kesav P (2013) Deep gray matter involvement in neurobrucellosis. Neurology 80(3):e28–e29
29. Samdani PG, Patil S (2003) Neurobrucellosis. Indian Pediatr 40:565–568
30. Santini C, Baiocchi P, Berardelli A, Venditti M, Serra P (1994) A case of brain abscess due to Brucella melitensis. Clin Infect Dis 19:977–978
31. Shakir RA, Al-Din AS, Araj GF, Lulu AR, Mousa AR, Saadah MA (1987) Clinical categories of neurobrucellosis. A report on 19 cases. Brain 110:213–223
32. Shoshan Y, Maayan S, Gomori MJ, Israel Z (1996) Chronic subdural empyema: a new presentation of neurobrucellosis. Clin Infect Dis 23:400–401
33. Solera J, Martínez-Alfaro E, Espinosa A (1997) Recognition and optimum treatment of brucellosis. Drugs 53:245–256
34. Solera J, Lozano E, Martinez-Alfaro E, Espinosa A, Castillejos ML, Abad L (1999) Brucellar spondylitis: review of 35 cases and literature survey. Clin Infect Dis 29:1440–1449
35. Solera J (2010) Update on brucellosis: therapeutic challenges. Int J Antimicrob Agents 36:S18–S20
36. Tajdini M, Akbarloo S, Hosseini SM, Parvizi B, Baghani S, Aghamollaii V, Tafakhori A (2014) From a simple chronic headache to neurobrucellosis: a case report. Med J Islam Repub Iran 28:12
37. Tappe D, Melzer F, Schmoock G, Elschner M, Lâm TT, Abele-Horn M, Stetter C (2012) Isolation of Brucella melitensis biotype 3 from epidural empyema in a Bosnian immigrant in Germany. J Med Microbiol 61:1335–1337
38. Tufan K, Aydemir F, Sarica FB, Kursun E, Kardes Ö, Cekinmez M, Caner H (2014) A extremely rare case of cervical intramedullary granuloma due to Brucella accompanied by Chiari Type-1 malformation. Asian J Neurosurg 9:173–176
39. Tunkel AR, Scheld WM (2005) Acute meningitis. In: Mandell G, Bennett J, Dolin R (eds) Principles and practice of infectious diseases, 6th edn. Churchill Livingstone, Philadelphia, pp 1084–1126
40. Turgut M, Cullu E, Sendur OF, Gürer G (2004) Brucellar spine infection-four case reports. Neurol Med Chir (Tokyo) 44:562–567
41. Turgut M, Sendur OF, Gürel M (2003) Brucellar spondylodiscitis in the lumbar region. Neurol Med Chir (Tokyo) 43:210–212
42. Young EJ (2010) Brucella species. In: Mandell GL, Bennett JE, Dolin R (eds) Principles and practice of infectious diseases, 7th edn. Churchill Livingstone, Philadelphia, pp 2921–2925

Brucella Meningitis

5

Teresa Somma, Chiara Caggiano, Enrico Tedeschi, Ahmet Tuncay Turgut, and Francesco Faella

Contents

T. Somma, MD (✉) • C. Caggiano, MD
Department of Neurosciences and Reproductive and Odontostomatological Sciences, School of Medicine and Surgery, Università degli Studi di Napoli Federico II, Naples, Italy
e-mail: teresa.somma85@gmail.com; c.caggiano88@gmail.com

E. Tedeschi, MD
Department of Advanced Biomedical Sciences, School of Medicine and Surgery, Università degli Studi di Napoli Federico II, Naples, Italy
e-mail: enrico.tedeschi@unina.it

A.T. Turgut, MD
Department of Radiology, Hacettepe University School of Medicine, Ankara, Turkey
e-mail: ahmettuncayturgut@yahoo.com

F. Faella, MD, PhD
I Division of Infectious Diseases, Department of Infectious Diseases, "D. Cotugno" Hospital, AORN "Dei Colli", Naples, Italy
e-mail: francesco.faella@ospedalideicolli.it

Abstract

Brucellosis is the most common zoonotic infection and is still endemic in many parts of the world.

Brucella is a Gram-negative, nonmotile, facultative aerobic coccobacillus. It possesses a unique ability to avoid the immune system and involves almost every organ system. The precise mechanisms by which *Brucella* enters the central nervous system (CNS) are unknown; probably, the bacteria may affect the CNS directly or indirectly causing meningitis or meningoencephalitis that can present with an acute or chronic onset and can occur either as the only site of infection or in the context of a systemic disease. Diagnostic criteria of *Brucella* meningitis are problematic and based on clinical features and laboratory exams on blood and cerebral fluid. The prognosis is better than other forms of chronic meningitis and the mortality is generally low, but the incidence of minor sequelae is high and will increase in case of a delay in treatment; this is done with tetracycline or doxycycline and streptomycin or rifampin or both.

M. Turgut et al. (eds.), *Neurobrucellosis: Clinical, Diagnostic and Therapeutic Features*,
DOI 10.1007/978-3-319-24639-0_5

Keywords
Brucella • Meningitis • Meningoencephalitis • Neurobrucellosis • Neurotropism

Abbreviations

CNS	Central nervous system
CSF	Cerebrospinal fluid
MAPK	Mitogen-activated protein kinases
MMP-9	Matrix metalloproteinases-9
RBT	Rose Bengal test
STA	Standard tube agglutination
TMP/SMZ	Trimethoprim-sulfamethoxazole
TNF-α	Tumor necrosis factor-α

5.1 Introduction

The neurobrucellosis is an uncommon disease; it can develop from a systemic brucellosis or due to direct central nervous system (CNS) infection. The clinical syndrome is diverse, but the meningeal involvement is present in most patients. The *Brucella* meningitis has not a pathognomonic presentation and the diagnostic criteria are problematic, so that in most cases the diagnosis and, consequently, the treatment are usually made 2–12 months after the onset of symptoms, with high risk of sequelae. In this chapter, we want to describe the different clinical presentations of *Brucella* meningitis and underline the criteria of the diagnosis to improve the prognosis of this disease.

5.2 Microbiology

Brucella is a genus of Gram-negative not shaped bacteria named after David Bruce (1855–1931). They are small (0.5–0.7 by 0.6–1.5 μm), nonmotile, without flagella or pili, nonencapsulated, non-spore-forming, facultative aerobic coccobacilli with a very slow growth in medium containing 5–10 % CO_2 [8]. *Brucella* spp. possesses a unique ability to invade both phagocytic and nonprofessional phagocytic cells and to reside, survive, and replicate in specialized endosomes called "brucellosomes," so that it avoids the immune system [8]. The bacterium recruits actin and activates small GTPases when internalized into cells, with the capacity to prevent apoptosis [8]. This ability explains why brucellosis is a systemic disease.

5.3 Epidemiology

Brucellosis is the most common zoonotic infection and is still endemic in many parts of the world, especially where there are not actual public health and domestic animal health programs. The most common neurological complication is meningitis or meningoencephalitis that can present with an acute or chronic onset and can occur either as the only site of infection or in the context of a systemic disease [15, 20, 32]. It represents 40–90 % of the cases of neurobrucellosis [15, 20, 32].

5.4 Etiopathogenesis

Brucella bacteria may affect the CNS directly or indirectly, by the action of cytokine or endotoxin on the neural tissue. The precise mechanisms by which *Brucella* enters the CNS are unknown. Direct invasion of the CNS is a rare occurrence and is present in less than 2 % of cases [8]. This organism can cause meningitis directly if there is a lesion of the hematoencephalic or the hematoliquoral barrier as following cranial injury [8, 25, 30, 32]. Otherwise, it is important to consider the "Trojan Horse theory" about the infection of the leptomeninges through invasion of immunologic cell system [8, 25, 30, 32]. Many studies show that *Brucella suis* prevents apoptosis of infected and uninfected monocytes. *Brucella* has more opportunity to cross the hematoencephalic barrier thanks to its property of lengthening the host cell's life [8, 11, 30]. It can also infect nonprofessional phagocytes like the endothelial cells composing the barrier. Infection of the CNS via neural route is not demonstrated [8, 11, 25].

The inflammatory response provoked in the CNS by *Brucella* can bring to an irreversible CNS damage and neuronal loss. Cytotoxic T lymphocytes and microglia activation play an immunopathologic role in the disease. The inflammatory response, prevalently tumor necrosis factor-α (TNF-α) mediated, elicited by lipoproteins (L-Omp19 and L-Omp2) of *Brucella abortus* in astrocytes and the production of matrix metalloproteinases-9 (MMP-9) and the mitogen-activated protein kinases (MAPK), may play a role in pathogenesis of damage of the brain, blood–brain barrier, and even neuron death [23, 30]. Miraglia et al. [23] suggest that the inhibition of such molecules, as TNF-α and MAPK, may represent pharmaceutical strategy to restrict MMP-9-mediated brain injury.

5.5 Anatomopathology

Pathological changes of the meninges are frequent. The acute and chronic inflammatory cell infiltration and connective cell proliferation cause a diffuse leptomeningeal thickening, especially in the basal areas. There are often lymphoplasmacytic infiltrate and/or meninx and brain inflammation with central necrosis, demyelination, gliosis, and the development of aneurysms [28]. Vascular inflammation can vary from minimal and mononuclear to massive and neutrophilic, and also possible is an inflammation of the perineurium of nerve roots in the peripheral nervous system [2].

5.6 Clinical Features

The clinical presentation of meningitis is various and is reported as non-pathognomonic from some authors. Meningitis can occur either as the only site of infection or in the context of systemic disease [21, 26, 29, 34].

Meningeal irritation findings in neurobrucellosis have been reported at <50 % (17–74 %). However the most common neurological symptoms are headache, nausea and/or vomiting, and nuchal rigidity. Kernig's sign, Brudzinski's sign, confusion, and altered consciousness are the chief signs. Onset of symptoms varies from abrupt to indolent. In children it was usually reported to have an acute presentation [3, 4, 9, 13, 15, 21, 26, 29, 34].

As with tuberculosis or sarcoidosis, the infection has a predilection for the base of the cranium, thereby involving the cranial nerves [14, 28, 33]. Cranial nerves II, III, VI, VII, and VIII are affected alone or in combination, with VIII being the most frequently involved, followed by VI and VII [14, 28, 33]. Consequently, visual loss, diplopia, facial weakness, and hearing loss are well-known complications.

Psychiatric manifestations, such as depression, amnesia, hallucinations, psychoses, and personality disturbances, are common. Various types of seizures have been reported and are thought to be due to cerebral vasospasm. Tremor and muscle rigidity can resemble Parkinson's disease, and an ascending paralysis resembling Guillain-Barré syndrome has been reported [18, 24].

Granulomatous inflammation within the subarachnoid space may stop the natural cerebrospinal fluid (CSF) reuptake by arachnoid villi, causing hydrocephalus [12, 29]. The meningovascular complications can be hemorrhage, transient ischemic attack, and venous thrombosis [17]. Brain localization may become chronic for the continuance of microorganism's intracellular effects or start-up of the immune mechanism, which can lead to myelin destruction [25, 28, 29].

5.7 Diagnosis

In the literature, there is not a common vision about the diagnostic criteria of *Brucella* meningitis. According to some authors, the diagnosis might be based on symptoms, whereas, according to others, the diagnosis is based on CSF characteristics [9, 12, 13, 15, 22]. In the Istanbul-2 study, Erdem et al. [9] suggested the case definitions of chronic *Brucella* meningitis were as follows:

1. The manifestation of clinical neurological symptoms for over 4 weeks
2. The presence of typical CSF evidences with meningitis (protein concentrations >50 mg/dL, pleocytosis over 10/mm^3, and glucose-to-serum glucose ratios <0.5)
3. Positive bacterial culture or serological test results for brucellosis in CSF (positive Rose Bengal test or serum tube agglutination) and in blood (positive Rose Bengal test and serum tube agglutination with a titer ≥1/160) or positive bone marrow culture
4. Nonappearance of any alternative neurological diagnosis

Diagnosis of *Brucella* meningitis is usually made 2–12 months after the onset of symptoms in most cases. Diagnosis usually depends on the presence of specific antibodies, because *Brucella* is very difficult to isolate in CSF (low bacteria density in CSF, slow and difficult growth in complex incubated medium, frequent use of antibiotics before referring to hospital, necessity of a prolonged period of incubation) and cultures of CSF and gram-stained smears positive in <20 % of cases [4, 9, 13, 14, 27].

In Mediterranean regions, *Brucella melitensis* is more commonly isolated than other *Brucella* spp., probably for its greater neurotropism. The yield of automated culture is higher than the conventional culture in CSF tests. *Brucella*-specific antibodies are usually not detected in the CSF unless the CNS is involved and the finding of brucellar antibody is always indicative of CNS infection [9, 13–15]. The presence of IgG in CSF indicates an intrathecal production of the antibody and also a passive diffusion from the blood [2]. There are four IgG subclasses targeting *Brucella*, with the IgG4 subclass predominating in three-fourths of patients with chronic brucellosis, followed by IgG1, IgG2, and IgG3 [2].

Based on the results of the Istanbul-2 study, the sensitivities of the principal tests were as follows: serum standard tube agglutination (STA), 94 %; CSF STA, 78 %; serum Rose Bengal test (RBT), 96 %; CSF RBT, 71 %; automated blood culture, 37 %; automated CSF culture, 25 %; and conventional CSF culture, 9 % [27]. According preliminary data, molecular diagnostic methods (real-time PCR) seem to be promising in the diagnosis and follow-up of neurobrucellosis [2].

The CSF abnormalities are >10 cells/μl with lymphomonocytic pleocytosis, protein levels >0.45 g/l, and glucose levels <40 mg/dl or 40 % of the blood glucose levels. Erdem et al. [9] in their study report CSF leukocyte counts of 215.99 ± 306.87, CSF protein levels of 330.64 ± 493.28 mg/dL, and CSF/blood glucose ratio of 0.35 ± 0.16. The pathogenesis of CSF hypoglycorrhachia is due to an increased glycolysis by leukocytes and bacteria and increased metabolic rate of the brain [31].

Even from a neuroimaging point of view, neurobrucellosis is a great mimicker: in *Brucella* meningitis brain magnetic resonance imaging may be normal or it may show intense meningeal enhancement, most frequently around the brain stem, possibly with granulomatous nodules and cranial nerve involvement (Figs. 5.1 and 5.2); also, scattered white matter lesions have been reported, as well as perivascular infiltration and vascular insult [1, 4, 19]. At electroencephalogram, no specific findings have been reported [6, 13, 31].

In the differential diagnosis of *Brucella* meningitis, all the infectious and noninfectious mononuclear meningitis have to be considered. *Brucella* meningitis should always be considered in the differential diagnosis of neurological and psychiatric cases that are encountered in endemic areas for brucellosis [15, 16, 20].

5.8 Prognosis

Brucella meningitis differs from other forms of chronic meningitis because it has a better prognosis; in fact mortality is generally lower, with disease being rarely fatal (<0.5) with proper management, and the cause of death is not always clearly related to brucellosis. On the contrary, patients who suffered from diffuse CNS involvement (severe

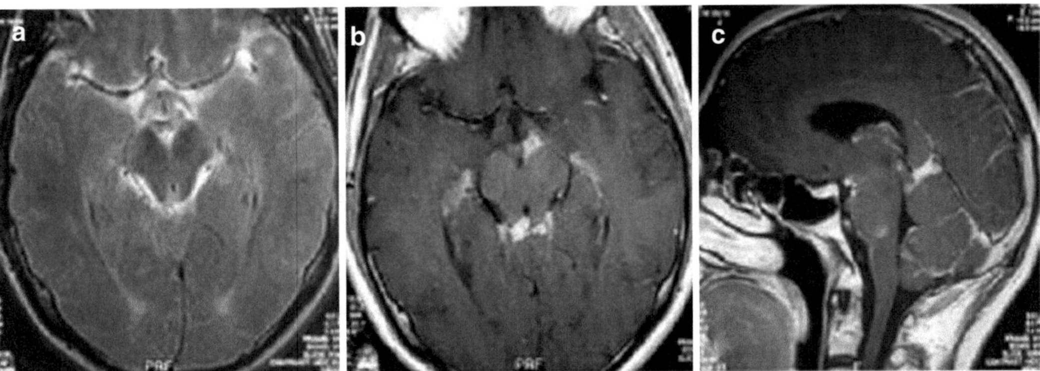

Fig. 5.1 Contrast-enhanced axial T2-FLAIR (**a**), axial (**b**), and sagittal (**c**) T1-weighted slices in a 31-year-old man with *Brucella* meningitis causing visual disturbances. Diffuse and intense enhancement in the basal cisterns after gadolinium administration, with evidence of enhancing granulomas in the interpeduncular and quadrigeminal cisterns. There is also perivascular enhancement along the course of the right middle cerebral artery. A small pontine capillary telangiectasia is evident in **c**

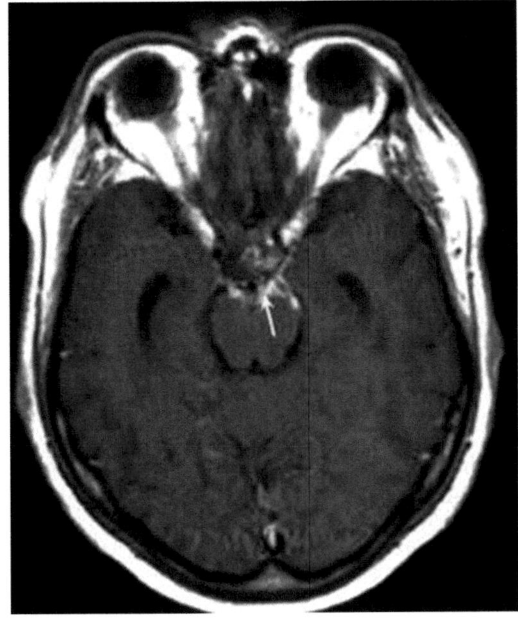

Fig. 5.2 Contrast-enhanced axial T1-weighted MRI in a 56-year-old man with *Brucella* meningitis causing intense headache and neck rigidity, in addition to bilateral abducens nerve palsy and amblyacousia. Note that the presence of basal enhancement of leptomeninges (*arrowhead*) after gadolinium administration (From Jochum et al. [19])

encephalic or spinal cord disease) had a worse prognosis, with mortality not negligible and frequent sequelae. Meningovascular complications, in particular mycotic aneurysms, ischemic stroke, venous thrombosis, and subarachnoid hemorrhage, are relatively common. The incidence of minor sequelae is high and will increase in case of a delay in treatment; however, only a few patients suffered important limitations in their normal activity [4, 20].

5.9 Treatment

There is still no agreement for choice of antibiotic, dose, and time of the treatment of neurological involvement by *Brucella* spp. [4]. Monotherapy can cause relapses, from 40 to 80 %; therefore, combined dual or triple combination therapy with doxycycline, rifampicin, trimethoprim-sulfamethoxazole (TMP/SMZ), streptomycin, or ceftriaxone for >2 months is recommended. Ciprofloxacin combined with other antibiotics is as effective as the standard regimen of doxycycline and rifampicin [5, 7, 10].

Cranial nerve palsies compared during acute infection usually resolve completely with therapy, whereas those with chronic CNS infection often have permanent neurological deficit [3, 4, 33]. Some authors suggest that antibiotic treatment has to be continued until improvement of clinical symptoms, glucose normalization in CSF, reduction of leukocytes less than 100 cells/mm^3, and the decrease of antibody titers [3].

Conclusion

- *Brucella* bacteria can cause meningitis directly or through invasion of immunologic cell system.
- Pathological changes of the meninges are frequent.
- The clinical presentation of meningitis is various; however, the most common neurological symptoms are headache, nausea, and/or vomiting, and the chief signs are nuchal rigidity, Kernig's sign, Brudzinski's sign, confusion, and altered consciousness.
- In the literature, diagnostic criteria are problematic, and the diagnosis is based on clinical and laboratory exams.
- The prognosis quoad vitam is better than the other forms of chronic meningitis; mortality is generally low, but the prognosis quoad valetudinem is low; the incidence of minor sequelae is high and will increase in case of a delay in treatment.
- Dual or triple combination therapy with doxycycline, rifampicin, TMP/SMZ, streptomycin, or ceftriaxone for >2 months is recommended.

References

1. Al-Sous MW, Bohlega S, Al-Kawi MZ, Alwatban J, McLean DR (2004) Neurobrucellosis: clinical and neuroimaging correlation. AJNR Am J Neuroradiol 25:395–401
2. Araj GF (2010) Update on laboratory diagnosis of human brucellosis. Int J Antimicrob Agents 36:S12–S17
3. Bouza E, García de la Torre M, Parras F, Guerrero A, Rodríguez-Créixems M, Gobernado J (1987) Brucellar meningitis. Rev Infect Dis 9:810–822
4. Ceran N, Turkoglu R, Erdem I, Inan A, Engin D, Tireli H, Goktas P (2011) Neurobrucellosis: clinical, diagnostic, therapeutic features and outcome. Unusual clinical presentations in an endemic region. Braz J Infect Dis 15:52–59
5. Conti R, Parenti F (1983) Rifampin therapy for brucellosis, flavobacterium meningitis, and cutaneous leishmaniasis. Rev Infect Dis 5:S600–S605
6. Corbel MJ (1997) Brucellosis: an overview. Emerg Infect Dis 3:213–221
7. Corbel MJ (1976) Determination of the in vitro sensitivity of Brucella strains to rifampicin. Br Vet J 132:266–275
8. Drevets DA, Leenen PJ, Greenfield RA (2004) Invasion of the central nervous system by intracellular bacteria. Clin Microbiol Rev 17:323–347
9. Erdem H, Kilic S, Sener B, Acikel C, Alp E, Karahocagil M, Yetkin F, Inan A, Kecik-Bosnak V, Gul HC, Tekin-Koruk S, Ceran N, Demirdal T, Yilmaz G, Ulu-Kilic A, Ceylan B, Dogan-Celik A, Nayman-Alpat S, Tekin R, Yalci A, Turhan V, Karaoglan I, Yilmaz H, Mete B, Batirel A, Ulcay A, Dayan S, Seza Inal A, Ahmed SS, Tufan ZK, Karakas A, Teker B, Namiduru M, Savasci U, Pappas G (2013) Diagnosis of chronic brucellar meningitis and meningoencephalitis: the results of the Istanbul-2 study. Clin Microbiol Infect 19:E80–E86
10. Farrell ID, Hinchliffe PM, Robertson L (1976) Sensitivity of Brucella spp to tetracycline and its analogues. J Clin Pathol 29:1097–1100
11. Gross A, Terraza A, Ouahrani-Bettache S, Liautard JP, Dornand J (2000) In vitro Brucella suis infection prevents the programmed cell death of human monocytic cells. Infect Immun 68:342–351
12. Gul HC, Erdem H, Bek S (2009) Overview of neurobrucellosis: a pooled analysis of 187 cases. Int J Infect Dis 13:e339–e343
13. Guven T, Ugurlu K, Ergonul O, Celikbas AK, Gok SE, Comoglu S, Baykam N, Dokuzoguz B (2013) Neurobrucellosis: clinical and diagnostic features. Clin Infect Dis 56:1407–1412
14. Haji-Abdolbagi M, Rasooli-Nejad M, Jafari S, Hasibi M, Soudbakhsh A (2008) Clinical and laboratory findings in neurobrucellosis: review of 31 cases. Arch Iran Med 11:21–25
15. Hatami H, Hatami M, Soori H, Janbakhsh AR, Mansouri F (2010) Epidemiological, clinical, and laboratory features of brucellar meningitis. Arch Iran Med 13:486–491
16. Hatami H, Saghari H (2003) Epidemiology of brucellosis. In: Hatami H (ed) Epidemiology and control of diseases related to bioterrorism Teharan Seda Publishing Co. 2nd edn. pp 195–260
17. Inan AS, Ceran N, Erdem I, Engin DO, Senbayrak S, Ozyurek SC, Goktas P (2010) Neurobrucellosis with transient ischemic attack, vasculopathic changes, intracerebral granulomas and basal ganglia infarction: a case report. J Med Case Rep 4:340
18. Jin K, Liu Y, Chen N, Kong L, Jiang L, Li J, Huang Z (2013) A case of brucellosis displaying Parkinsonian-like tremor. J Infect Dev Ctries 7:1008–1011
19. Jochum T, Kliesch U, Both R, Leonhardi J, Bär KJ (2008) Neurobrucellosis with thalamic infarction: a case report. Neurol Sci 29:481–3
20. Karsen H, Tekin Koruk S, Duygu F, Yapici K, Kati M (2012) Review of 17 cases of neurobrucellosis: clinical manifestations, diagnosis, and management. Arch Iran Med 15:491–494
21. McLean DR, Russell N, Khan MY (1992) Neurobrucellosis: clinical and therapeutic features. Clin Infect Dis 15:582–590
22. Mehmet RM, Rustu YF, Hanefi B, Mursel D, Fusun A, Mehmet I (2013) Direct pelvic access percutaneous

nephrolithotomy in management of ectopic kidney stone: a case report and literature review. Ren Fail 35:1440–1444

23. Miraglia MC, Scian R, Samartino CG, Barrionuevo P, Rodriguez AM, Ibanez AE, Coria LM, Velasquez LN, Baldi PC, Cassataro J, Delpino MV, Giambartolomei GH (2013) Brucella abortus induces TNF-alpha-dependent astroglial MMP-9 secretion through mitogen-activated protein kinases. J Neuroinflammation 10:47
24. Molins A, Montalban J, Codina A (1987) Parkinsonism in neurobrucellosis. J Neurol Neurosurg Psychiatry 50:1707–1708
25. Pappas G, Akritidis N, Bosilkovski M, Tsianos E (2005) Brucellosis. N Engl J Med 352:2325–2336
26. Ranjbar M, Rezaiee AA, Hashemi SH, Mehdipour S (2009) Neurobrucellosis: report of a rare disease in 20 Iranian patients referred to a tertiary hospital. East Mediterr Health J 15:143–148
27. Sanchez-Sousa A, Torres C, Campello MG, Garcia C, Parras F, Cercenado E, Baquero F (1990) Serological diagnosis of neurobrucellosis. J Clin Pathol 43:79–81
28. Seidel G, Pardo CA, Newman-Toker D, Olivi A, Eberhart CG (2003) Neurobrucellosis presenting as leukoencephalopathy: the role of cytotoxic T lymphocytes. Arch Pathol Lab Med 127:e374–e377
29. Shakir RA, Al-Din AS, Araj GF, Lulu AR, Mousa AR, Saadah MA (1987) Clinical categories of neurobrucellosis. A report on 19 cases. Brain 110:213–223
30. Tolomeo M, Di Carlo P, Abbadessa V, Titone L, Miceli S, Barbusca E, Cannizzo G, Mancuso S, Arista S, Scarlata F (2003) Monocyte and lymphocyte apoptosis resistance in acute and chronic brucellosis and its possible implications in clinical management. Clin Infect Dis 36:1533–1538
31. Tunkel AR (2010) Approach to the patient with central nervous system infection. In: Mandell GL, Bennett JE, Dolin R (eds) Mandell, Douglas, and Bennett's principles and practice of infectious diseases, 7th edn. Churchill Livingstone Elsevier, Philadelphia, pp 1183–1188
32. Turel O, Sanli K, Hatipoglu N, Aydogmus C, Hatipoglu H, Siraneci R (2010) Acute meningoencephalitis due to Brucella: case report and review of neurobrucellosis in children. Turk J Pediatr 52:426–429
33. Vinod P, Singh MK, Garg RK, Agarwal A (2007) Extensive meningoencephalitis, retrobulbar neuritis and pulmonary involvement in a patient of neurobrucellosis. Neurol India 55:157–159
34. Young EJ (2010) Brucella species. In: Mandell GL, Bennett JE, Dolin R (eds) Mandell, Douglas, and Bennett's principles and practice of infectious diseases, 7th edn. Churchill Livingstone, Philadelphia, pp 2921–2925

Brucellar Encephalitis

6

Güliz Uyar Güleç and Ahmet Tuncay Turgut

Contents

Abstract

Brucellosis involving the central nervous system is endemic in many parts of the world, especially in the Mediterranean region and Middle East. The most frequent clinical syndrome is acute meningoencephalitis with generalized and focal signs, but neurobrucellosis may be overlooked owing to its nonspecific clinical findings. In this chapter, clinical manifestations and microbiological laboratory findings of brucellar encephalitis, as well as the treatment and the detection of various complications, were reviewed. In particular, clinical suspicion is the most important clue in the diagnosis and treatment of cases with brucellosis. It is very important to keep in mind the likelihood of neurobrucellosis in patients with unexplained neurological and psychiatric symptoms in endemic parts of the world.

Keywords

Neurobrucellosis • Non-granulomatous encephalitis • Meningoencephalitis

Abbreviations

CNS	Central nervous system
CSF	Cerebrospinal fluid
ELISA	Enzyme-linked immunosorbent assay

G.U. Güleç, MD (✉)
Department of Infectious Diseases, Adnan Menderes University School of Medicine, Aydın, Turkey
e-mail: gulizuyar@yahoo.com

A.T. Turgut, MD
Department of Radiology, Hacettepe University School of Medicine, Ankara, Turkey
e-mail: ahmettuncayturgut@yahoo.com

M. Turgut et al. (eds.), *Neurobrucellosis: Clinical, Diagnostic and Therapeutic Features*,
DOI 10.1007/978-3-319-24639-0_6

HKBA	Heat-killed bacteria
IL-6	Interleukin 6
MCP-1	Monocyte chemoattractant protein-1
PCR	Polymerase chain reaction
RBT	Rose Bengal test
STA	Serum tube agglutination
TMP/SMZ	Trimethoprim/sulfamethoxazole
TNF	Tumor necrosis factor

6.1 Introduction

Brucellosis is a zoonosis spread throughout the world. The symptoms associated with the disease are related to clinical manifestations of various acute and chronic infectious entities and may mimic various diseases. Neurobrucellosis is an unusual complication of brucellosis and occurs in less than 5 % of the patients. Clinically, the spectrum of neurobrucellosis involves central and peripheral subtypes. The entity can present as meningitis, encephalitis, myelitis-radiculoneuritis, brain abscess, epidural abscess, meningovascular complications, peripheral neuropathy, and psychosis [17, 21]. Neurobrucellosis is usually present as meningitis or meningoencephalitis.

Encephalitis implies the presence of an inflammatory process in the brain tissue. As a result of this inflammation, clinical signs of neurological dysfunction arise. The majority of pathogens reported to cause encephalitis are the viruses. There are several epidemiological clues that determine the etiology such as the prevalence of disease in the local community, travel history, animal contact, season of the year, recreational activities, occupational exposure, insect contact, vaccination history, and immune status of the patient [30]. Encephalitis caused by *Brucella* species is usually associated with meningitis as a component in clinical cases [32].

6.2 Immunopathology of Brucellar Encephalitis

Neurobrucellosis is an inflammatory disorder. As *Brucella* lacks exotoxins, exoproteases, or cytolysins, in order to explain the central nervous system (CNS) damage mechanisms in neurobrucellosis, several processes have been proposed; among these the most accepted are the direct action of the bacterium, the effect of pro-inflammatory cytokines, and a demyelinating immunopathological pathway [4].

The entities of encephalitis and myelitis are directly associated with the presence of the bacterium in the cerebral tissue and the spinal cord. In spite of the fact that the brain is rarely biopsied in patients with brucellosis, and the reported number of microscopic descriptions of CNS involvement is relatively few, concomitant presence of diffuse white matter involvement and astrogliosis and reactive microgliosis has consistently been described in the literature [4].

The role of pro-inflammatory cytokines in the immunopathology of neurobrucellosis has been presented in a study [14]. *Brucella abortus* and its lipoproteins activate the innate immunity which initiates an inflammatory response in the CNS of mice, and this leads to astrogliosis which is characteristically associated with neurobrucellosis [14]. Heat-killed bacteria (HKBA) and the L-Omp19 lipoprotein elicit two features of astrogliosis, namely, astrocyte apoptosis and proliferation, and apoptosis depends on tumor necrosis factor (TNF) signaling [14]. In vitro, *B. abortus* infection of astrocytes and microglia induced the secretion of interleukin 6 (IL-6), IL-1, TNF, and monocyte chemoattractant protein-1 (MCP-1), but HKBA and L-Omp19 also induced the same cytokine and chemokine secretion pattern [14].

In the literature, a case of meningoencephalitis with a diffuse involvement pattern of the white matter mimicking leukoencephalopathy has been described [28]. The inflammatory infiltrate was mainly composed of T cells [28]. Cell surface markers including CD4 and CD8 immunophenotyping of the T cell infiltrates in the white matter and cortex showed that the T cells were CD8 lymphocytes predominantly [28]. Based on their findings, the authors hypothesized that the clinical and radiological abnormalities were mediated, at least in part, by immunopathogenic mechanisms related to direct cytotoxic T lymphocyte-mediated injury of the white matter and the cerebral cortex [28].

6.3 Clinical Features

Neurobrucellosis may present with neurological and psychiatric symptoms. Therefore some patients are referred to neurology or psychiatry physicians as well as infectious disease departments.

The clinical presentation of two or more clinical syndromes may appear in the same patient [24]. Diffused or localized meningitis or acute, subacute, relapsing, or chronic meningoencephalitis has been described [27]. Clinically, acute brucellosis cases typically present with the findings of chills, fever, fatigue, sweating, weight loss, and back pain. On the other hand, subacute cases show less severe symptoms. In the chronic cases, patients usually present malaise, nervousness, emotional lability, depression, and generalized musculoskeletal pain [10, 34].

In a retrospective evaluation of 1028 cases with brucellosis, these were divided into four groups: acute (0–2 months), subacute (2–12 months), chronic (>12 months), and relapse. CNS involvement was present in 58 cases [5]. With regard to clinical findings, 49 cases were evaluated as acute, eight as subacute, one as chronic, and no relapse cases [5]. Of these, 45 patients (77.6 %) had meningitis or meningoencephalitis, seven (12.1 %) had encephalitis, and the remaining had other neurological conditions [5].

In a study by Yetkin et al. [33], fever and headache were detected as the major presenting complaints. According to the findings of Güven's study [18], the presence of headache, blurred vision, loss of hearing, and confusion was found to be significantly higher in cases with neurobrucellosis than in cases without brucellosis. In another study, the cases were classified into two clinical categories: the first group had meningovascular complications such as fever and neck stiffness, and the second group had prominent signs of diffuse brain or spinal cord involvement [6]. Neurological findings in meningoencephalitis cases were papilledema, intentional tremor, hearing loss, dysmetria, ataxia, diplopia, motor aphasia, hemiparesis, and confusion [6]. Karsen et al. [22] have reported three cases of meningoencephalitis and 13 cases of meningitis. Symptoms of cases were headache (in all patients), fever (38 %), and nausea-vomiting (33 %). Neurological (hemiparesis, aphasia, dizziness, facial paralysis, diplopia, ataxia, tremor, etc.) and psychiatric symptoms were also present in some patients.

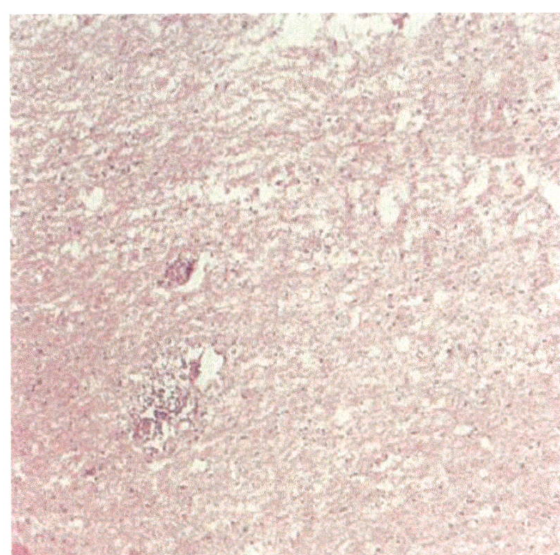

Fig. 6.1 Non-granulomatous encephalitis. A hematoxylin and eosin (H&E)-stained brain section shows scattered lymphocytic infiltrates and perivascular lymphocytic cuffing (From Erdem et al. [13], with permission)

There is no doubt that unusual clinical forms of neurobrucellosis can also be seen. A case of encephalitis caused by *B. melitensis*, mimicking a cerebral tumor, was described. The solitary mass lesion was clinically and radiologically indistinguishable from a brain tumor, but there was no evidence of meningeal inflammation [13]. The diagnosis was established by isolating *B. melitensis* in a blood culture, and a positive serum tube agglutination (STA) test on the cerebrospinal fluid (CSF) at 1:320 titers and paraffin sections of the cerebral mass depicted non-granulomatous encephalitis consisting of diffuse lymphocytic infiltrates and perivascular lymphocytic cuffing (Fig. 6.1) [13].

6.4 Diagnosis

The diagnosis requires the combination of several approaches. All patients must be questioned about epidemiological risk factors for brucellosis. Clinical examination, routine hematological and biochemical laboratory tests, and radiological investigations are elements of the primary approach.

The diagnosis of brucellar meningoencephalitis requires the demonstration of the findings related to meningeal inflammation, abnormal CSF findings, and direct or indirect evidence of *Brucella* in the CSF [20, 25, 29].

Lumbar puncture is suggested in all cases with symptoms and clinical findings consistent with neurobrucellosis, unless contraindicated. Analysis findings of CSF reveal lymphocytic pleocytosis, increased CSF protein level, and normal or decreased CSF/plasma glucose ratio [31].

Culture, when positive, is accepted as the gold standard for the laboratory diagnosis of brucellosis. Importantly, the speed of recovery is dependent on the culture method used and the type of specimen used. In this regard, the conventional method requiring a long incubation time of 6 weeks has a yield of 5–20 % in chronic, focal, and complicated cases [2]. In a study automated culture systems yielded the pathogen from the CSF significantly higher than the conventional culture [11].

As culturing of *Brucella* takes time, laboratory diagnosis very often relies on detecting specific serum antibodies. In the serological diagnosis of brucellosis, Rose Bengal test (RBT), microagglutination test, STA, indirect Coombs (antihuman globulin) test, complement fixation, enzyme-linked immunosorbent assay (ELISA), and immunocapture agglutination techniques have been used [2, 15].

Serological tests such as serum STA, RBT, and ELISA as well as CSF RBT, STA, and ELISA were applied to 177 patients with chronic brucellar meningitis or meningoencephalitis in a multicenter, retrospective study [11]. The sensitivities of the tests were 94 % for serum STA, 96 % for serum RBT, 78 % for CSF STA, and 71 % for CSF RBT [11]. No significant difference was detected between the sensitivities of CSF RBT and CSF STA ($p=0.163$) and the serum RBT and the serum STA ($p=0.500$), whereas the differences for either serum and CSF RBT or serum and CSF STA were significant statistically ($p<0.001$) [11].

A total of 31 neurobrucellosis cases, 14 with meningoencephalitis, were evaluated in a study. STA was performed on 16 CSF samples; 14 samples were found positive ranging from 1/20 to 1/1280. In one patient, neurobrucellosis was diagnosed despite negative CSF culture and serology, just based on the clinical response with anti-*Brucella* treatment. The authors suggest that it is better to use CSF Coombs test, in addition to CSF STA test and culture, because CSF STA test may be negative in patients with suspicious neurobrucellosis [19].

In another case series of 11 patients, all the initial blood STA titers were lower than 1/200, and the CSF STA titers were under 1/100 on initial examination. All of the cases had positive CSF serology [17].

Molecular assays, like conventional polymerase chain reaction (PCR) and real-time PCR, have been utilized for investigation of patients with brucellosis. They can be used for direct detection of *Brucella* from clinical specimens, to monitor treatment response, for the identification and differentiation of recovered *Brucella* spp. [9, 23]. The sensitivity of these assays ranges from 50 to 100 % and the specificity from 60 to 98 % [2]. In a study, real-time PCR was applied to CSF samples of three meningoencephalitis and three meningitis patients. PCR assays were positive in all six cases of neurobrucellosis, whereas the sensitivity of seroagglutination and cultures of CSF samples were 66.6 % and 33.3 %, respectively. It was concluded by the authors that the method may be a very useful tool and even could be considered as the new gold standard for the diagnosis of neurobrucellosis [7].

Radiological findings in neurobrucellosis can be due to an inflammatory process, white matter changes, or vascular injury. But radiology may be entirely normal [26]. Imaging abnormalities may mimic other neurological diseases such as multiple sclerosis, acute disseminated encephalomyelitis, or Lyme disease. Granuloma formation or meningeal enhancement can occur due to inflammation (Fig. 6.2) [1, 32]. Anatomically, brucellosis may involve CNS parenchyma at any location including the cerebellum, spinal cord, and cerebellar white matter (Fig. 6.3) [13, 25].

6.5 Treatment

The crucial therapeutic component of all forms of human brucellosis is the administration of effective antibiotics for an adequate length of time. Importantly, the treatment of CNS complications of brucellosis may be problematic because it is needed to achieve high concentrations of drugs in the CSF.

A variety of drugs have activity against *Brucella* spp., though the results of in vitro susceptibility tests are not always consistent with clinical efficacy. The treatment recommended by the World Health Organization for uncomplicated brucellosis in adults is doxycycline 100 mg twice daily for 6 weeks and streptomycin 1 g/day intramuscularly administered for 2–3 weeks. Rifampicin is recommended as principal alternative therapy [8]. In clinical practice doxycycline plus rifampicin an all-oral regimen eliminates the need for parenteral administration and may allow for better compliance [3].

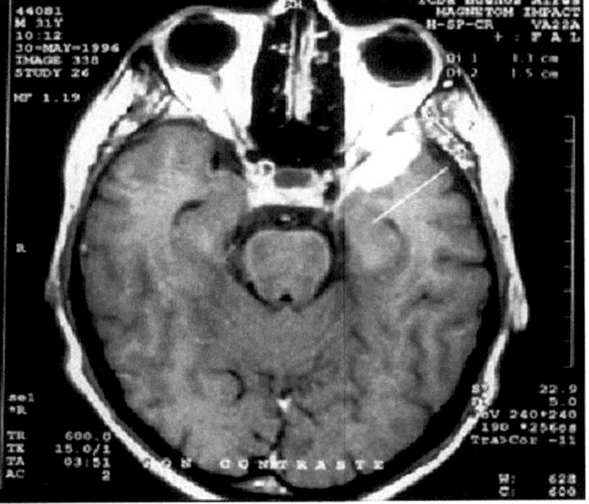

Fig. 6.2 Cerebral magnetic resonance image of a patient with neurobrucellosis due to *Brucella suis*. Areas of increased signal consistent with granulomas can be seen in the left parietal and temporal lobes (From Wallach et al [32], with permission)

The paucity of therapeutic data precludes any recommendations to be offered for the time being for neurobrucellosis. Since tetracyclines and aminoglycosides do not penetrate the blood/brain barrier well, it is recommended that drugs which achieve this, such as rifampicin, trimethoprim/sulfamethoxazole (TMP/SMZ), ciprofloxacin, or ceftriaxone, be added to the standard regimen of doxycycline plus streptomycin [8, 12].

There is no data in the literature on whether brucellar meningitis or meningoencephalitis can be treated with oral antibiotics or whether an intravenous extended-spectrum cephalosporin should be added to the regimen. In various studies, ceftriaxone was found to be the most effective extended-spectrum cephalosporin for *Brucella* species. In addition the use of ceftriaxone alone in patients with brucellosis has been known to be associated with frequent therapeutic failures and relapses.

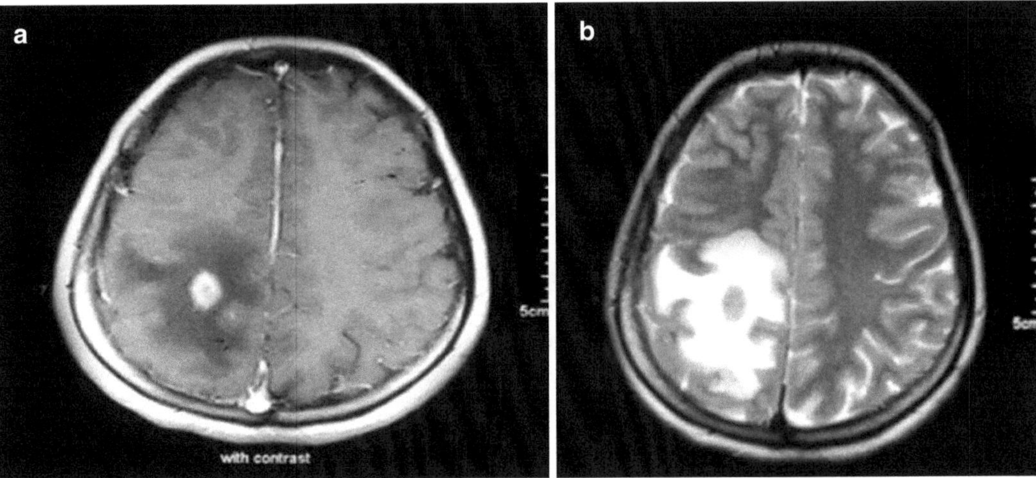

Fig. 6.3 A nodule in the right parietal region surrounded by vasogenic edema on T1- weighted (**a**) and T2-weighted (**b**) gadolinium-enhanced axial images (From Erdem et al. [13], with permission)

In a retrospective study including 215 adult patients, the first group (P1, $n = 120$) received ceftriaxone, rifampicin, and doxycycline [12]. The second protocol (P2, $n = 44$) consisted of TMP/SMZ, rifampicin, and doxycycline. In the third protocol (P3, $n = 51$), however, the patients started with P1 and transferred to P2 when ceftriaxone was stopped [12]. The treatment period was shorter with the ceftriaxone-based regimens ($p = 0.002$), and the efficacy of this regimen was found to be better when a relapse and therapeutic failure were considered [12].

The optimal duration of treatment for neurobrucellosis has not been reported, though a minimum of 6–8 weeks, and possibly longer, depending on the clinical response, has been recommended by most authorities [8]. The duration of treatment ranged from 3 months to 1 year in various clinical case studies [1, 6, 18, 33].

A total of 35 publications and 187 neurobrucellosis cases from Turkey were evaluated in a review [16]. The duration of antibiotic therapy was reported for 56 patients in the publications as 2–15 months, median 5 months [16]. In this study, ceftriaxone, doxycycline, rifampicin, streptomycin, TMP/SMZ, gentamicin, and ofloxacin were the drugs used in different combinations and over different intervals [16].

Conclusion

Brucellar meningoencephalitis frequently has a subtle nature and cannot be diagnosed easily. It should be kept in mind that all cases can easily be confused with other infectious diseases like viral encephalitis, tuberculosis, and neurological or psychiatric disorders without infectious origin. In this regard, accurate and timely diagnosis of the disease is crucial in the rational management of patients. Importantly, neuroimaging and neurophysiologic evaluation in combination with the microbiological diagnostic tools are helpful for both the diagnosis and the detection of complications of the disease. Finally, the clinicians practicing in endemic areas in particular should keep in mind the likelihood of neurobrucellosis in patients with unexplained neurological and psychiatric symptoms.

References

1. Al-Sous MW, Bohlega S, Al-Kawi MZ, Alwatban J, McLean DR (2004) Neurobrucellosis: clinical and neuroimaging correlation. AJNR Am J Neuroradiol 25:395–401
2. Araj GF (2010) Update on laboratory diagnosis of human brucellosis. Int J Antimicrob Agents 36:S12–S17
3. Ariza J, Bosilkovski M, Cascio A, Colmenero JD, Corbel MJ, Falagas ME, Memish ZA, Roushan MR, Rubinstein E, Sipsas NV, Solera J, Young EJ, Pappas G (2007) Perspectives for the treatment of brucellosis in the 21st century: the Ioannina recommendations. PLoS Med 4, e317
4. Baldi PC, Giambartolomei GH (2013) Immunopathology of Brucella infection. Recent Pat Antiinfect Drug Discov 8:18–26
5. Buzgan T, Karahocagil MK, Irmak H, Baran AI, Karsen H, Evirgen O, Akdeniz H (2010) Clinical manifestations and complications in 1028 cases of brucellosis: a retrospective evaluation and review of the literature. Int J Infect Dis 14:e469–e478
6. Ceran N, Turkoglu R, Erdem I, Inan A, Engin D, Tireli H, Goktas P (2010) Neurobrucellosis: clinical, diagnostic, therapeutic features and outcome. Unusual clinical presentations in an endemic region. Braz J Infect Dis 15:52–59
7. Colmenero JD, Queipo-Ortuno MI, Reguera JM, Baeza G, Salazar JA, Morata P (2005) Real time polymerase chain reaction: a new powerful tool for the diagnosis of neurobrucellosis. J Neurol Neurosurg Psychiatry 76:1025–1027
8. Corbel MJ (2006) Brucellosis in humans and animals. World Health Organization Publications, Geneva, pp 36–41
9. Debeaumont C, Falconnet PA, Maurin M (2005) Real-time PCR for detection of Brucella spp. DNA in human serum samples. Eur J Clin Microbiol Infect Dis 24:842–845
10. Doğanay M, Meşe Alp E (2008) Brucellosis (in Turkish). In: Topcu AW, Söyletir G, Doğanay M (eds) Infection diseases and microbiology (in Turkish), 3rd edn. Nobel Tıp Kitabevleri, İstanbul, pp 897–909
11. Erdem H, Kılıç S, Sener B, Açıkel C, Alp E, Karahocagil M, Yetkin F, Inan A, Kecik-bosnak V, Gul HC, Tekin-Koruk S, Ceran N, Demirdal T, Yılmaz G, Ulu-Kılıç A, Ceylan B, Doğan-Çelik A, Nayman-Alpat S, Tekin R, Yalci A, Turhan V, Karaoglan I, Yilmaz H, Mete B, Batirel A, Ulcay A, Dayan S, Sezalnal A, Ahmed SS, Tufan ZK, Karakas A, Teker B, Namiduru M, Savasci U, Pappas G (2012) Diagnosis of chronic brucellar meningitis and meningoencephalitis: the results of the Istanbul-2 study. Clin Microbiol Infect 19:E80–E86
12. Erdem H, Ulu-Kilic A, Kilic S, Karahocagil M, Shehata G, Eren-Tulek N, Yetkin F, Celen MK, Ceran N, Gul HC, Mert G, Tekin-Koruk S, Dizbay M, Inal AS, Nayman-Alpat S, Bosilkovski M, Inan D, Saltoglu N, Abdel-Baky L, Adeva-Bartolome MT, Ceylan B, Sacar S, Turhan V, Yilmaz E, Elaldi N,

Kocak-Tufan Z, Ugurlu K, Dokuzoguz B, Yilmaz H, Gundes S, Guner R, Ozgunes N, Ulcay A, Unal S, Dayan S, Gorenek L, Karakas A, Tasova Y, Usluer G, Bayindir Y, Kurtaran B, Sipahi OR, Leblebicioglu H (2012) Efficacy and tolerability of antibiotic combinations in neurobrucellosis: results of the Istanbul study. Antimicrob Agents Chemother 56:1523–1528

13. Erdem M, Namiduru M, Karaoglan I, Kecik VB, Aydin A, Tanriverdi M (2012) Unusual presentation of neurobrucellosis: a solitary intracranial mass lesion mimicking a cerebral tumor: a case of encephalitis caused by Brucella melitensis. J Infect Chemother 18:767–770
14. Garcia Samartino C, Delpino MV, Pott Godoy C, Di Genaro MS, Pasquevich KA, Zwerdling A, Barrionuevo P, Mathieu P, Cassataro J, Pitossi F, Giambartolomei GH (2010) Brucella abortus induces the secretion of proinflammatory mediators from glial cells leading to astrocyte apoptosis. Am J Pathol 176:1323–1338
15. Gomez MC, Nieto JA, Rosa C, Geijo P, Escribano MA, Munoz A, Lopez C (2008) Evaluation of seven tests for diagnosis of human brucellosis in an area where the disease is endemic. Clin Vaccine Immunol 15:1031–1033
16. Gul HC, Erdem H, Bek S (2009) Overview of neurobrucellosis: a pooled analysis of 187 cases. Int J Infect Dis 13:e339–e343
17. Gul HC, Erdem H, Gorenek L, Ozdag MF, Kalpakci Y, Avci IY, Besirbellioglu BA, Eyigun CP (2008) Management of neurobrucellosis: an assessment of 11 cases. Intern Med 47:995–1001
18. Guven T, Ugurlu K, Ergonul O, Celikbas AK, Gok SE, Comoglu S, Baykam N, Dokuzoguz B (2013) Neurobrucellosis: clinical and diagnostic features. Clin Infect Dis 56:1407–1412
19. Haji-Abdolbagi M, Rasooli-Nejad M, Jafari S, Hasibi M, Soudbakhsh A (2008) Clinical and laboratory findings in neurobrucellosis: review of 31 cases. Arch Iran Med 11:21–25
20. Hatipoglu CA, Yetkin A, Ertem GT, Tulek N (2004) Unusual clinical presentations of brucellosis. Scand J Infect Dis 36:694–697
21. Karaoglan I, Namiduru M, Akcali A, Cansel N (2008) Different manifestations of nervous system involvement by neurobrucellosis. Neurosciences 13:283–287
22. Karsen H, Tekin Koruk S, Duygu F, Yapici K, Kati M (2012) Review of 17 cases of neurobrucellosis: clinical manifestations, diagnosis, and management. Arch Iran Med 15:491–494
23. Kattar MM, Zalloua PA, Araj GF, Samaha-Kfoury J, Shbaklo H, Kanj SS, Khalife S, Deeb M (2007) Development and evaluation of real-time polymerase chain reaction assays on whole blood and paraffin-embedded tissues for rapid diagnosis of human brucellosis. Diagn Microbiol Infect Dis 59:23–32
24. Kyebambe PS (2005) Acute brucella meningomyeloencephalo-spondylosis in a teenage male. Afr Health Sci 5:69–72
25. McLean DR, Russell N, Khan MY (1992) Neurobrucellosis: clinical and therapeutic features. Clin Infect Dis 15:582–590
26. Montazeri M, Sadeghi K, Khalili H, Davoudi S (2013) Fever and psychosis as an early presentation of Brucella-associated meningoencephalitis: a case report. Med Princ Pract 22:506–509
27. Obiako OR, Ogoina D, Danbauchi SS, Kwaifa SI, Chom ND, Nwokorie E (2010) Neurobrucellosis- a case report and review of literature. Niger J Clin Pract 13:347–350
28. Seidel G, Pardo CA, Newman-Toker D, Olivi A, Eberhart CG (2003) Neurobrucellosis presenting as leukoencephalopathy: the role of cytotoxic T lymphocytes. Arch Pathol Lab Med 127:e374–e377
29. Shakir R (1986) Neurobrucellosis. Postgrad Med J 62:1077–1079
30. Tunkel AR, Glaser CA, Bloch KC, Sejvar JJ, Marra CM, Roos KL, Hartman BJ, Kaplan SL, Scheld WM, Whitley RJ (2008) The management of encephalitis: clinical practice guidelines by the Infectious Diseases Society of America. Clin Infect Dis 47:303–327
31. Turel O, Sanli K, Hatipoglu N, Aydogmus C, Hatipoglu H, Siraneci R (2010) Acute meningoencephalitis due to Brucella: case report and review of neurobrucellosis in children. Turk J Pediatr 52:426–429
32. Wallach JC, Baldi PC, Fossati CA (2002) Clinical and diagnostic aspects of relapsing meningoencephalitis due to Brucella suis. Eur J Clin Microbiol Infect Dis 21:760–762
33. Yetkin MA, Bulut C, Erdinç FŞ, Oral B, Tulek N (2006) Evaluation of the clinical presentations in neurobrucellosis. Int J Infect Dis 10:446–452
34. Young EJ (2010) Brucella species. In: Mandell GL, Bennett JE, Dolin R (eds) Principles and practice of infectious diseases, 7th edn. Churchill Livingstone, Philadelphia, pp 2921–2925

Brucella Abscess and Granuloma of the Brain

7

Fuad Sami Haddad†

Contents

Abstract

A thorough search of the literature reveals a total of 21 cases of brain *Brucella* abscess and brucelloma. In this chapter, these were reviewed and tabulated and their incidence, the ways of brain invasion, and their distribution as to sex, age, lateralization, localization, multiplicity, size, signs and symptoms, laboratory findings, and pathology were discussed.

Keywords

Brucella abscess • Brucelloma

Abbreviations

ESR	Erythrocyte sedimentation rate
CNS	Central nervous system
CSF	Cerebrospinal fluid
CT	Computed tomography
MRI	Magnetic resonance imaging
STA	Serum tube agglutination

7.1 Introduction

Although the author had reported, in 2006, on a series of 21 personal cases of *Brucella* spondylitis [20], his first and only encounter with a brain *Brucella* abscess was in 1995 when such an

† Author was deceased at the time of publication.

F.S. Haddad, MD, FACS, FRCS, ABNS
Department of Surgery, American University of Beirut, Beirut, Lebanon
e-mail: fshaddad@aub.edu.lb

M. Turgut et al. (eds.), *Neurobrucellosis: Clinical, Diagnostic and Therapeutic Features*,
DOI 10.1007/978-3-319-24639-0_7

abscess was evacuated from the remaining frontal lobe of a patient who had been hemispherectomized 23 years earlier for infantile intractable seizures (Fig. 7.1) [19]. He had been fed raw milk in an attempt "to improve his resistance against disease." At that time a thorough search of the medical literature revealed only ten such abscesses. At present, an additional 16 references on *Brucella* abscess or "brucelloma" (the word brucelloma is not found in the medical dictionaries. It has been coined to denote a granuloma due to *Brucella* infection) of the brain were found in the available world literature (two authors reported each two cases) [34] (see Table 7.1). The entire material shall be analyzed in this chapter.

7.2 Incidence

Central nervous system (CNS) complications associated with *Brucella* infection are rare but varied. The commonest are encephalitis, meningitis, radiculitis, and myelitis. On the other hand, brain abscess is one of the rarest. We were able to collect only 24 publications in which *Brucella* abscess or brucelloma of the brain was reported. Some of the studies dealing with neurobrucellosis do not report the presence of brain brucelloma nor abscess probably because neither computed tomography (CT) scan nor magnetic resonance imaging (MRI) of the brain was obtained in their patients [21, 22]. Had these tests been available or had they been performed, most probably more brucellomata would have been described. Furthermore a great number of brucelloma and *Brucella* abscess have never been reported. This is why the published incidence is inferior to the real one.

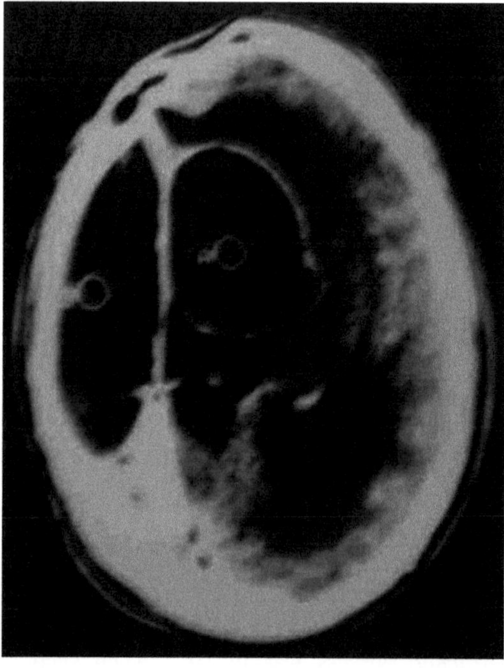

Fig. 7.1 Abscess in the remaining hemisphere of a hemispherectomized patient

This incidence is variably recorded. Of 400 cases of brucellosis, 13 presented with neurobrucellosis and none had an abscess nor a brucelloma [3]; Benjamin and Annobil [7] found only two cases of neurobrucellosis in 157 *Brucella* infections, none of whom had a brain brucelloma or abscess; Lubani et al. [30] report on nine children suffering from neurobrucellosis, none of whom had a brain brucelloma; Tanir et al. [37] reported on 90 cases of childhood brucellosis with only two cases of neurobrucellosis not having a brain brucelloma nor *Brucella* abscess. Kochar et al. [29] reported on 175 serologically confirmed cases of brucellosis and found 33 (18.86 %) involving the nervous system. Al-Eissa [1] reported on 112 cases suffering from brucellosis, only one of whom had a cerebellar *Brucella* abscess; out of 430 cases of brucellosis, Demiroğlu et al. [12] recorded one case of cerebellar abscess; Gul et al. [14], reviewing the entire Turkish literature over a 10-year period, reported four cases of brain abscesses out of 187 cases of neurobrucellosis; Galanakis et al. [13] reported one brain abscess out of 52 childhood brucellosis in Greece.

These lesions may occur at any stage of the disease: in the acute, subacute, or chronic phases. Benjamin and Annobil [7] define these stages as follows: the acute phase refers to the first 7 days of the disease, the subacute phase is from the 8th to the 30th day, and the chronic phase over 30 days. Their symptoms may start while the patient is on medicinal treatment: Guvenc et al.'s [19] patient was receiving penicillin and streptomy-

Table 7.1 A review of *Brucella* abscess or "brucelloma" of the brain in the available world literature

Reference and date of publication	Age in years	Sex	Symptoms	Signs	Number of lesions	Location	Pathology	Treatment	Result
Ayala-Gaytan et al. 1989 [6]	19	M	Headache, vomiting, fever, and joint pain	Left cerebellar syndrome and bilateral papilledema	1	Left cerebellar hemisphere	Multiloculated abscess	Surgical removal and medical	Cured
Guvenc et al. 1989 [19]	4	M	Headache, weakness, fever, nausea, and vomiting	Hepatosplenomegaly, mild papilledema	6	Both hemispheres and all lobes	Abscesses 2×2 to 4×4 cm	Aspiration and medical	Cured
Kalelioglu et al. 1990 [24]	12	M	NM	NM	1	NM	Abscess	Aspiration and medical	Cured
Al-Eissa 1993 [1]	3	M	Fever, vomiting, irritability, and unsteady gait	Bilateral Babinski, nystagmus	1	Right cerebellum	Abscess	Aspiration and medical	Cured
Santini et al. 1994 [33]	41	F	Chills, fever, night sweats	Splenomegaly, stiff neck, aphasia, right hemiparesis, and coma	2	L temporal and L parietal	Abscess	Medical	Cured
Galanakis et al. 1996 [13]	5	M	Fever, vomiting, and headache	Aphasia, right hemiparesis followed by coma	1	NA	Abscess	Medical	Cured
Stranjalis et al. 2000 [36]	60	F	Gradual visual loss and headache	NA	1	Chiasmatico-frontal	Multiloculated abscess	Aspiration and medical	Improved
Trifiletti et al. 2000 [39]	60	M	Polydipsia, headache, fever, and asthenia	Nystagmus, hyperreflexia, limb dysmetria, diabetes insipidus	Multiple	Bilateral frontobasilar	Masses	Medical	Cured
Martinez-Chamoro et al. 2002 [31]	14	M	Seizures, no fever, no vomiting, no headache	Mild hypoesthesia of left arm	1	Right parietal surrounded with edema	Nodular lesion	Surgical removal and medical	Cured
Sohn et al. 2003 [34]	26	M	Periorbital pain, headache, and seizures	Neurological examination was "non-focal"	1	Left frontal	5×5 mass	Biopsy and medical	Cured
Idem [34]	15	M	Headache, nausea, vomiting	Decreased vision	Several	Left occipitoparietal	Granuloma	Biopsy and medical	Improved
Al-Sous et al. 2004 [4]	30	F	Headache, deafness	Papilledema, sensory ataxia, areflexia	1	Suprasellar	Granuloma	Medical	Cured
Kizilkilic et al. 2005 [27]	30	M	Headache, fever, nausea, vomiting, gait disturbance, and vertigo	Right dysdiadochokinesia, dysmetria, and ataxia	1	Right inferior cerebellar peduncle	Abscess	Medical	Cured

(continued)

Table 7.1 (continued)

Reference and date of publication	Age in years	Sex	Symptoms	Signs	Number of lesions	Location	Pathology	Treatment	Result
Haddad et al. 2006 [20]	31	M	Seizures, headache, chills, fever, vomiting	Unconscious, localizing to pain, neck rigidity	1	Left frontal parasagittal	Multiloculated abscess	Surgical and medical	Died
Koc[a] 2006 [28]	70	M	Headache, confusion, and visual disturbance	NA	3	Right occipital	Multiloculated abscess	Craniotomy and medical	Cured
Miguel et al. 2006 [32]	13	F	Nonfebrile seizures	Fever (38°), no meningeal signs	1	Left parietal	Ring lesion	Medical	Cured
Carrasco- Moro et al. 2006 [9]	54	M	Refractory epilepsy			Right temporal	Abscess	Surgical and medical	Cured
Keihani-Douste et al. 2006 [25]	12	M	Back pain, headache, nausea, of 6 months duration	Quadriplegia and incontinence	Multiple	Brain and spinal intramedullary	Abscesses	Medical	Improved
Haji-Abdolbagi et al. 2008 [22]	NA	NA	NA	NA	1	NA	Abscess	NA-	NA
Gul et al.[b] 2009 [15]	12	F	NA	NA	4	3 cerebral and 1 cerebellar	Hyperintense lesions	Medical	Improved
Tonekaboni et al. 2009 [38]	13	M	Visual impairment, unilateral hearing loss		1	Suprasellar and optic chiasm	Mass	Medical	Improved
Solmaz et al. 2010 [35]	10	M	Fever, malaise, anemia, weakness, dysarthria, and anorexia	Fever and cervical lymphadenopathy	1	Left frontal	Abscess	Medical	Cured
Ceran et al. 2011 [10]	NA	NA	NA	NA	1	NA	Granuloma	NA	NA
Demiroğlu et al. 2011 [12]	*NA*	*NA*	NA	MA	1	Cerebellum	Abscess	*NA*	*NA*
Budnik et al. 2012 [8]	3	F	Fever, arthralgia, and seizure	Negative neurological examination, fever 38 °C, blood culture + for *Brucella*	1	Left parietal	Ring lesion surrounded by edema	Surgical resection and medical	Cured
Guven et al. 2013 [18]	NM	NM	NM	NM	NM	NM	Abscesses	NM	NM
Idem [18]	NM	NM	NM	NM	NM	NM	Abscesses	NM	NM

NM not mentioned in the text
[a]The case of Gundes (2004) and that of Koc (2006) appear to be the same case
[b]Gul has no personal cases. He reviewed all the Turkish literature up until 2009 and found three cerebral and one cerebellar cases. Some of these may have been reported by other Turkish authors, cited in this table, preceding his report

cin, Santini et al. [33] tetracycline and streptomycin, and Solmaz et al. [35] doxycycline, rifampin, and streptomycin, or after having received a course of treatment with complete systemic recovery, Ayala-Gaytán et al. [6] trimethoprim/sulfamethoxazole for 10 days with resolution of symptoms and followed by chloramphenicol and tetracycline; Martinez-Chamorro et al. [31] had his patient on doxycycline and rifampin for 6 weeks. Stranjalis et al. [36] had a "successful" treatment for brucellosis.

In one case, in which the brain lesion was multiple, there was a concomitant spinal intramedullary lesion [25].

7.3 Routes of Brain Invasion

The spread of infection in general takes one of three routes: the direct, the blood, or the lymphatic routes. In the brain there is no lymphatic circulation. In case the spread is a direct spread from the meninges, which is the assumption of Martinez-Chamorro et al. [31], many more brain lesions should be found because there is a lot more infections of the meninges than there are *Brucella* abscesses or brucellomata. Furthermore, in the majority of cases, the mass is not in direct contact with the meninges, and none of the reported cases of *Brucella* abscess or brucelloma had concomitant meningitis. Nevertheless, it still remains a possible route of transmission. The last route of spread, and the most plausible one, is the vascular one. The distribution of the masses in the brain is certainly more in favor of an arterial spread than a venous one.

7.4 Distribution

7.4.1 Sex

The male-to-female ratio in neurobrucellosis has been variably reported from one series to another. In our series it is 77.27 % in favor of males. Of 11 cases of neurobrucellosis reported by Gul et al. [14], the male-to-female ratio was 10:1 (90.1 %) and that by Ariza et al. [5], reviewing 56 cases of general brucellosis, 80.5 % in favor of males. With the exception of the previous two reports, our set of patients reveals a higher ratio than the ones reported in the general neurobrucellosis population by Guven et al. [18] of 66.6 % of males, by Ceran et al. [10] 61.1 %, by Haji-Abdolbagi et al. [22] 61 %, by Gul et al. [14] 57.1 %, and by Gür et al. [17] 51 %. This predominance of males in brain brucelloma and abscess has not been explained.

7.4.2 Age

Although neurobrucellosis is considered as rare in childhood [11, 26, 30, 35], the median age of the patients in our series (see Fig. 7.2) is 24.2 years which is on the younger side of the average age of the general neurobrucellosis population reported elsewhere: Gul et al. [14] (187 cases) report it at 40.3, Guven et al. [18] (128 cases) at 42, and Al Freihi et al. [3] (70 cases) at 35. There is a distinct shift toward the younger ages in the cases of brain *Brucella* abscess and brucelloma with a definite peak between the ages of 11 and 15 years; many authors claim that neurobrucellosis is rare in children [10, 30], and Tanir et al. [37] puts the ratio at 20–25 % of all cases. The age range of our cases is from 3 to 70 years which, again, is lower than the range in the general neurobrucellosis population of 10–77 [14], 13–77 [18], and 17–71 [4]. Haji-Abdolbagi et al. [22] report these figures at 13–72.

7.4.3 Lateralization

Seven lesions were in the left hemisphere, six in the right, and three in the midline. In three cases they were bilaterally found.

7.4.4 Location

When single, their preferred location is in the interface of the cortical gray matter and white matter, similar to metastatic tumors, a character-

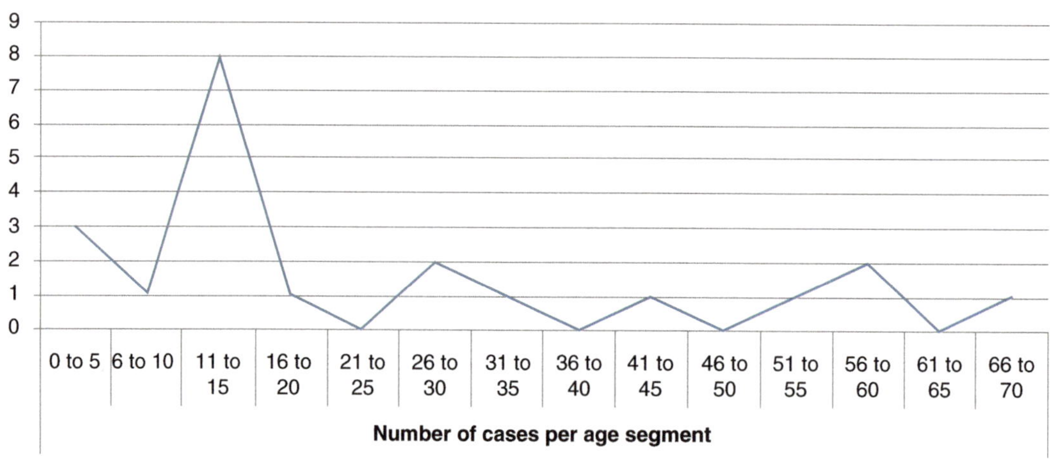

Fig. 7.2 Number of patients suffering from brucelloma per 5-year sections of age

istic of arterial dissemination; when multiple they were all deeply embedded in the cerebral hemispheres, none was outside that site. The majority were located in the anterior portion of the cerebral hemispheres, that is, mostly in the distribution of the carotid flow (5 frontal, 5 parietal, 2 temporal, and 2 suprasellar). Four were located in the cerebellar hemispheres and two in the occipital lobe. It is interesting to note that in the case of Keihani-Douste et al. [25], there were multiple brain abscesses one of them in the brain stem (the only one found in our series in this location) and another spinal intramedullary lesion.

7.4.5 Multiplicity

Of the 23 patients where the number of lesions was mentioned, in 16 there was one single lesion. Guvenc et al. [19] report a 4-year-old boy with six abscesses which were drained and cured. This greater number of single lesion is difficult to explain, especially that the spread to the brain is presumably an arterial one. Why is it that when a flood of active emboli reaches the brain, through the arterial blood flow, only one granuloma or one abscess forms? Is there a defense mechanism that arises in the brain to prevent the formation of other lesions?

7.4.6 Size

These lesions vary in size from 1 mm to 6 cm in diameter. When they are multiple they tend to have the same size [10] as if they were the product of one single bolus of emboli.

7.5 Symptoms and Signs

7.5.1 Symptoms

The major symptoms in these cases are fever [1, 2, 6, 8, 13, 19, 23, 25–27, 29, 32, 33, 35, 36, 39], headache [4, 6, 8, 13, 16, 25, 27, 28, 33, 36, 39], vomiting [1, 6, 8, 10, 13, 16, 20, 27], seizures [8, 9, 20, 28, 31, 32], weight loss [1, 6, 25, 39], excessive sweating [25, 33], anorexia [35], and malaise [35]. Other focal symptoms are related to the location of the mass in the brain, like aphasia [10], visual impairment [38], and hearing loss [38] which has been reported as the commonest CNS affection besides meningitis.

7.5.1.1 Fever

A total of 13 patients suffered from a low-grade fever, most probably as a consequence of the systemic disease. It may accompany the course of the disease (38 °C) [8, 19], and it may be of the intermittent type [6].

7.5.1.2 Headache

In their paper, it "can occur early in the course of the disease or as late as 1 year after the onset of systemic symptoms," says Haji-Abdolbagi et al. [22]. In our collection, whenever symptoms were recorded, 14 cases out of 22 patients suffered from headache (63.63 %). On the other hand, in Ceran et al. [10] series of general neurobrucellosis, 15 out of 18 patients had headache (83.34 %), yet these patients did not suffer from a brain abscess or a brucelloma. Therefore, in our cases, headache is not always the reflection of increased intracranial pressure, but could be due to the fever.

7.5.1.3 Vomiting

Vomiting was mentioned in seven cases, and it was associated with headache in six cases. No description of the type of vomiting was reported (whether projectile or not).

7.5.1.4 Neck Pain and Rigidity

Neck pain and rigidity may occur [29, 33]. This is due to meningeal irritation, and not necessarily meningitis. In the neurobrucellosis series of Ceran et al. [10], 11 out of 18 cases had neck stiffness. In our group of patients, only the above two cases were reported to suffer from neck rigidity.

7.5.1.5 Seizures

Seizures may be the first symptom of a *Brucella* abscess [9] or its only symptom [31]. They may be focal [31] or generalized [32, 34]; they may respond to medicinal treatment [8, 32] or may be refractory to such [9].

7.5.1.6 Loss of Vision

Loss of vision occurs due to direct involvement of the optic nerves as in the cases of Tonekaboni et al. [36, 38] (this will be discussed under cranial nerve involvement) or involvement of the visual radiations [16, 28, 34].

7.5.2 Signs

Most patients were awake and well oriented at the time of surgery; some were confused [28] or disoriented [16] and two were unconscious [20, 33]. All 18 cases of neurobrucellosis in Ceran et al.'s paper had meningeal involvement, yet 12 out of these were admitted for other complaints [10]. Bilateral papilledema was recorded twice [4, 6]. The other signs depended on the location of the lesion: aphasia and right hemiparesis were described [33], cerebellar findings [6], and ataxic gait with consistent falling to the left [1].

Hepatosplenomegaly was observed in three cases [1, 6, 33], yet this is most probably another feature of the generalized brucellosis and is not a specific result of the *Brucella* brain abscess. Galanakis et al. [13] observed splenomegaly more often than hepatomegaly.

Cervical lymphadenopathy was described three times [1, 6, 35].

7.6 Laboratory Findings

Most changes in the laboratory findings in brain brucelloma reflect the changes due to the systemic disease and may not be directly related to the brain lesion. They shall be recorded here for the sake of completeness.

7.6.1 Blood

At times no alterations are found [18]. On the other hand, serum agglutination titers are usually elevated reaching levels up to 1:5120. Blood culture grew *Brucella melitensis* in 15 cases [32] and *B. abortus* in 2 cases [35]. IgG and IgM for *Brucella* spp. are also elevated. Erythrocyte sedimentation rate may be mildly elevated [1] or may be normal [38].

7.6.2 Cerebrospinal Fluid

Cerebrospinal fluid (CSF) may be normal [18]. A depressed glucose concentration, an elevated protein concentration, and a marked leukocytosis with predominance of lymphocytes (540 with 60 % lymphocytes) [1] are the usual parameters of this disease [31, 39]. CSF agglutination titers may be elevated [20, 27, 35], but not always so.

CSF culture is often sterile but may grow the bacteria in 0–30 % of cases [32, 33]. Serum tube agglutination (STA) is usually elevated (1:15120) [13]. Gram-stained smears are negative [1].

7.6.3 Bacteriology

The results of blood culture were recorded in 11 cases and were positive for *B. melitensis* in 2 cases [6, 28], for *Brucella* spp. in 2 cases [8, 32], and for *B. abortus* in 1 case [35] and were negative in 6 cases [13, 20, 27, 31, 33, 36]. The CSF culture was recorded in 8 cases and all showed no growth. Cultures from the specimen were obtained in 6 cases with 3 growing *B. melitensis* [6, 28, 33]; in one case the growth was *Brucella* without specifying the type [22], and in another case there were two organisms, namely, *B. abortus* and *Staphylococcus aureus* [24]. In one case the culture remained negative [1]. STA titers are usually elevated (1:1208) [35].

7.6.4 Pathology

The majority of the cerebral lesions were abscesses with a granulomatous outer layer formed of epithelioid histiocytes and lymphocytes with an important leukocytic infiltration. Their centers are filled with necrotic tissue forming a mass of pus. The granuloma does not have a liquefied center [34]. Which pathology precedes the other is not clear. Does the center of the granuloma liquefy and form an abscess or does the liquid part of the abscess get absorbed and thus forms a granuloma? Most probably it is the first supposition that is the correct one as this is what usually happens in other parts of the body. This opinion is shared by Al-Eissa [1]. These lesions are surrounded by moderate focal edema [31].

7.7 Radiological Findings

The MRI was found to be more sensitive and more revealing than the CT scan [4]. CT scan and MRI of the brain show a mass with a central liquefaction in most cases (abscess). The outer circular rim does enhance. Occasionally the central portion is absent and the entire lesion is one single mass (brucelloma). These lesions are frequently surrounded by edema [16, 31]. Santini et al. [33] described a lesion "with hypodense linear areas but without ring enhancement." These lesions may be confused with other pyogenic abscesses like tuberculous and metastatic conditions [1].

Conclusions

1. Brain *Brucella* abscess or granuloma is a rare condition. Only 26 reports of such lesions were found in the medical literature.
2. They have not been reported as associated with *Brucella* abscess in other organs except in one case in the spine.
3. They tend to occur in the younger age group.
4. The lesion is more frequently single than multiple.
5. They usually occur in the hemispheres; they have not been seen in the brain stem. One case arose in a cerebellar peduncle and another in the optic nerve.
6. The symptom triad for cerebral brucelloma or *Brucella* abscess is: fever, headache, and vomiting. These may be the characteristics of brucellosis in general.
7. There are no specific signs related to brain brucelloma or *Brucella* abscess.
8. Radio imaging is the main diagnostic tool and in particular magnetic resonance imagery, yet they have to be differentiated from tuberculomas or other pyogenic abscesses.
9. The medical and surgical treatment of these conditions will be discussed in Chaps. 20 and 21 of this book, respectively.

References

1. Al-Eissa YA (1993) Unusual suppurative complications of brucellosis in children. Acta Paediatr 82:987–992
2. Al Deeb SM, Yaqub BA, Sharif HS, Phadke JG (1989) Neurobrucellosis: clinical characteristics, diagnosis and outcome. Neurology 39:498–501

3. Al-Freihi HM, Al-Mohaya SA, Al-Mohsen MA, Ibrahim EM, Al-Souhaibani MO, Twum-Danso K, Idrissi HY (1986) Brucellosis in Saudi Arabia: diverse manifestations of an important cause of pyrexial illness. Ann Saudi Med 6:95–99
4. Al-Sous MW, Bohlega S, Al-Kawi MZ, Alwatban J, McLean DR (2004) Neurobrucellosis: clinical and neuroimaging correlation. AJNR Am J Neuroradiol 25:395–401
5. Ariza J, Gudiol F, Pallares R, Rufi G, Fernandez-Viladrich P (1985) Comparative trial of rifampin-doxycycline versus tetracycline-streptomycin in the therapy of human brucellosis. Antimicrob Agents Chemother 28:548–551
6. Ayala-Gaytán JJ, Ortegon-Baqueiro H, de la Maza M (1989) Brucella melitensis cerebellar abscess. J Infect Dis 160:730–732
7. Benjamin B, Annobil SH (1992) Childhood brucellosis in southwestern Saudi Arabia: a 5-year experience. J Trop Pediatr 38:167–172
8. Budnik I, Fuchs I, Shelef I, Krymko H, Greenberg D (2012) Case report: unusual presentations of pediatric neurobrucellosis. Am J Trop Med Hyg 86:258–260
9. Carrasco-Moro R, Pedrosa-Sánchez M, Garcia Navarrete E, Pascual-Garvi JM, Minervini-Marín M, Sola RG (2006) Refractory epilepsy as the presenting symptom of a brucellar brain abscess. Revista Neurología 43:729–732
10. Ceran N, Turkoglu R, Erdem I, Inan A, Engin D, Tireli H, Goktas P (2011) Neurobrucellosis: clinical, diagnostic, therapeutic features and outcome. Unusual clinical presentations in an endemic region. Braz J Infect Dis 15:52–59
11. Cooper CW (1991) The epidemiology of human brucellosis in a well defined urban population in Saudi Arabia. J Trop Med Hyg 94:416–422
12. Demiroğlu YZ, Turunç T, Karaca S, Arlıer Z, Alışkan H, Colakoğlu S, Arslan H (2011) Neurological involvement in brucellosis; clinical classification, treatment and results. Mikrobiyol Bul 45:401–410
13. Galanakis E, Bourantas KL, Leveidiotou S, Lapatsanis PD (1996) Childhood brucellosis in north-western Greece: a retrospective analysis. Eur J Pediatr 155:1–6
14. Gul HC, Erdem H, Bek S (2009) Overview of neurobrucellosis: a pooled analysis of 187 cases. Int J Infect Dis 13:e339–e343
15. Gul HC, Erdem H, Gorenek L, Ozdag MF, Kalpakci Y, Avci IY, Besirbellioglu BA, Eyigum CP (2008) Management of neurobrucellocis: an assessment of 11 cases. Intern Med 47:995–1001
16. Gündes S, Meric M, Willke A, Erdenlig S, Koc K (2004) A case of intracranial abscess due to Brucella melitensis. Int J Infect Dis 8:379–381
17. Gür A, Geyik MF, Dikici B, Nas K, Cevik R, Sarac J, Hosoglu S (2003) Complications of brucellosis in different age groups: a study of 283 cases in southeastern Anatolia of Turkey. Yonsei Med J 44:33–44
18. Guven T, Ugurlu K, Ergonul O, Celikbas AK, Gök SE, Comoglu S, Baykam N, Dokuzoguz B (2013) Neurobrucellosis: clinical and diagnostic features. Clin Infect Dis 56:1407–1412
19. Guvenc H, Kocabay K, Okten A, Bektas S (1989) Brucellosis in a child complicated with multiple brain abscesses. Scand J Infect Dis 21:333–336
20. Haddad FS, Bitar E, Haddad GF (2006) A rare, late complication in a hemispherectomized patient: a brucella abscess in the contra lateral hemisphere. Pan Arab J Neurosurg 10:70–74
21. Haddad FS, Fahl M, Haddad SF (1989) Brucellar spondylitis: review of 21 cases. J Med Liban 37:4–8
22. Haji-Abdolbagi M, Rasooli-Nejad M, Jafari S, Hasibi M, Soudbakhsh A (2008) Clinical and laboratory findings in neurobrucellosis: review of 31 cases. Arch Iran Med 11:21–25
23. Hatipoglu CA, Yetkin A, Ertem GT, Tulek N (2004) Unusual clinical presentations of brucellosis. Scand J Infect Dis 36:695–698
24. Kalelioğlu M, Ceylan S, Koksal I, Kuzeyli K, Akturk F (1990) Brain abscess caused by Brucella abortus and Staphylococcus aureus in a child. Infection 18:386–387
25. Keihani-Douste Z, Daneshjou K, Ghasemi M (2006) A quadriplegic child with multiple brain abscesses: case report of neurobrucellosis. Med Sci Monit 12:CS119–CS122
26. Khuri-Bulos N, Daoud AH, Azab SM (1993) Treatment of childhood brucellosis: results of a prospective trial on 113 children. Pediatr Infect Dis J 12:377–381
27. Kizilkilic O, Turunc T, Yildirim T, Demiroglu YZ, Hurcan C, Uncu H (2005) Successful medical treatment of intracranial abscess caused by Brucella spp. J Infect 51:77–80
28. Koc K (2006) Brucellar brain abscess and bilateral arachnoid cysts, unilaterally complicated by subdural haematoma. J Clin Neurosci 13:485–487
29. Kochar DK, Agarwal N, Jain N, Sharma BV, Rastogi A, Meena CB (2000) Clinical profile of neurobrucellosis-a report on 12 cases from Bikaner (North-West India). J Assoc Physicians India 48:376–380
30. Lubani MM, Dudin KI, Araj GF, Manandhar DS, Rashid FY (1989) Neurobrucellosis in children. Pediatr Infect Dis J 8:79–82
31. Martınez-Chamorro E, Muñoz A, Esparza J, Muñoz MJ, Giangaspro E (2002) Case report; focal cerebral involvement by neurobrucellosis: pathological and MRI findings. Eur J Radiol 43:28–30
32. Miguel PS, Fernandez G, Vasallo FJ, Hortas M, Lorenzo JR, Rodriguez I, Ortiz-Rey JA, Anton I (2006) Neurobrucellosis mimicking cerebral tumor: case report and literature review. Clin Neurol Neurosurg 108:404–406
33. Santini C, Baiocchi P, Berardelli A, Venditti M, Serra P (1994) A case of brain abscess due to Brucella melitensis. Clin Infect Dis 19:977–978
34. Sohn AH, Probert WS, Glaser CA, Gupta N, Bollen AW, Wong JD, Grace EM, McDonald WC (2003) Human neurobrucellosis with intracerebral granuloma caused by a marine mammal Brucella spp. Emerg Infect Dis 9:485–488

35. Solmaz Ç, Mustafa H, Melda S (2010) Brucellar brain abscess in a child. J Pediatr Inf 4:89–91
36. Stranjalis G, Singounas E, Boutsikakis I, Saroglou G (2000) Chronic intracerebral Brucella abscess. Case illustration. J Neurosurg 92:189
37. Tanir G, Tufekci SB, Tuygun N (2009) Presentation, complications, and treatment outcome of brucellosis in Turkish children. Pediatr Int 51:114–119
38. Tonekaboni SH, Karimi A, Armin S, Khase LA, Sabertehrani AS (2009) Neurobrucellosis: a partially treatable cause of vision loss. Pediatr Neurol 40:401–403
39. Trifiletti RR, Restivo DA, Pavone P, Guifrida S, Parano E (2000) Diabetes insipidus in neurobrucellosis. Clin Neurol Neurosurg 102:163

Pseudotumor Cerebri in Neurobrucellosis

Fuad Sami Haddad†

8

Contents

Abstract

All the available cases of pseudotumor cerebri related to brucellosis were reviewed. They were ten in number. Their case histories were summarized and their etiology, symptoms, and signs as well as their management were discussed.

Keywords

Abscess • *Brucella* • Granuloma • Intracranial pressure • Neurobrucellosis • Pseudotumor cerebri

Abbreviations

CSF Cerebrospinal fluid
CT Computed tomography
MRI Magnetic resonance imaging

8.1 Introduction

Few papers report symptoms similar to those described in Chap. 7 of the book, in the absence of brucelloma or *Brucella* abscess. In other words there is evidence of increased intracranial pressure in patients suffering from brucellosis, without any obvious or visible intracranial mass or meningeal inflammation. A total of ten such cases have been collected under the title of *Brucella* pseudotumor cerebri (see Table 8.1).

† Author was deceased at the time of publication.

F.S. Haddad, MD, FACS, FRCS, ABNS
Department of Surgery, American University of Beirut, Beirut, Lebanon
e-mail: fshaddad@aub.edu.lb

M. Turgut et al. (eds.), *Neurobrucellosis: Clinical, Diagnostic and Therapeutic Features*,
DOI 10.1007/978-3-319-24639-0_8

Table 8.1 A review of ten cases with pseudotumor cerebri in world literature

Reference and date of publication	Age in years	Sex	Symptoms	Signs	Neck rigidity	Neuroimaging	Blood evaluations	CSF evaluations
Tekeli et al. 1999 [14]	22	F	Uncrossed diplopia, headache	Intracranial hypertension			Culture positive for *Brucella*	Culture positive for *Brucella*
Bessisso et al. 2001 [3]	8	M	Fever, headache, neck pain for 1 month	Bilateral papilledema	Present	CT and MRI of brain normal	*Brucella* titer 1/1280	Pressure 360 mmHg, WBC 5/mm^3, protein 0.63 g/dl, culture neg, *Brucella* titer 1/320
Idem [3]	3	F	VP shunt for hydrocephalus at age of 3 weeks	Fever, weight loss, right upper quadrant abdominal mass, aphasia	Present	Dilated ventricles and periventricular edema	1/5120, *B. melitensis* cultured	WBC 75/mm^3, protein 2 g/dl, sugar 0.5 mmol/dl, *B. melitensis* cultured
Emadoleslamia and Mahmoudianb 2007 [6]	11	F	Headache, vomiting, transient right hemiparesis, blurred vision	Confused, right hemiparesis, bilateral papilledema	Absent	MRI of brain normal	Wright 1/320, serum sugar 90 mg/ml	Pressure 32 cm H_2O, glucose 20 mg/dl, no cells, normal protein
Panagariya et al. 2007 [11]	30	F	Headache, vomiting, no fever	Bilateral papilledema, enlarged bilateral blind spot	NM	MRI of brain normal	ESR 15 mm	Opening pressure 370 mm, WBC 35/mm^3, protein 60 mg%, sugar 38 mg%
Tanir et al. 2009 [13]	13	F	NM	Increased intracranial pressure	NM	MRI of brain normal	Wright 1/160	Raised pressure, negative culture
Sinopidis et al. 2010 [12]	4	M	Vomiting and headaches	Left side papilledema, left abducens nerve palsy	Absent	MRI of brain normal	Wright 1/320	Pressure 48 mmHg, 162 cell/ml, glucose 32 mg/dl, protein 60 mg/dl, culture negative

Reference and date of publication	Age in years	Sex	Symptoms	Signs	Neck rigidity	Neuroimaging	Blood evaluations	CSF evaluations
Işıkay 2011 [10]	15	F	Blurred vision, diplopia, fatigue, headache, nausea and vomiting	Bilateral papilledema	NM	CT and MRI of brain normal	Serum agglutination 1/2560, culture negative	Rose Bengal and Wright negative; culture negative
Yilmaz et al. 2011 [15]	15	F	Headache, vomiting,	Papilledema, left abducens nerve palsy	NM	MRI of brain normal	ESR 4 mm, Wright 1/160	Pressure 340 mm of H_2O, Wright 1/80, culture: *B melitensis*
Akhondian et al. 2014 [1]	11	F	Headache, transient right hemiparesis	Blurred vision, confusion, bilateral papilledema	Absent	MRI of brain normal	Wright 1/320	Pressure 32 cm H_2O, no cells, normal protein, glucose 20 mg/dl

F female, *M* male, *ESR* erythrocyte sedimentation rate per 1st hour, *MRI* magnetic resonance imaging, *CT* computed tomography, *NM* not mentioned

8.2 Definition

For the purpose of this paper, pseudotumor cerebri shall be defined as a case of increased intracranial pressure without evidence of an intracranial mass or infection. The neuroimaging of the brain should include a magnetic resonance imaging (MRI) and/or a computed tomography (CT) scan and should neither show an intracranial mass nor evidence of infection. This condition has also been called "primary idiopathic intracranial hypertension" [4, 8].

8.3 Etiology

It is well known that tetracyclines and their derivatives may produce a picture identical to pseudotumor cerebri [5, 7]. Before inculpating brucellosis as the reason for that condition, one should be sure that the patient is not taking this drug or one of its derivatives.

The mechanism of this increase in cerebral pressure in the absence of a mass lesion or inflammation is supposed to be due to an immune-mediated response causing a blockage in the cerebrospinal fluid (CSF) absorption at the level of the villi due to vascular inflammation of these villi [9].

In one case the intracranial hypertension was due to the distal blockage of a ventriculoperitoneal shunt system placed 2 years earlier for congenital hydrocephalus [3].

8.4 Review of the Literature (See Table 8.1)

Al Deeb et al. [2] report on 4 cases of pseudotumor cerebri out of 400 cases suffering from brucellosis (these cases were not included in Table 8.1, because no individual description of these cases is given).

Tekeli et al. [14] reported on a 22-year-old female who developed a sudden onset of diplopia accompanied by increased intracranial pressure. Microbiological tests of CSF and sera revealed neurobrucellosis. The patient received therapy for this condition, and her symptoms due to increased intracranial pressure disappeared.

In 2001, Bessisso et al. [3] reported on two cases of pseudotumor cerebri (see Table 8.1). He comments, "Intracranial pressure may be raised in neurobrucellosis as a consequence of the basilar meningitis impeding the flow of CSF or pseudotumor cerebri or cerebritis" [3].

In 2002, Güngör et al. [9] published a report on a female 35 years of age who presented with bilateral papilledema and laboratory findings confirming neurobrucellosis. She recovered fully after an anti-*Brucella* treatment.

In 2007, Panagariya et al. [11] described the case of a 30-year-old lady who suffered continuous headache and morning vomiting for 1 month. There were no fever, no seizures, and no altered sensorium [11]. On examination she had bilateral papilledema, no other neurological deficit, and no sign of meningeal irritation [11]. Her sedimentation rate was 15 mm in the first hour and she had a normal MRI [11]. Visual perimetry revealed a bilateral enlargement of the blind spots and a left inferior nasal scotoma [11]. Opening CSF pressure was 370 mm of H_2O, and the CSF showed 30–35 lymphocytes per mm^3, a protein of 60 mg%, and a sugar of 38 mg% [11]. Serology for *Brucella* demonstrated IgG of 295 and IgM titers of 130 U/l [11]. The headache and papilledema disappeared on anti-*Brucella* treatment, and the abnormal blood and CSF pictures reverted to normal [11].

In a retrospective evaluation of 90 children with brucellosis, Tanir et al. [13] reported an interesting pediatric neurobrucellosis case with increased intracranial pressure but negative CSF culture and normal cranial MRI.

In 2011, Yilmaz et al. [15] reported on a 15-year-old girl with headache, vomiting, diplopia, and papilledema possibly due to intracranial hypertension but normal cranial MRI. In this case, *Brucella melitensis* grew on CSF culture [15].

Afterward, Işıkay et al. [10] also reported on a 15-year-old girl admitted with diplopia, vision loss, headache, nausea, vomiting, and bilateral papilledema but normal eye movements. Also, neuroimaging was normal and blood and CSF cultures were negative; patient responded well to anti-*Brucella* treatment [10].

Recently, Sinopidis et al. [12] described the case of a 4-year-old boy admitted "because of persistent headache and vomiting." He also experienced fever and difficulty in walking, and examination revealed papilledema in the left eye and left third nerve palsy [12]. There were no meningeal signs and laboratory examination confirmed the suspected diagnosis of brucellosis [12]. An MRI was normal and he improved on anti-*Brucella* treatment and recovered completely within 7 months [12].

More recently, Akhondian et al. [1] present the case of an "11-year-old female patient [who] was hospitalized with a severe headache, complaint that was worsening over a period of 2 months … and the day after, [she experienced a] transient right hemiparesis that lasted less than 1 h" as well as blurred vision and bilateral papilledema. Laboratory findings revealed serum agglutination Wright test positive at 1/320 and 2-mercaptoethanol *Brucella* agglutination test positive at 1/160 [1]. A lumbar puncture showed a clear CSF with increased opening pressure (32 cm of H_2O), and CSF examination was within normal range [1]. She recovered completely following anti-*Brucella* treatment [1]. This case appears to be, word to word, identical to the case of Emadoleslamia and Mahmoudianb [6] (2007) and had received an identical treatment [6]. In the discussion, they will be considered as the same case adding up the total number of cases to ten.

8.5 Symptoms

Headache is the commonest symptom and was present in seven out of ten cases. It is usually the first symptom and lasts until the patient is cured. It may be constant or recurrent in nature and is more severe in the morning.

On the other hand, fever and vomiting were mentioned each in three cases and only once in the same patient.

Moreover, diplopia was reported three times. And, transient hemiparesis was reported twice.

8.6 Signs

Papilledema was the most constant sign and was reported in all ten cases. Two patients were confused at the time of surgery. Hemiplegia was reported once and so was aphasia.

8.7 Management

The treatment of these cases is to treat the original cause, i.e., the neurobrucellosis. This treatment shall be fully discussed in Chap. 20. Once the original cause is cured, the intracranial pressure returns to normal.

Conclusion

In conclusion it is fair to say that cases of pseudotumor cerebri secondary to neurobrucellosis are very uncommon. We were able to collect only ten such cases from the literature, a value which does not represent 4 % of patients suffering from neurobrucellosis as claimed by Panagariya et al. [11].

References

1. Akhondian J, Ashrafzadeh F, Beiraghi Toosi M, Hashemi N (2014) A rare presentation of neurobrucellosis in a child with recurrent transient ischemic attacks and pseudotumor cerebri (a case report and review of literature). Iran J Child Neurol 8:65–69
2. Al Deeb SM, Yaqub BA, Sharif HS, Phadke JG (1989) Neurobrucellosis: clinical characteristics, diagnosis and outcome. Neurology 39:498–501
3. Bessisso MS, Elsaid MF, Elshazli SSE, Abdelrahman HM, Al Ali MG, Ali AR, Aljaber HM (2001) Case report: neuro-brucellosis in children. Neurosciences 6:67–69
4. Binder DR, Horton JC, Lawton MT, McDermott MW (2004) Idiopathic intracranial hypertension. Neurosurgery 54:538–552
5. Chiu AM, Chiu AM, Chuenkongkaew WL, Cornblath WT, Trobe JD, Digre KB, Dotan SA, Musson KH, Eggenberger ER (1998) Minocycline treatment and pseudotumor cerebri syndrome. Am J Ophthalmol 126:116–121
6. Emadoleslamia M, Mahmoudianb T (2007) A case of pseudotumor cerebri and brucellosis. Pediatr Infect Dis J 2:251–253

7. Giles C, Soble A (1971) Intracranial hypertension and tetracycline therapy. Am J Ophthalmol 72: 981–982
8. Glaser JS (1999) Neuro-ophthalmology, 3rd edn. JB Lippincott, Philadelphia
9. Güngör K, Bekir NA, Namiduru M (2002) Case report: pseudotumor cerebri complicating brucellosis. Ann Ophthalmol 34:67–69
10. Işıkay S, Yılmaz K, Okumuş S (2011) Increased intracranial pressure associated with neurobrucellosis: a case report. Gaziantep Med J 17:100–102
11. Panagariya A, Sharma B, Mathew V (2007) Pseudotumor like presentation of neurobrucellosis. J Assoc Physicians India 55:301–302
12. Sinopidis X, Kaleyias J, Mitropoulou K, Triga M, Kothare SV, Mantagos S (2012) An uncommon case of pediatric neurobrucellosis associated with intracranial hypertension. Case Rep Infect Dis 2012:1–3
13. Tanir G, Tufekci SB, Tuygun N (2009) Presentation, complications, and treatment outcome of brucellosis in Turkish children. Pediatr Int 51:114–119
14. Tekeli O, Tomac S, Gürsel E, Hasiripi H (1999) Divergence paralysis and intracranial hypertension due to neurobrucellosis. A case report. Binocul Vis Strabismus Q 14:117–118
15. Yilmaz S, Serdaroglu G, Gokben S, Tekgul H (2011) A case of neurobrucellosis presenting with isolated intracranial hypertension. J Child Neurol 26:1316–1318

Cerebrovascular Involvement in Neurobrucellosis and Mycotic Aneurysms

9

Dheeraj Khurana, Roopa Rajan, Ahmet Tuncay Turgut, and Venugopalan Y. Vishnu

Contents

D. Khurana, MD (✉) • R. Rajan, MD
V.Y. Vishnu, MD
Department of Neurology, Postgraduate Institute of Medical Education and Research, Chandigarh, India
e-mail: dherajk@yahoo.com; roops84@gmail.com; vishnuvy16@yahoo.com

A.T. Turgut, MD
Department of Radiology, Hacettepe University School of Medicine, Ankara, Turkey
e-mail: ahmettuncayturgut@yahoo.com

Abstract

Cerebrovascular manifestations are uncommon features of brucellosis especially as the presenting feature. The major mechanisms of stroke in neurobrucellosis are mycotic aneurysm, embolism from cardiac vegetations, and Brucella-associated vasculitis. Spread of inflammation from adjacent meninges may lead to cerebral venous sinus thrombosis. Common clinical presentation includes stroke, transient ischemic attack, seizures, and symptoms of increased intracranial pressure along with features of meningeal irritation and systemic features. Neurotuberculosis, primary central nervous system lymphoma, demyelination, neurosyphilis, and vasculitis are the common differential diagnoses. There are no evidence-based guidelines for the management of cerebrovascular complications of neurobrucellosis. The usual clinical practice is medical management followed by surgical/endovascular treatment if required.

Keywords

Neurobrucellosis • Mycotic aneurysm • Stroke • Transient ischemic attack

Abbreviations

BA Basilar artery
CNS Central nervous system

M. Turgut et al. (eds.), *Neurobrucellosis: Clinical, Diagnostic and Therapeutic Features*, DOI 10.1007/978-3-319-24639-0_9

CSF	Cerebrospinal fluid
CVT	Cerebral venous sinus thrombosis
ICH	Intracerebral hemorrhage
MCA	Middle cerebral artery
SAH	Subarachnoid hemorrhage
TIA	Transient ischemic attack

9.1 Introduction

Brucellosis is a common zoonosis that presents with protean manifestations involving multiple organ systems. While neurological involvement is commonly encountered in brucellosis, involvement of the cerebral vessels is uncommon. Central nervous system (CNS) involvement in Brucella melitensis infection was documented in the late nineteenth and early twentieth centuries, immediately after the discovery of an organism responsible for Malta fever by Bruce in 1887 [10].

The earliest description of cerebrovascular brucellosis was the seminal report of a mycotic basilar artery (BA) aneurysm in a 26-year-old male treated for systemic brucellosis in 1931 [16]. This young man presented with episodes of transient numbness and aphasia, followed by occipital headache and episodes of delirium, subsequently succumbed to his illness. The cerebrospinal fluid (CSF) examination revealed a lymphocytic pleocytosis, a positive agglutination titer, and a serum and CSF cultures and guinea pig inoculation identified the organism as Brucella melitensis var porcine. It was the autopsy which revealed an aneurysm of BA with extensive subarachnoid hemorrhage (SAH), while the histopathological examination showed meningeal, perivascular, as well as adventitial chronic inflammation and fibrosis.

In the current era, reports of cerebrovascular involvement in brucellosis are largely confined to case reports and series. In a review of 187 cases of neurobrucellosis detected in Turkey, stroke was identified in 3.2 % including four patients with ischemic stroke, one with SAH and one with subdural hemorrhage [14]. Intracranial mycotic aneurysms have been sporadically reported [5]. Ischemic strokes and transient ischemic attacks (TIAs) are known to occur in brucellosis [8, 9]. Rarely, cerebral venous sinus thrombosis (CVT) may complicate Brucella meningoencephalitis [34].

9.2 Pathology

The pathogenesis of cerebrovascular involvement in brucellosis is multifactorial. Current understanding suggests that two independent mechanisms predominate [1]. Mycotic aneurysms may develop secondary to infective embolism from brucellar endocarditis, with subsequent rupture and SAH. Infective microemboli from cardiac vegetations may also cause ischemic strokes [6]. Another mechanism is Brucella-associated vasculitis resulting in lacunar infarct, intracerebral hemorrhage (ICH), and venous thromboses. Angiographic evidence of vasculopathy in the form of multiple cutoffs, vascular contour irregularities, and stenosis has been reported [1]. Histopathological examination of a surgically treated intracranial aneurysm revealed features consistent with necrotizing vasculitis [5].

Direct invasion of Brucella in the cerebral vessels has not been demonstrated. However, it has been reported in few patients with Brucella aortitis, although the resulting vasculopathy is thought to be primarily immunologically mediated [2]. In addition to aorta, vasculitis of other large, medium, and small arteries and veins may also occur in brucellosis. Dermal biopsies have revealed granulomatous vasculitis. Cryoglobulinemia with leukocytoclastic cutaneous vasculitis has also been reported in brucellosis [33]. Spread of inflammation from adjacent meninges is usually responsible for CVT. Thus, cerebrovascular involvement in brucellosis represents the outcome of heterogeneous pathogenic mechanisms.

9.3 Clinical Features

Patients with brucellosis may present acutely as a medical emergency, although symptoms due to cerebrovascular involvement are like a stroke of any other cause. Most patients are in the age group of 20–30 years, belonging to the category of young stroke, while cerebrovascular brucellosis has been reported in children and older adults as well [8]. Neurological deficits depend on the arterial territory involved. Both anterior and posterior circulations seem to be equally involved [6–8]. Lacunar infarction of the thalamus has also been reported (Fig. 9.1) [20].

Clinical clues suggesting headache, nuchal rigidity, and cranial nerve palsies may be present due to meningitic process. Stroke as a presenting manifestation of neurobrucellosis is uncommon in which case the diagnosis may not be suspected [6]. TIAs are also a common manifestation; in one series two out of four patients who developed TIA had no prior history of brucellosis [9]. McLean et al. [26] described a total of 18 patients with neurobrucellosis, of which four patients had a stroke: two ischemic strokes and two ICH presumably due to mycotic aneurysm. Nevertheless, neither angiogram nor autopsy was performed. Al Deeb et al. [4] in their series of 13 patients with neurobrucellosis reported a single patient with ischemic stroke who had hypodensities in CT scan with a normal DSA. Pascual et al. [28] reported two patients with vascular involvement as TIA or SAH, and both patients had normal angiograms. Vogt et al. [32] described a patient with neurobrucellosis and multiple subcortical infarcts, but angiogram was not done. Hernandez et al. [17] have reported neurobrucellosis patients with stroke. Recently, Adaletli et al. [1] have reported a patient with stroke and an angiogram showing evidence of vasculopathy like occlusion of branches of the right middle cerebral artery (MCA), vascular cutoff signs, vascular contour irregularities, and stenosis. Gul et al. [14], in their pooled analysis of 187 cases, reported six cases (3.2 %), one case each of SAH and subdural hematoma and four cases of ischemic stroke. Jochum et al. [20] have reported a case of neurobrucellosis who had a thalamic infarct as a complication, but no angiography was done on this patient.

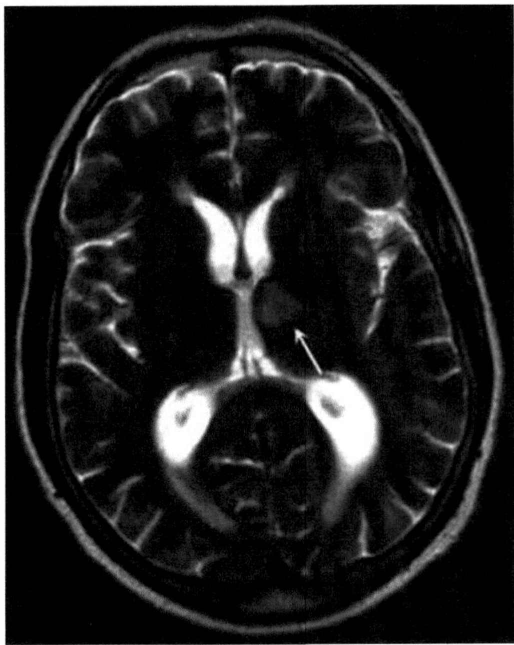

Fig. 9.1 Contrast-enhanced axial T2-weighted cranial MRI of a male patient with meningoencephalitis. Note the presence of fresh infarction of the left thalamus (*arrowhead*) (From Jochum et al. [20] with permission)

In 2006, Bingöl et al. [9] have described four cases of neurobrucellosis presenting as TIAs. Inan et al. [18] have reported TIA and stroke as the presenting feature in neurobrucellosis. Akhondian et al. [3] have described an 11-year-old child with neurobrucellosis who had TIA as the presenting manifestation, but angiogram was not done on this patient.

In a large series of patients with neurobrucellosis, headache, fever, weight loss, sweating, and back pain were the most common presenting symptoms [14]. Meningeal irritation, hypesthesia, confusion, and hepatosplenomegaly were the most commonly encountered physical signs. Presence of systemic features such as arthralgia, fever, meningeal irritation, peripheral nervous system involvement, and cranial neuropathies or hearing loss in young patients presenting with symptoms suggestive of cerebrovascular accident in endemic regions should trigger a high degree of suspicion for neurobrucellosis.

Brucella-related cerebral aneurysms may present with SAH or maybe detected incidentally on neuroimaging. Aneurysms involving the BA, anterior cerebral artery, and MCA have been reported [5, 19, 21, 25]. In patients presenting with SAH, history of fever and other systemic complaints prompts consideration of a mycotic aneurysm due to an infective etiology. McLean et al. [26]

described two patients with ICH due to a presumed mycotic aneurysm. Of the eight reported cases, three involved the BA which is an uncommon site for mycotic aneurysms, and these have been postulated to be due to basilar meningitis [26].

Patients with hemorrhagic infarcts secondary to CVT may present with seizures [13]. Other rare presentations thought to be due to cerebral venous sinus involvement are headache, papilledema, and raised intracranial pressure, without any focal deficits, mimicking pseudotumor cerebri [27]. Since most descriptions of cerebrovascular brucellosis are restricted to small case series or case reports, manifestations cannot be categorized as being typical and may vary.

9.4 Differential Diagnosis

Neurological involvement in brucellosis is rare, especially as a presenting feature; the differential diagnosis includes other infectious, neoplastic, and inflammatory conditions which can have a similar presentation. As mentioned above, the cerebrovascular manifestations in neurobrucellosis are attributable to multiple mechanisms including mycotic aneurysms, infective emboli from the heart, vasculitis, and even adjacent inflammation of the cerebral sinuses, from the meninges causing CVT. In any young patient with a stroke with features of chronic meningitis or arachnoiditis, from an endemic region, neurobrucellosis should be considered. In tropical countries like India, a high index of suspicion of neurobrucellosis is mandatory in those patients with a history of traveling to the Middle east/Gulf countries and in those who consume raw milk, but a patient presenting with pure cerebrovascular manifestations should be subjected to the standard evaluation for a young stroke. Concurrent systemic features and evidence of meningitis clinically or by CSF analysis should arouse suspicion. The common differential diagnoses which would be considered are neurotuberculosis, demyelination, primary CNS lymphoma, vasculitis, and neurosyphilis.

9.4.1 Tuberculosis

Tuberculosis can present in a very similar manner and may be difficult to distinguish since endemic regions of both these infections overlap significantly. Erdem et al. [11] have shown that Thwaites or Lancet scoring systems used for tubercular meningitis may lead to a misdiagnosis of neurobrucellosis as tubercular meningitis in endemic countries. In fact, many patients with neurobrucellosis may be treated as misdiagnosis of tuberculosis, and neurobrucellosis is suspected only when the patient worsens in spite an adequate antitubercular treatment [22]. The CSF picture composed of raised protein value, low sugar and lymphocytic pleocytosis, as well as stroke and cranial nerve palsies represents a close overlap of both these chronic infections. A brucellosis serology would be valuable in this situation to confirm the diagnosis.

9.4.2 Demyelination

Neurobrucellosis with stroke-like presentations may mimic a demyelinating disease on neuroimaging. The involvement of the deep gray matter is unusual and may resemble closely an acute disseminated encephalomyelitis (Fig. 9.2) [29]. Nevertheless, the presentation with systemic features would be suggestive of a secondary cause of demyelination.

9.4.3 Lymphoma

Lymphoma can present with chronic meningitis and demyelination-like lesions, while intravascular lymphoma can even have stroke-like episodes.

9.4.4 Neurosyphilis

Even in this era, neurosyphilis cannot be forgotten as it is the great mimicker, and its neurovascular complications may closely mimic neurobrucellosis.

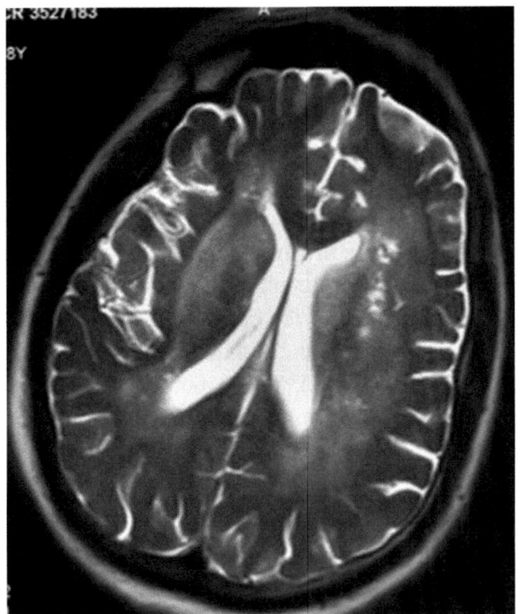

Fig. 9.2 Axial T2-weighted cranial MRI showing bilateral periventricular and basal ganglia hyperintensities

9.5 Investigations

9.5.1 CSF Examination

The evaluation of a suspected case of neurobrucellosis is usually tailored to the presenting clinical features. CSF examination shows an elevated protein, reduced glucose concentration, and moderate leukocytosis with predominant lymphocytes [26]. The rate of isolation of Brucella spp. from CSF is low (<20 %); hence, the diagnosis of neurobrucellosis depends on the specific antibodies in the CSF [24]. Even though the positive culture is the gold standard for definitive diagnosis, low yield and longtime consumed makes it less practical as a viable option for diagnosis in clinical practice.

9.5.2 Neurophysiologic Evaluation

Brainstem auditory evoked responses which can detect subtle vestibulocochlear involvement may provide vital clue for diagnosis since vestibulocochlear nerve is the most common cranial nerve involved in neurobrucellosis [15, 23].

9.5.3 Neuroimaging

Cranial CT scan and MRI should be done to identify and localize the lesion. Angiography (CT angiography and full four-vessel angiography if required in cases of suspected mycotic aneurysms) and echocardiography to identify brucellar endocarditis will add to the evidence for vascular involvement of neurobrucellosis. CT venography or MR venography in CVT is diagnostic.

9.6 Management

The management protocol for brucellosis has been discussed elsewhere (Chaps. 20 and 21). We have restricted our discussion to specific management principals of cerebrovascular complications of neurobrucellosis.

9.6.1 Mycotic Aneurysm

There have been eight reported cases of mycotic aneurysms related to neurobrucellosis. Hansmann et al. [16] described the first case with an autopsy finding of mycotic aneurysm due to neurobrucellosis. Jabbour et al. [19] described a proximally located BA aneurysm which disappeared following successful medical therapy. SAH with normal angiogram has been described in one patient [28]. Kaya et al. [21] reported a thrombosed distal dissecting aneurysm of the BA which resolved with medical management. Mycotic aneurysm with neurobrucellosis has been treated surgically after failed medical management [5, 12]. Ranjbar et al. [30] have described 20 patients with neurobrucellosis, among which one patient had a stroke due to a mycotic aneurysm rupture. There was no mention of angiogram in this patient. Thus, of the eight cases, only two cases of aneurysm warranted invasive management. Amiri et al. [5] used surgical option, endovascular or surgical excision, only after an inadequate response to medical management. They opined that the factors determining the choice between endovascular and surgical excisions were morphology and location of the aneurysm, possibility of sacrificing the parent artery, status of valve replacement surgery, vasospasm, the severity and location of ICH, and general medical condition of the patient [5]. There is currently insufficient evidence to make recommendations for the management of mycotic aneurysm due to brucellosis. The practical approach would be to adopt an invasive line of management when there is no or inadequate response to conservative medical management.

9.6.2 Subdural Hemorrhage

In 2004, a 49-year-old patient with subdural hemorrhage associated with neurobrucellosis has been reported by Ertem et al. [31]. Furthermore, Gul et al. [14] in their pooled analysis of 187 cases have reported a patient with subdural hematoma.

9.6.3 Ischemic Stroke and Transient Ischemic Attack

None of the reported cases of TIA associated with neurobrucellosis used any antiplatelets or anticoagulants. The patients were treated with antibiotics. Although there is no evidence to support use of antiplatelets, the use of short-term antiplatelets with antibiotics should be appropriate.

9.6.4 Cerebral Venous Sinus Thrombosis

In 1999, Zaidan et al. [34] first reported a CVT related to brucellar meningitis, who was treated with anticoagulants and antibiotics. Faraji et al. [13] have reported a case of neurobrucellosis with CVT as the presenting feature who also received anticoagulants. Though there is a controversy on the role of anticoagulants in septic CVT, both cases in the literature have been treated with anticoagulants.

9.6.5 Endovascular Treatment for Stroke

Ay et al. [7] reported a case of young stroke, right MCA infarct, with distal right MCA stenosis that was treated with stenting before a diagnosis of neurobrucellosis was made by positive blood and CSF culture. They reported that angiogram repeated during the reevaluation of the patient was normal [7].

Most of the cases with ischemic stroke had normal angiogram, and the mechanism was attributed to the involvement of deep penetrating branches. Adaletli et al. [1] have reported occlusion of branches of the right MCA, vascular cut-off signs, vascular contour irregularities, and stenosis. Afterward, this patient was managed with methylprednisolone and antibiotics [1].

9.6.6 Corticosteroids

The use of corticosteroids in neurobrucellosis is not the standard of care, but they have been used for complications of brucellosis like optic neuritis and arachnoiditis. Infectious vasculitic involvement in neurobrucellosis may be an indication for steroids. Jochum et al. [20] have used prednisolone, while methylprednisolone was used by Adaletli et al. [1]

Conclusion

Cerebrovascular complications of neurobrucellosis are unusual, ranging from occlusive strokes to SAHs and intracranial aneurysms. Many cases maybe misdiagnosed as tuberculosis since both share endemic areas and clinical features. A high index of suspicion is warranted, and more often, the diagnosis would be missed unless a vascular imaging, CT angiography, or MR angiography is carried out in the appropriate clinical setting.

References

1. Adaletli I, Albayram S, Gurses B, Ozer H, Yilmaz MH, Gulsen F, Sirikci A. 2006Vasculopathic changes in the cerebral arterial system with neurobrucellosis. AJNR Am J Neuroradiol 27:384–386
2. Aguado JM, Barros C, Gomez Garces JL, Fernández-Guerrero ML (1987) Infective aortitis due to Brucella melitensis. Scand J Infect Dis 19:483–484
3. Akhondian J, Ashrafzadeh F, Toosi MB, Hashemi N (2014) A rare presentation of neurobrucellosis in a child with recurrent transient ischemic attacks and

pseudotumor cerebri (a case report and review of literature). Iran J Child Neurol 8:65–69
4. Al Deeb SM, Yaqub BA, Sharif HS, Phadke JG (1989) Neurobrucellosis: clinical characteristics, diagnosis, and outcome. Neurology 39:498–501
5. Amiri RS, Hanif H, Ahmadi A, Amirjamshidi A (2014) Brucella-related multiple cerebral aneurysms: report of a case and review of the literature. Surg Neurol Int 5:152
6. Antela A, San José MD, Fortún J, Casanova M, López Vélez R, Guerrero A (1992) Endocarditis caused by Brucella melitensis on a mitral valve prosthesis presenting as an ischemic cerebrovascular accident. Enferm Infecc Microbiol Clin 10:486–488
7. Ay S, Tur BS, Kutlay Ş (2010) Cerebral infarct due to meningovascular neurobrucellosis: a case report. Int J Infect Dis 14(Suppl 3):e202–e204
8. Bahemuka M, Shemena AR, Panayiotopoulos CP, al-Aska AK, Obeid T, Daif AK (1988) Neurological syndromes of brucellosis. J Neurol Neurosurg Psychiatry 51:1017–1021
9. Bingol A, Togay-Isikay C (2006) Neurobrucellosis as an exceptional cause of transient ischemic attacks. Eur J Neurol 13:544–548
10. Bruce D (1887) Note on the discovery of a microorganism in Malta fever. Practitioner 39:161–170
11. Erdem H, Senbayrak S, Gencer S, Hasbun R, Karahocagil MK, Sengoz G, Karsen H, Kaya S, Civljak R, Inal AS, Pekok AU, Celen MK, Deniz S, Ulug M, Demirdal T, Namiduru M, Tekin R, Guven T, Parlak E, Bolukcu S, Avci M, Sipahi OR, Nayman-Alpat S, Yaşar K, Pehlivanoğlu F, Yilmaz E, Ates-Guler S, Mutlu-Yilmaz E, Tosun S, Sirmatel F, Şahin-Horasan E, Akbulut A, Johansen IS, Simeon S, Batirel A, Öztoprak N, Cag Y, Catroux M, Hansmann Y, Kadanali A, Turgut H, Baran AI, Gul HC, Karaahmetoglu G, Sunnetcioglu M, Haykir-Solay A, Denk A, Ayaz C, Kose S, Gorenek L (2015) Tuberculous and brucellosis meningitis differential diagnosis. Travel Med Infect Dis 13:185–191
12. Erdogan B, Sener L, Ozsahin K, Savas L, Caner H (2005) An unusual case of ruptured distal anterior cerebral artery aneurysm associated with brucellosis. J Infect 51:e79–e82
13. Faraji F, Didgar F, Talaie-Zanjani A, Mohammadbeigi A (2013) Uncontrolled seizures resulting from cerebral venous sinus thrombosis complicating neurobrucellosis. J Neurosci Rural Pract 4:313–316
14. Gul HC, Erdem H, Bek S (2009) Overview of neurobrucellosis: a pooled analysis of 187 cases. Int J Infect Dis 13:e339–e343
15. Guven T, Ugurlu K, Ergonul O, Celikbas AK, Gok SE, Comoglu S, Baykam N, Dokuzoguz B (2013) Neurobrucellosis: clinical and diagnostic features. Clin Infect Dis 56:1407–1412
16. Hansmann GH, Schenken JR (1932) Melitensis meningoencephalitis: mycotic aneurysm due to Brucella melitensis var. Porcine. Am J Pathol 8:435–444
17. Hernández MA, Anciones B, Frank A, Barreiro P (1988) Neurobrucellosis and cerebral vasculitis. Neurologia 3:241–243
18. Inan AS, Ceran N, Erdem I, Engin DO, Senbayrak S, Ozyurek SC, Goktas P (2010) Neurobrucellosis with transient ischemic attack, vasculopathic changes, intracerebral granulomas and basal ganglia infarction: a case report. J Med Case Rep 4:340
19. Jabbour R, Khalifeh R, Al Kutoubi A, Atweh S (2003) Dissecting aneurysm of the basilar trunk in a young man. Arch Neurol 60:1016–1018
20. Jochum T, Kliesch U, Both R, Leonhardi J, Bär KJ (2008) Neurobrucellosis with thalamic infarction: a case report. Neurol Sci 29:481–483
21. Kaya S, Velioglu M, Colak A, Kutlay M, Demircan MN, Tekin T, Cetinkal A (2008) Brucella-related cerebral aneurysms/subarachnoidal hemorrhage: a short review featuring a case report. Neurosurg Rev 31:337–341
22. Kesav P, Venugopalan Y, Khurana D (2014) Fatal disseminated neurobrucellosis. QJM 107:321–322
23. Kesav P, Vishnu VY, Khurana D (2013) Is neurobrucellosis the Pandora's Box of modern medicine? Clin Infect Dis 57:1056–1057
24. Kizilkilic O, Calli C (2011) Neurobrucellosis. Neuroimaging Clin N Am 21:927–937
25. Korri H, Awada A, Ali Y, Choucair J (2008) Brucellar meningitis complicated by aneurysmal subarachnoid hemorrhage. Rev Neurol (Paris) 164:1052–1055
26. McLean DR, Russell N, Khan MY (1992) Neurobrucellosis: clinical and therapeutic features. Clin Infect Dis 15:582–590
27. Panagariya A, Sharma B, Mathew V (2007) Pseudotumour-like presentation of neurobrucellosis. J Assoc Physicians India 55:301–302
28. Pascual J, Combarros O, Polo JM, Berciano J (1988) Localized CNS brucellosis: report of 7 cases. Acta Neurol Scand 78:282–289
29. Rajan R, Khurana D, Kesav P (2013) Deep gray matter involvement in neurobrucellosis. Neurology 80: e28–e29
30. Ranjbar M, Rezaiee AA, Hashemi SH, Mehdipour S (2009) Neurobrucellosis: report of a rare disease in 20 Iranian patients referred to a tertiary hospital. East Mediterr Health J 15:143–148
31. Tuncer-Ertem G, Tülek N, Yetkin MA (2004) Case report: subdural hemorrhage in neurobrucellosis. Mikrobiyol Bul 38:253–256
32. Vogt T, Hasler P (1999) A woman with panic attacks and double vision who liked cheese. Lancet 354:300
33. Yrivarren J, Lopez L (1987) Cryoglobulinemia and cutaneous vasculitis in human brucellosis. J Clin Immunol 7:471–474
34. Zaidan R, Al Tahan AR (1999) Cerebral venous thrombosis: a new manifestation of neurobrucellosis. Clin Infect Dis 28:399–400

Brucellar Psychosis

10

Hamid Reza Naderi

Contents

Abstract

The cognitive and mood disorders among neurobrucellosis patients are well documented. While neurobrucellosis is typically diagnosed by abnormal cerebrospinal fluid (CSF) analysis and detected specific antibodies in CSF, it is prudent to consider any case with unexplained psychological or mental disorder in the course of an active brucellosis as brucellar psychosis. The psychological manifestations of brucellosis can present in various clinical forms, and prompt antibrucellar antibiotic therapy should be started following the diagnosis of the infection by strong serological tests and/or isolation of the organism. The subject is especially concerning in the endemic areas where brucellosis is prevalent or whenever there is a history of exposure to Brucella species. The psychotic manifestations of a patient with active brucellosis improve by antibrucellar treatment, even without antipsychotic therapy.

Keywords

Neurobrucellosis • Psychosis • Cerebrospinal fluid • Antibrucellar treatment

Abbreviations

2-ME	2-Mercaptoethanal
Bid	Twice a day

H.R. Naderi, MD
Department of Infectious Diseases,
Mashhad University of Medical Sciences,
Mashhad, Iran
e-mail: naderihr@mums.ac.ir

M. Turgut et al. (eds.), *Neurobrucellosis: Clinical, Diagnostic and Therapeutic Features*,
DOI 10.1007/978-3-319-24639-0_10

CSF	Cerebrospinal fluid
CNS	Central nervous system
DS	Double strength
DSM-IV	Criteria Diagnostic and Statistical Manual of Mental Disorders-IV
EEG	Electroencephalogram
ELISA	Enzyme-linked immunosorbent assay
HDRS	Hamilton Depression Rating Scale
LPS	Lipopolysaccharides
MAG	Microagglutination test
MMPI	Minnesota Multiphasic Personality Inventory
MMSE	Mini-Mental State Examination
Qhs	Every night at bedtime
SAT	Standard agglutination test
TMP–SMZ	Trimethoprim–sulfamethoxazole

10.1 Introduction

Edward Browne described a curious case in his famous "Arabian Medicine" back in 1920. He wrote: "A certain prince of the House of Buwayh was afflicted with melancholia and suffered from the delusion that he was a cow. Every day he would low like a cow, causing annoyance to everyone and crying 'Kill me, so that a good stew may be prepared from my flesh'; until matters reached such a pass that he would eat nothing, while the physicians were unable to do him any good. Finally, Avicenna was persuaded to take the case in hand. First of all he sent a message to the patient bidding him be of good cheer because the butcher was coming to slaughter him, whereat, the sick man rejoiced. Some time afterwards Avicenna, holding a knife in his hand, entered the sick-room, saying 'Where is this cow, that I may kill it?' The patient lowed like a cow to indicate where he was. By Avicenna's orders he was laid on the ground bound hand and foot. Avicenna then felt him all over and said: 'He is too lean, and not ready to be killed; he must be fattened'. Then they offered him suitable food, of which he now partook eagerly, and gradually he gained strength, got rid of his delusion, and was completely cured" [10]. According to the Diagnostic and Statistical Manual of Mental Disorders-IV (DSM)-IV criteria for specification of mental disorders, we shall assume that this case was an acute psychotic disorder not otherwise specified [33]. The diagnosis requires the presence of delusions, false implausible beliefs, hallucinations, or false perceptions that may be visual, auditory, or tactile [9] about which there is inadequate information to make a specific diagnosis or any disorder with psychotic symptoms that does not meet the criteria for any specific psychotic disorder [33]. The patient treated by Avicenna was a nobleman with no recorded preceding event for triggering his sudden bizarre behavior, and he was completely cured within 1 month of feeding and medication. Hence, it is likely that he suffered from a psychotic disorder due to a treatable medical illness, and it would not be farfetched to regard Avicenna's case as the first possible case of toxic or septic encephalopathy presenting as acute psychosis described in the literature.

It has long been suggested that infection can affect the levels of neurotransmitters which is associated with septic encephalopathy development. During an infectious illness, the central nervous system (CNS) is one of the first organs affected and reciprocal interactions between the immune system and the CNS are considered to be major components of the host response in the process [12]. The evidence proposed immune and inflammatory cascades in conjunction with infection may play a role in the pathology [19]. Theoretically, circulating cytokines synthesized by an infectious trigger can diffuse through the blood–brain barrier, or they can act on their receptors in the CNS to modulate brain function [12]. However, one major limitation is related to the difficulty of proving causality. The interactions between infectious agents and host factors resulting in mental disturbance generally do not follow Koch's postulates, which require that there be a one-to-one correspondence between the two entities [43]. According to Yolken and Torrey [43], the relationship between infectious agents and chronic diseases often does not follow the straightforward associations defined by Koch's postulates but rather a number of factors, including the timing of infection, the nature of the infecting strain, and the genetic makeup of the host, can compromise the situation leading the infected subject to diverse clinical outcomes. Recently, Hayes et al. [19] examined molecular changes in the cerebrospinal fluid from patients with schizophrenia and at-risk mental status for psychosis exploring how infectious agents such as Toxoplasma gondii and herpes simplex type 1 affect these molecular changes, and they found the possible relationship of some inflammatory molecular signatures in the CSF to these disease-associated infections.

One of the earliest researchers who believed that microbial agents might be etiologically linked to psychotic disorders was Emil Kraepelin. In 1896, he addressed the dementia praecox as "a tangible morbid process of the brain caused by an autointoxication" [43]. Since then, numerous reports throughout the world have been published to present cases with infection-related psychoses supporting the infectious theory. Tuberculosis, typhoid fever, syphilis, toxoplasmosis, herpes simplex and cytomegalovirus infection, and cysticercosis are just a few infamous infectious diseases that have been linked to psychiatric disorders [3, 18, 20, 22, 26, 37, 39]. Interestingly, brucellosis caused by different *Brucella* spp. (B. abortus, B. canis, B. melitensis, and B. suis) is one of these infectious agents in which neuropsychiatric manifestations have raised much attention during the past decades. Neurobrucellosis was first reported by Hughes in 1896 [27]. The psychiatric changes in neurobrucellosis occur rarely, and there are few reports of brucellar psychosis in the literature [2, 4, 14, 23, 28].

10.2 Brucellar Psychosis

Although rarely seen, the spectrum of psychosomatic manifestations of patients with brucellosis is very diverse, and many authors presented cases with mental disabilities that ranged from subtle cognitive dysfunctions detected only by neuropsychological evaluation to apparent psychosis or schizophreniform disorders. The psychiatric manifestations, while rarely reported, were depression, amnesia, agitation, nightmares, personality disorders, euphoria, nervousness, loss of perception, disturbance of spontaneous and voluntary attention, disturbances in process of thinking with poverty of content, hallucination, delirium, convulsion, dysarthria, psychosis, and night raving [14, 17, 23, 30]. In a study by Shehata et al. [35], 38.5 % of patients with brucellosis without apparent neurological symptoms had depression or cerebellar affection, in addition to significant impairments in some cognitive function, as mental control, logical memory, and visual reproduction in comparison with control group. In this study, depression was detected in seven patients (29.2 %); three of them have evident neurobrucellosis, whereas four were apparently without any neuropsychiatric involvement [35]. Depression is significantly more present in patients with brucellosis without marked neurological symptoms than in patients with apparent neurological manifestations. The explanation of that could be relied on the mechanism of depression in these patients whose altered moods point to different mechanisms such as direct effect of the organism or its products on the meninges and brain [1, 35]. Alapin [2], in his extensive review of neurological aspects of brucellosis, wrote that "many papers underline the commonness of neurological and psychotic complications with infection by B. melitensis. There is an option that B. abortus produce a much lower percentages of neuro-psychiatric complications than B. melitensis or B. suis" [2, 38]. Roger and Poursines [31] classified the neuropsychiatric manifestations of brucellosis as "psychotic encephalitis of the pseudo-tumoral form" and "different psychological disorders" with psychasthenia as the most common form for a late course of chronic brucellosis.

According to Alapin [2], multiple cases were diagnosed as neurasthenia, psychasthenia, or depression during the course of chronic brucellosis without an acute period. Evans [15] called this state "a ramshackle feeling" (in French: patraquement) and Janbon and Bertrand "subjective syndrome of chronic brucellosis." Those subjective symptoms were headaches, tiredness/fatigability both physical and mental, insomnia in the evening as well as early awakening, increased nervous sensibility, sexual troubles, as well as pains and aches without easy explanation. Those symptoms sometimes increased to complete psychic asthenia, incapacity of concentration, troubles of memory, irritability, exaggeration of emotions, and depressive states. Such a state is much more expressed in persons who, even before infection, showed immaturity or inadequacy of personality [2].

While these authors represented depression as the most common manifestation of brucella mental disturbances, some like Imboden believed that depressive mood is part of a fatigue syndrome accompanied by any chronic illness rather than a specific representation of neurobrucellosis, which manifests significantly more often in cases who suffer from other psychological traumatic experiences and personality or mood disorders. In one study, he compared eight patients with brucellosis who had recovered in 2 or 3 months, with 16 who were still symptomatic after 1 year with such complaints as fatigue, headache, nervousness, and vague aches and pains. All, but one, were males. There were no differences between the two groups in medical findings at onset or at time of reexamination. The 16 who were still ill, however, differed significantly from the eight who had recovered with respect to incidence of psychologically traumatic events in early life (69 % vs. 25 %), a seriously disturbed life situation within 1 year before or after the acute infection (69 % vs. 0 %), and significantly higher scores on an index of morale loss derived from the Minnesota Multiphasic Personality Inventory (MMPI) [21]. He described a patient who was visited 2 years after a treated acute brucellosis. He was an emigrant who suffered from depression, extreme fatigue, headaches, introversion, and asociality. His younger siblings were dead, and his parents left him alone and returned to their homeland before his illness. Another patient with the diagnosis of chronic brucellosis and symptoms of depression and lassitude was a heavy drinker who became a member of a religious order after his father died. His mood disorder did not improve even after the successful treatment of brucellosis. The authors debated whether these disturbed life-associated mood disorders were related to the diagnosis of brucellosis [25]. Conversely, Eren et al. [14] studied 34 neurobrucellosis cases and 30 patients with brucellosis without neurological involvement. The patients were evaluated by two psychiatrists, and the Hamilton Depression Rating Scale (HDRS) and Mini-Mental State Examination (MMSE) or Folstein tests were performed before the therapy and 1 and 2 weeks after the therapy. The psychiatrists interviewed the neurobrucellosis patients and diagnosed mild depression due to a general medical condition (neurobrucellosis) according to DSM-IV criteria in all of the cases. The mean score of MMSE among neurobrucellosis patients was 21.7 before the therapy. The improvement began in the first week of the therapy and reached a mean score of 24.3 at the end of the second week ($p \leq 0.001$). The mean HDRS test score among neurobrucellosis patients was ten before the therapy and improved to 8.2 1 week later ($p = 0.006$) and to 5.2 2 weeks later ($p = 0.001$). On the other hand, among the brucellosis patients without neurological involvement, no significant changes of MMSE and HDRS test scores were observed. The test scores of neurobrucellosis patients were also compared with the scores of the patients without neurological involvement before the therapy. Test scores of HDRS were significantly different in two groups ($p = 0.035$), whereas test scores of MMSE were not ($p = 0.351$). They also found that the improvement in the MMSE scores in neurobrucellosis was significant ($p \leq 0.001$), whereas in control group, it was not. The mild depression that was detected in neurobrucellosis patients after the psychiatric examination was improved at the end of 2 weeks ($p = 0.001$). On the other hand, among the brucellosis patients without neurological involvement, depression was not detected as HDRS test scores were within normal ranges. The significant difference between the HDRS scores in two groups ($p = 0.035$) supports the depression seen in neurobrucellosis. While no improvement of the scores was noticed among the patients without neurological involvement, the authors concluded that the cognitive and emotional disturbances among neurobrucellosis improve by antibiotic therapy, without any antidepressive or antipsychotic therapy [14]. Finally, it seems that although previous traumatic stress disorders during childhood as well as the current life-disturbing events can affect the extent and severity of the mood swings in brucella patients, the deleterious impact of the infection itself on their psychological symptoms and mental disabilities is a matter of serious concern.

10.3 Case Records

A wide variety of psychiatric symptoms ranging from memory deficits and mild personality changes to severe depression and frank psychosis have been described in patients with brucellosis. Alapin [2] claimed that the difference in severity of cases is due to such pathogenetic factors as extreme virulence of *Brucella* spp., constitutional somatopsychic predisposition of individuals, and the time of exposure to infectious process.

Almost all authors have pointed out that neuropsychiatric manifestations of brucellosis can display in every stage of the disease: as a presenting symptom in acute brucellosis [32], during the exacerbations mostly with febrile course [32, 38], or in chronic course, mainly many years after infection [2].

Alapin [2] presented two interesting cases with active brucellosis and paranoid personality disorder, which had persecutory delusions:

"He showed confusional state, was agitated, expressed multiple persecutory delusions and several ideas of reference ("they think that I am a Nazi … I am followed . . . trains were stopped to prevent my being on time", etc.). During further observation he became lucid and then he was able to explain that during the acute phase he had visual and auditory illusions and hallucinations. The delusional syndrome slowly receded when treated with chlorpromazine but returned later … The CSF was normal and the electroencephalogram (EEG) showed rather a normal trace. The diagnosis of brucella encephalopathy with chronic paranoid psychosis and brucella peripheral poly-neuropathy was made."

"The patient, first veterinary surgeon, then medical practitioner, was treated for brucellosis 10 years earlier. In 1965, he produced persecutory delusions and ideas of reference. His EEG confirmed diffuse pathology of the trace and serological investigation proved an active brucellosis. Neither familial, personal data nor further 3 years' long observation of the patient suggest the probability of schizophrenia". He concluded that: "the fact that in about a third of our patients we could find distinct proofs of an allergo-inflammatory involvement of the CNS and the fact that the peripheral nervous system is involved in about 25 % of cases seems to suggest rather the direct impact of toxins on the autonomic nervous system and therefore brucellosis has to be looked upon as an illness leading to a multi-factorial (somato-psychic-psychosomatic) pathogenesis of psychoses, pseudo-neurotic syndrome and other manifestations in the nervous system of a patient infected with brucella" [2]. Tuncel et al. [40] reported three cases with psychosis due to neurobrucellosis. One of them represents a typical case of evident psychosomatic disorder.

"A 49-year-old woman presented with gait disturbance, behavior change and seizure … The patient has experienced a gradual, slowly progressive neurocognitive decline such amnesia and difficulty performing activities of daily living, and gait disturbance for 2 years. General physical examination was normal. Vital parameters were normal. Neurologically, she was conscious, but uncooperative. There were cognitive impairment in verbal fluency, loss of recent memory, copying of written figures, attention and calculation (MMSE: 16/30), dysarthria, ataxia, bilateral sensorineural hearing loss, weakness of upper proximal extremities (Medical Research Council grade: 4/5). Brucella tube agglutinin was positive at 1/2560 titers in blood and positive at spot and 1/2560 titers in CSF. The patient was treated with ceftriaxone, rifampicin (600 mg/daily), doxycycline (200 mg/daily) and trimethoprim/sulfamethaxazole (TMP–SMZ) (320/1600 mg/daily). In the control examination after 2 weeks and 1 month, her mental status (respectively; MMSE: 19/30, 27/30) and physical performance were gradually partly improved" [40].

Previously, Alapin [2] described 6 cases of brucellosis who suffered from bouts of epilepsy (four with grand mal, one with petit mal, and one with absence). In five of these patients, EEG was performed, and the results confirmed the diagnosis of epilepsy, while three patients treated for brucellosis lost their epileptic fits and their EEG tracing improved greatly, two of them could stop their antiepileptic drugs completely [2].

Ghaffarinejad et al. [16] reported a case with psychotic behavior and bizarre hallucinations as a part of chronic brucellosis:

"A 26-year-old man, married, shepherd, from Baft city, Kerman, (south of Iran) was admitted to Kerman psychiatric hospital because of acute psychotic symptoms. He had neither positive previous nor family history of psychiatric disorders. At that time he had resting tremor and cogwheel rigidity in neurological examination. Wright agglutination test of blood was positive (1/640) and 2-mercaptoethanal (2-ME) reduction test of blood was positive (1/320) as well. He was treated with doxycycline, rifampin, and co-trimoxazole. He was highly restless and impulsive, and had episodic unreasonable crying … This condition was changed rapidly and replaced by impulsions of laughing when the topic was changed by interviewer. He reported to be able to see and hear the voices of three fairy females who seduced and invited him for dance. He had uninhibited sexual impulses. His cognition was intact and had only partial insight. Two months after starting the treatment with 6 mg risperidone and 6 mg trihexyphenidyl, frequency of his impulsive behavior, delusions, and hallucinations were decreased, but his style of speech remained unchanged. Despite proper treatment with antibiotic, 2-ME test of blood remains positive (1/320)" [16].

The authors suggested that in patients with atypical psychosis in endemic areas, physicians should consider the possibility of chronic brucellosis" [16].

Montazeri et al. [29] reported a female patient whose delusional disorder completely vanished after she was treated for brucellosis without any antipsychotic drug prescription:

"A 36-year-old woman was admitted to hospital, because of acute onset of fever and decreased level of consciousness. Her problem began 3 days prior to admission with hallucination, delusions and fever. She was single and unemployed, living in a small town, without previous history of brucellosis in herself and her family … On admission, she had disorientation to time and place. She was agitated and had visual hallucination and grandiose delusion. Despite her high temperature (39 °C) other vital signs were normal … At this time serology tests for brucellosis became positive including: Wright agglutination test = 1/40, Coombs Wright = 1/80, Brucella ELISA IgG = 146.6 U/ml (normal < 8 U/ml). With probable diagnosis of neurobrucellosis, triple therapy was started … Within a week, the patient's symptoms including fever and psychosis improved and she became completely alert without any neurological problems and regained ability to talk and eat. After 3 months, she became completely well. She received 6 months' treatment totally with clinical follow-ups showing no problem at 3 months and at the end of 6 months" [29].

According to Alapin [2], brucellar schizophreniform psychosis with paranoid personality disorder was reported by Annesley in 1968. This case also became symptom-free after treatment for brucellosis without any psychotherapeutic intervention:

"A married woman of 41 was admitted to hospital after becoming paranoid, hallucinated and violent. She gave a history of three miscarriages subsequent to the birth of her last child.

There was no previous history of mental illness, nor of serious physical illness … In October she was admitted to a general hospital, and she was treated with 'Bradosol' lozenges for a sore throat, iron and an ascorbic acid preparation, improved and was discharged home after 8 days. A week later she was readmitted to the same hospital with complaints of giddiness, headaches, sweating and weakness. She now had a fever of 100. It was noticed that she was apprehensive and suspicious … She now began to show clear paranoid symptoms. She believed that the patients and nurses were trying to trick and poison her and thought they were altering her appearance. She searched the other patients' beds for radios which she said were being used to influence her thoughts … She complained that the patients were all hostile to her. She heard them saying she had recently had a baby, and asked where the child could be. She was reluctant to eat, as she believed her food was being tampered with. She was diagnosed as suffering from a schizophreniform psychosis secondary to organic illness …

Tests for brucella agglutinins gave a titer of 1/160. Her paranoid symptoms improved spontaneously after a week, but she continued to complain of food having an unpleasant taste for a fortnight after starting antibiotics. Her treatment consisted of tetracycline, 0.5 g six hourly with streptomycin, 1 g daily, for 3 weeks. No phenothiazines were given. She was physically and mentally well when followed up a month later. She remarked on her feeling of relief at being able to sit down without any backache. Malaise, weakness and headache had remitted and she had put on weight. She was having no difficulty in running her home and this improvement was confirmed by her husband" [2].

Nonetheless, some cases of brucella psychosis need antipsychotic therapy indeed, as a 66-year-old farmer presented by Bidaki et al. [8]:

"He had behavioral abnormalities such as restlessness, impulsivity, and episodic crying. His speech was incoherent. It seemed that he was driving in a car and he believed that nurses injected the worms in his serum. His cognition was impaired and had poor insight. Three day after the treatment with risperidone (1 mg qhs), haloperidole (2.5 mg bid) and sodium-valproate (200 mg OD), his impulsive behavior, restlessness, and psychotic symptoms decreased and finally were resolved." The authors concluded that psychotic symptoms probably follow after acute brucellosis and response to antipsychotic therapy is favorable in this condition [8].

Sheybani et al. [36] reported three patients with brucellosis manifested as psychiatric disorder, one of whom represents a true case of relapsing psychosis:

"A 60-year-old peasant man without any significant past psychiatric history was admitted to the hospital, because of a gradual onset of fever accompanied by headache, nausea and vomiting and a progressive confusional state which started about 1 week before presentation … He was conscious but disoriented with visual and auditory hallucinations of seeing someone who wasn't present and hearing voices without external stimulus. His mental impairment persisted even though the patient was afebrile, and a lumbar puncture was performed to evaluate for encephalitis … He was discharged from hospital with some improvement after 2 weeks. Some weeks later, he was readmitted because of relapsed mental illness, presented again as bizarre behavior and a variety of hallucinations. This time, serologic markers of brucellosis in serum and CSF requested which confirmed the diagnosis of neurobrucellosis. He was treated with TMP–SMZ (2DS tablets/bid) and rifampin (600 mg/bid) for 6 months with no evidence of mental disturbance at the end of therapy" [36].

In another two patients, acute mental disturbance and bizarre behavior were the main features and systemic signs and symptoms of brucellosis were subtle or absent:

"An 18-year-old girl was referred to the hospital because of a presumed sepsis syndrome superimposed on an acute psychosis manifested as a personality disorder, for which she had been admitted in a psychiatry center two days before. She thought that she was a dog … On the 3rd day of her admission, while the mental status didn't change, both the serum and CSF serological assays for acute brucellosis gave significant positive results, as well as the blood culture which isolated B. abortus a few days later. She was treated with intramuscular streptomycin (1 g/daily), oral rifampin (600 mg/daily) and doxycycline (100 mg/ bid) without any antipsychotic therapy, and she improved dramatically after about 10 days. The oral drugs continued for 5 months, when her CSF-Wright test resulted negative. She was followed for several months thereafter, only to be assured that there was no problem with her mental status" [36].

"A 24-year-old man was referred to hospital, with a possible diagnosis of rabies encephalitis. The young man, a rancher living in a village near the city, had been bitten by a stray dog few days before his mental disturbance began. According to his father, one night the patient returned from grassland uneasy and restless. He was febrile and he said irrelevant things about himself and the others. He saw some people who were not present and he laughed, cried, bawled, biting himself and insulting the others. He had a kind of hydrophobia. He became irritated, and he drew back and started to whimper, when someone was offering him something to drink. He had neither photophobia/aerophobia nor sialorrhea. He was just extremely agitated and fidgety. Concerning the possible diagnosis of rabies encephalitis, ribavirin and amantadin started and the patient also received rabies human immunoglobulin. His CSF analysis was normal, but serologic markers of the patient confirmed the acute brucellosis with CNS involvement. Doxycycline (100 mg/ bid), rifampin (600 mg/daily) and TMP–SMZ (2DS tablets/ bid) were prescribed and the patient was discharged from hospital with a normal mental status." The authors suggested that brucellosis should be considered in patients with unexplainable psychiatric problems, when there is a history of possible exposure to *Brucella* spp. [36].

Finally, Angle [5] as well as Angle and Algie [6] reported an unusual case whose psychotic symptoms exaggerated following receiving brucella vaccination as a therapeutic intervention that was suggested before:

"A white male aged 23 was admitted to the hospital January 8, 1936, in a state of violent catatonic excitement … He was sent to a hospital where it was found that his blood serum agglutinated B. abortus in a dilution of 1/640. It was learned that he had been a habitual drinker of raw milk. His condition was diagnosed as undulant fever. After a short period of observation he was sent home. January 6, he was despondent, irritable, and, at times, mildly delirious. On this date he was given 0.25 cc of B. abortus vaccine intramuscularly. This was followed in a few hours by increased fever, chills, and a more severe delirium. The reaction subsided promptly but recurred the next day following the administration of 0.5 cc of the vaccine. He was mildly confused when seen in consultation January 8. It was decided that he should be sent to the hospital for observation. The family history was entirely negative for mental disturbance … The serum agglutinated B. abortus in a dilution of 1/1280 … Early in the fourth week his temperature again increased to 104 °F and was accompanied by increased agitation but the temperature subsided to normal in a few days and the agitation decreased … He had lost more than 40 pounds during his illness. Repeated neurological examinations revealed no evidence of any focal lesion of the brain or spinal cord… He continued to be hyperactive and hallucinated. He was very destructive to his clothing and bedding and was frequently nude… From the early part of May, his mental condition cleared up rapidly and he was dismissed June 15, apparently normal. Since his return he has been seen frequently. There has been no psychotic tendency … At present he is working in a packing plant. So far there has been no indication of a return of his undulant fever … Although the early symptoms of psychosis had preceded the administration of the vaccine, they developed much more rapidly following its use. The symptoms of general intoxication, likewise, were greatly intensified. We were so impressed by this fact that we considered it unwise to continue the vaccine therapy."

Based on his findings, he suggested that the presence of a psychosis should be added to the list of contraindications to the use of vaccine already reported [6].

10.4 Diagnostic Challenges

Neurological aspects of brucellosis have been classified in two major groups: (I) those related to the acute toxic febrile state that occurs in any acute illness and (II) those related to actual invasion and localization of the pathogen in the CNS. The incidence of neurological complications in brucellosis has been reported to be 1.7–10 %; it was 2.35 % in Akdeniz et al. [1] cases. Diagnosis of classical neurobrucellosis is usually made through the detection of specific antibodies in the CSF; organisms can be cultured from the CSF in no more than 25 % of cases [23]. The primary immune response is an increase in IgM followed by an increase in IgG and IgA, with often only IgG and IgA antibodies being detected in chronic cases. Although ELISA, which is a test used in the detection of these antibodies, is a specific and sensitive method, standard agglutination test (SAT) has more widespread use in diagnosis. Fundamentally, ELISA has no advantage over SAT or Coombs tests [23].

Interestingly, in toxic febrile neurobrucellosis, the presence of antibodies to brucella in the CSF is not expected. Because the antigen involved in the agglutination is in the form of lipopolysaccharides (LPS) which is responsible for the development of immune response and also activates the classical and alternative complement pathways [24], thus, only when the pathogen directly enters into the CSF, LPS stimulates the immune system and gives rise to pleocytosis, antibody production, hyperproteinorrachia, and hypoglycorrhachia in the CSF. In contrast (i.e., in the absence of invasion), LPS does not exist in the CSF and consequently does not give rise to antibody response. In this condition, pleocytosis is not seen, and agglutination does not occur and biochemistry of the CSF does not change [23].

While some experts suggest that ELISA (IgG, IgM, and IgA profiles) is the test of choice in the diagnosis of patients with brucellosis, especially those with chronic or CNS infection [34], others are concerned about the fact that ELISA assays suffer from poor sensitivity and specificity when compared with agglutination tests [23].

Regarding the fact, preliminary results have not demonstrated any advantage of the ELISA over the SAT or Coombs test. It should be pointed out that the antibrucellar Coombs test in CSF is of great value in the diagnosis of neurobrucellosis. The rate of positive reactions obtained with the rose bengal test in cerebrospinal fluid seems to be similar to that of the microagglutination test and inferior to that obtained by the Coombs test; and the serological study of both serum and CSF is essential for the diagnosis of neurobrucellosis [34].

To conclude, the diagnosis of brucellar psychosis is based upon the presence of an unexplained psychotic behavior accompanied by the evidence of systemic brucellar infection and/or the presence of inflammatory alteration in the CSF [17].

Brucellosis is an aggressive disease which requires immediate treatment, and prompt antibrucellar antibiotic therapy is effective in most cases [42]. Toxic febrile neurobrucellosis responds rapidly to medications, as it develops in a short period. Treatment does not differ from systemic brucellosis; however, most authorities recommend two or three drugs which cross the blood–brain CSF barrier (such as doxycycline, rifampin, and trimethoprim–sulfamethoxazole). The duration of therapy for neurobrucellosis is generally prolonged, varying from 1 to 19 months [7, 13]. The antibiotic treatment of systemic brucellosis, particularly the CNS form, is still a considerable problem. This is in part due to the intracellular location of the microorganism and in part to the fact that successful treatment requires bactericidal levels of the antibiotic in the CSF. Tetracyclines, sulfonamides, TMP–SMZ, streptomycin, and rifampicin are reputed to be the best drugs for brucellosis. The high possibility for relapses makes combination therapy necessary [11]. Brucella antibody titers have been recommended to assess the therapeutic efficacy and resolution of the diseases [41].

Conclusion

Neurobrucellosis is typically diagnosed by abnormal cerebrospinal fluid analysis and detected specific antibodies in CSF. Nonetheless, it is advised that any case with unexplained psychological or mental disorder in the course of an active brucellar infection (confirmed by strongly positive serological test results and/or culture positivity of blood or bone marrow aspirates) should be regarded as a case of brucellar psychosis and should be treated accordingly. Given that the systemic signs of the disease may be absent and the patients may not even have fever, the psychological manifestations of brucellosis can present in various clinical forms, and regarding the undulant course of the disease and its marked tendency to relapse, the matter is especially concerning in endemic areas, where brucellosis is prevalent. However, brucellosis should be considered in patients who experience vague psychosomatic disorders, when there is a history of possible exposure to *Brucella* spp., even in countries where the disease is not endemic.

References

1. Akdeniz H, Irmak H, Anlar O, Demiröz AP (1998) Central nervous system brucellosis: presentation, diagnosis and treatment. J Infect 36:297–301
2. Alapin B (1976) Psychosomatic and somato-psychic aspects of brucellosis. J Psychosom Res 20: 339–350

3. Ali G, Rashid S, Kamli MA, Shah PA, Allaqaband GQ (1997) Spectrum of neuropsychiatric complications in 791 cases of typhoid fever. Trop Med Int Health 2:314–318
4. Amato E, Anasagasti I, Poza JJ, Yerobi JA (1989) Acute psychosis as a manifestation of brucellosis. Enferm Infecc Microbiol Clin 7:231–232
5. Angle FE (1935) Treatment of acute and chronic brucellosis (undulant fever): Personal observation of one hundred cases over a period of seven years. JAMA 105:939–942
6. Angle FE, Algie WH (1937) Major psychosis in undulant fever. Ann Intern Med 10:1890–1892
7. Araj GF, Lulu AR, Khateeb MI, Saadah MA, Shakir RA (1988) ELISA versus routine tests in the diagnosis of patients with systemic and neurobrucellosis. APMIS 96:171–176
8. Bidaki R, Yassini SM, Maymand MT, Mashayekhi M, Yassini S (2013) Acute psychosis due to brucellosis: a report of two cases in a rural Iran. Int J Infect Microbiol 2:29–31
9. Bostic J, Prince JB (2008) Chapter 69. Child and adolescent psychiatric disorders. In: Stern: Massachusetts general hospital comprehensive clinical psychiatry, 1st edn. Mosby, Philadelphia, p 953
10. Browne EG (1921) Arabian medicine. Cambridge University Press, Cambridge, pp 88–89
11. Bucher A, Gaustad P, Pape E (1990) Chronic neurobrucellosis due to Brucella melitensis: case report. Scand J Infect Dis 22:223–226
12. Dal-Pizzol F, Tomasi CD, Ritter C (2014) Septic encephalopathy: does inflammation drive the brain crazy? Rev Bras Psiquiatr 36:251–258
13. Drevets DA, Leenen PJM, Greenfield RA (2004) Invasion of the central nervous system by intracellular bacteria. Clin Microbiol Rev 17:323–347
14. Eren S, Bayam G, Ergonul O, Celikbas A, Pazvantoglu O, Baykam N, Dokuzoguz B, Dilbaz N (2006) Cognitive and emotional changes in neurobrucellosis. J Infect 53:184–189
15. Evans AC (1961) Chronic brucellosis: the unreliability of diagnostic tests. J Am Med Womens Assoc 16:942–945
16. Ghaffarinejad AR, Safarzadeh F, Sedighi B, Sadeghieh T (2008) Psychosis as an early presentation of neurobrucellosis. Iran J Med Sci 33:57–59
17. Gul HC, Erdem H, Bek S (2009) Overview of neurobrucellosis: a pooled analysis of 187 cases. Int J Infect Dis 13:e339–e343
18. Hamdani N, Daban-Huard C, Lajnef M, Richard JR, Delavest M, Godin O, Le Guen E, Vederine FE, Lépine JP, Jamain S, Houenou J, Le Corvoisier P, Aoki M, Moins-Teisserenc H, Charron D, Krishnamoorthy R, Yolken R, Dickerson F, Tamouza R, Leboyer M (2013) Relationship between Toxoplasma gondii infection and bipolar disorder in a french sample. J Affect Disord 148:444–448
19. Hayes LN, Severance EG, Leek JT, Gressitt KL, Rohleder C, Coughlin JM, Leweke FM, Yolken RH, Sawa A (2014) Inflammatory molecular signature associated with infectious agents in psychosis. Schizophr Bull 40:963–972
20. Hung HC, Chu JL, Lu T (2013) Psychotic disorder due to neurosyphilis. J Neuropsychiatry Clin Neurosci 25:E67–E68
21. Imboden JB, Canter A, Cluff LE, Trever RW (1959) Brucellosis. III. Psychologic aspects of delayed convalescence. Arch Intern Med 103:406–414
22. James BO, Agbonile IO, Okolo M, Lawani AO, Omoaregba JO (2013) Prevalence of Toxoplasma gondii infection among individuals with severe mental illness in Nigeria: a case control study. Pathog Glob Health 107:189–193
23. Karsen H, Akdeniz H, Karahocagil MK, Irmak H, Sünnetçioğlu M (2007) Toxic-febrile neurobrucellosis, clinical findings and outcome of treatment of four cases based on our experience. Scand J Infect Dis 39:990–995
24. Lapaque N, Moriyon I, Moreno E, Gorvel JP (2005) Brucella lipopolysaccharide acts as a virulence factor. Curr Opin Microbiol 8:60–66
25. Madkour MM, Al-Moutaery KR, Al-Deeb S, Al-Swailem R, Al-Okaily F (2001) Neurobrucellosis. In: Madkour's brucellosis. Springer, Berlin/Heidelberg, pp 166–178
26. Mathuranath PS, Radhakrishnan K (2009) Chapter 21. Neurological tuberculosis. In: Tuberculosis, 2nd edn. Jaypee Brothers Medical Publishers, New Delhi, p 307
27. McLean DR, Russell N, Kahn MY (1992) Neurobrucellosis: clinical and therapeutic features. Clin Infect Dis 15:582–590
28. Mohr JA, Wilson JD (1973) Schizophreniform psychosis with chronic brucellosis. J Okla State Med Assoc 66:319–321
29. Montazeri M, Sadeghi K, Khalili H, Davoudi S (2013) Fever and psychosis as an early presentation of Brucella-associated meningoencephalitis: a case report. Med Princ Pract 22:506–509
30. Pascual J, Combarros O, Polo JM, Berciano J (1988) Localized CNS brucellosis: report of 7 cases. Acta Neurol Scand 78:282–289
31. Roger H, Poursines Y (1951) Psychotic forms of meningo-neuro-brucellosis. Ann Med Psychol (Paris) 109:145–169
32. Roger H (1954) Brucellar paraplegia. Encéphale 43:246–279
33. Sadock B, Kaplan HI, Sadock VA (2007) Chapter 14. Other psychotic disorders. In: Kaplan & Sadock's synopsis of psychiatry: behavioral sciences/clinical psychiatry, 10th edn. Lippincott Williams and Wilkins, Philadelphia, p 519
34. Sanchez-Sousa A, Torres C, Campello MG, Garcia C, Parras F, Cercenado E, Baquero F (1990) Serological diagnosis of neurobrucellosis. J Clin Pathol 43:79–81
35. Shehata GA, Abdel-Baky L, Rashed H, Elamin H (2010) Neuropsychiatric evaluation of patients with brucellosis. J Neurovirol 16:48–55
36. Sheybani F, Sarvghad MR, Bojdi A, Naderi HR (2012) Brucellar psychosis. Arch Iran Med 15:723–725

37. Shirts BH, Prasad KM, Pogue-Geile MF, Dickerson F, Yolken RH, Nimgaonkar VL (2008) Antibodies to cytomegalovirus and Herpes simplex virus 1 associated with cognitive function in schizophrenia. Schizophr Res 106:268–274
38. Spink WW (1956) Brucellosis; epidemiology, clinical manifestations, diagnosis. Semin Int 5:15–17
39. Srivastava S, Chadda RK, Bala K, Majumdar P (2013) A study of neuropsychiatric manifestations in patients of neurocysticercosis. Indian J Psychiatry 55: 264–267
40. Tuncel D, Uçmak H, Gokce M, Utku U (2008) Neurobrucellosis. Eur J Gen Med 5:245–248
41. Turgut M, Cullu E, Sendur OF, Gürer G (2004) Brucellar spine infection-four case reports. Neurol Med Chir (Tokyo) 44:562–567
42. Turgut M, Sendur OF, Gürel M (2003) Brucellar spondylodiscitis in the lumbar region. Neurol Med Chir (Tokyo) 43:210–212
43. Yolken RH, Torrey EF (2008) Are some cases of psychosis caused by microbial agents? A review of the evidence. Mol Psychiatry 13:470–479

Radiological Appearance of Brucellosis of the Brain and Its Coverings

11

Roula Hourani and Huwayda Murad

Contents

R. Hourani, MD (✉) • H. Murad, MD
Department of Diagnostic Radiology, American University of Beirut Medical Center, Beirut, Lebanon
e-mail: rh64@aub.edu.lb; mourad.howayda@gmail.com

Abstract

The aim of this chapter is to describe the neuroimaging findings of neurobrucellosis. Neurobrucellosis can present with different clinical and neuroradiological signs. The imaging findings are variable and mainly divided into four categories: normal imaging, inflammatory changes in the brain and meninges, white matter changes, and vasculopathic lesions. The different radiological patterns of neurobrucellosis will be discussed thoroughly on CT and MRI. Knowledge of the multiple radiologic findings of neurobrucellosis will enable radiologists and neurologist to include neurobrucellosis in the differential diagnosis and may allow reliable diagnosis.

Keywords

Brain • Brucellosis • Computed tomography • Magnetic resonance imaging • Neuroimaging

Abbreviations

2D	Two dimensional
CNS	Central nervous system
CT	Computed tomography
DSA	Digital substraction angiography
FLAIR	Fluid-attenuated inversion recovery
MRI	Magnetic resonance imaging

M. Turgut et al. (eds.), *Neurobrucellosis: Clinical, Diagnostic and Therapeutic Features*,
DOI 10.1007/978-3-319-24639-0_11

11.1 Introduction

Brucellosis is an endemic zoonosis in the Mediterranean and Middle East area. It is the most common zoonotic infection around the world with 500,000 new cases per year, representing a serious health problem in developing countries [16]. Involvement of nervous system by *Brucella* spp. is known as "neurobrucellosis" and it may affect the central and/or peripheral nervous system [12, 13, 17]. Involvement of the central nervous system (CNS) by the causative organism is one of the rare complications, since *Brucella* exhibit a great affinity for the meninges, with an estimated incidence of 0.5 to 25 % of adults with systemic brucellosis and only 0.8 % in the pediatric population [8].

11.2 Neuroimaging Findings

In patients with altered mental status or focal neurologic deficits, brain computed tomography (CT) is warranted. Although the CT scan is generally normal, it may disclose evidence of subarachnoid hemorrhage, cerebral abscess formation, or leptomeningitis caused by *Brucella* spp. Magnetic resonance imaging (MRI) is the imaging modality of choice; it is more sensitive compared to CT with capability to demonstrate parenchymal brain lesions and leptomeningeal involvement. Administration of contrast material is necessary for the evaluation of leptomeningeal disease.

In cases with neurobrucellosis, nonspecific clinical and neuroradiological signs and symptoms may be confused with some neurologic diseases [5, 7]. Because of the rarity of this disease, even in endemic region, neurobrucellosis remains a challenging diagnostic problem. As a rule, a high index of suspicion is required for correct diagnosis in patients from endemic areas [4, 12]. Neuroimaging findings are variable, described on both CT and MRI [2, 11]. Radiologically, they are divided into several types: normal imaging, inflammation, white matter changes, and vascular lesions [5].

11.2.1 Normal Imaging

It is important to know that MRI or CT of the brain may be normal despite positive clinical findings, when brucellosis of CNS presents as acute meningoencephalitis.

11.2.2 Inflammation

Neurobrucellosis can be present as basal meningitis with involvement of several cranial nerves in about 50 % of cases. Meningoencephalitis can cause intracranial hypertension and in rare cases hydrocephalus. The imaging findings of uncomplicated meningitis are usually normal or may demonstrate enhancement of the meninges or nerve roots on postcontrast images. Abnormal enhancement is mostly seen in the suprasellar region, basal and dural meninges, and perivascular region. Sometimes, granulomatous formation results from inflammation. Predominantly, in all types of meningitis, contrast MRI is more sensitive compared to CT. The best sequences are contrast-enhanced T1-weighted and fluid-attenuated inversion recovery (FLAIR) images that show meningeal enhancement. The differential diagnosis includes other infectious etiology like tuberculosis, fungal infection, and sarcoidosis. In the early phase of parenchymal infection cerebritis, MRI shows abnormal T2 signal in the cortex and subcortical white matter. During the late stage of abscess formation, imaging demonstrates ring enhancing lesion with central necrosis and central restricted diffusion with surrounding vasogenic edema. Granuloma can present as a focal brain mass, cortical and/or subcortical in location with "target" appearance after contrast administration consistent of a central nodular enhancement with thin peripheral enhancing rim, surrounded by vasogenic edema; findings are similar to brain abscess [11]. Neurobrucellosis may present clinically and radiologically as a brain mass-mimicking tumor. CT and MRI reveal an irregular enhancing mass with surrounding vasogenic edema. In the literature, 14 cases of neurobrucellosis presented as abscess, where two of them were misdiagnosed as brain tumor [12]. The location of the abscess or granulomas is variable and in most cases, the final diagnosis was made by surgery and histopathology. An enzyme-linked immunosorbent assay is the test of choice to detect IgM antibodies in the serum and CSF.

11.2.3 White Matter Changes

White matter changes may be related to an autoimmune reaction; they are noted as hyperintense lesions on T2-weighted and FLAIR images. The white matter changes have different patterns on brain MRI as diffuse, periventricular, and peripheral affecting the subcortical U-fibers in the "arcuate" zone or focal demyelinating lesions; they may mimic a wide variety of conditions such as demyelinating disease like multiple sclerosis and acute disseminated encephalomyelitis and other infections: cytomegalovirus, human immunodeficiency virus, and human papillomavirus (Figs. 11.1 and 11.2) [6]. Nevertheless, involvement of the corpus callosum and enhancement of the lesions have not been described in neurobru-

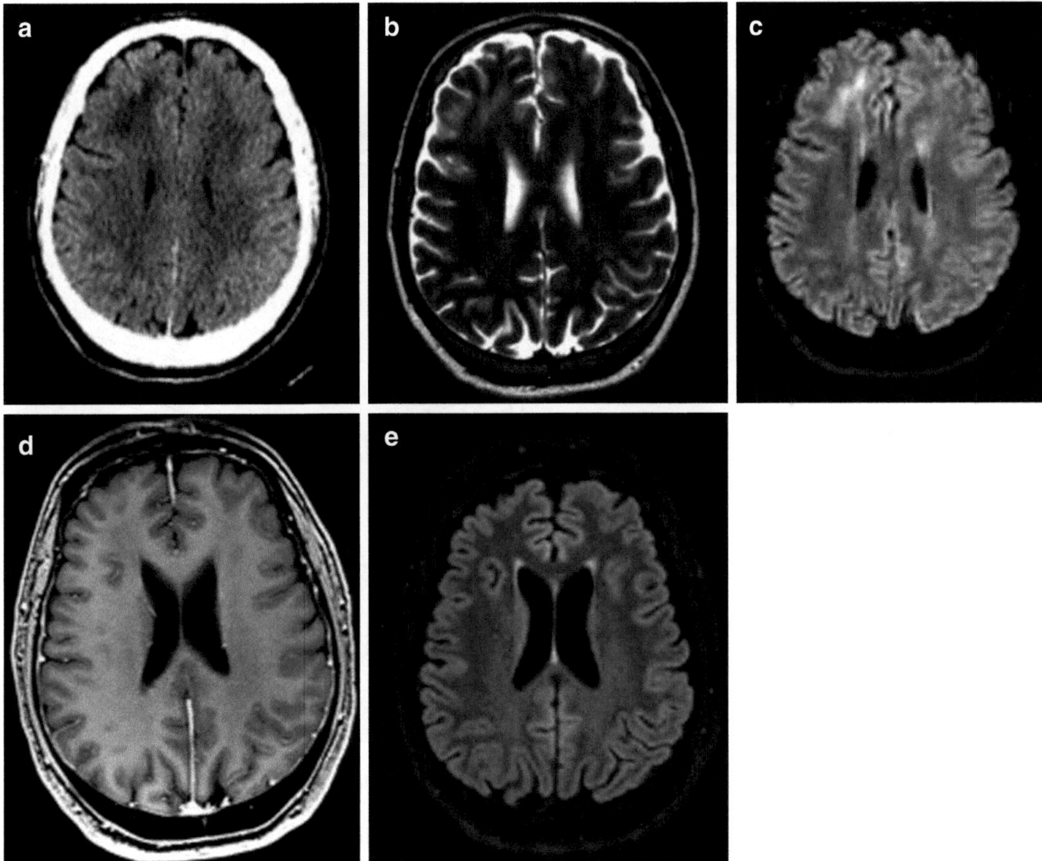

Fig. 11.1 A 37-year-old male presents with fever, expressive aphasia, and altered mental status. (**a**) CT brain shows subcortical white matter hypodensities involving the anterior frontal lobes. Brain MRI: (**b**) axial T2, (**c**) FLAIR, and (**d**) enhanced T1-weighted images demonstrate sheetlike area of high T2 signal in the subcortical white matter of the anterior frontal lobes. There is no evidence of abnormal parenchymal or meningeal enhancement following contrast administration (**d**). DSA was performed to rule out vasculitis and was normal (not shown here). (**e**) Follow-up MRI: axial FLAIR, 5 months after treatment, demonstrates complete resolution of the previous abnormal signal in the subcortical white matter

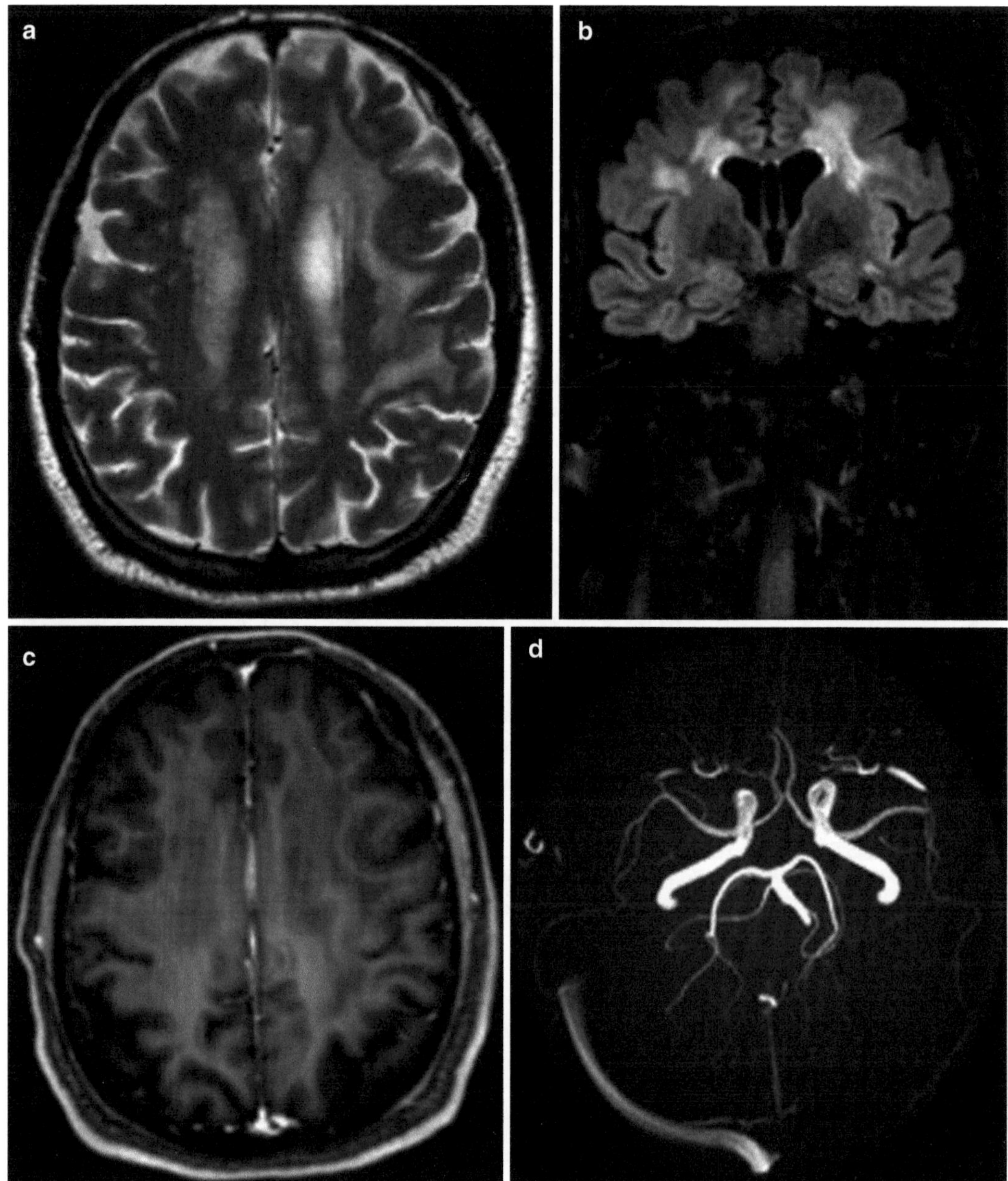

Fig. 11.2 A 55-year-old male previously healthy, presenting with right-sided acute transient numbness. Brain MRI: (**a**) axial T2 and (**b**) coronal FLAIR images of the brain show extensive abnormal high signal intensity lesions in the cerebral white matter predominately subcortical involving the U-fibers (*arrow*) (**a**) as well as the centrum semiovale. (**c**) Axial T1 after gadolinium administration: These lesions show no enhancement after contrast administration. (**d**) Brain MRA shows normal intracranial vessels with no evidence of significant obstructive pathology or aneurysmal formation

cellosis. Posterior fossa lesions have been described in few papers [3, 14, 15]. Radiographic white matter changes usually persist on follow-up imaging despite effective treatment, representing sequelae of demyelination [2].

11.2.4 Vascular Lesions

Vasculopathic change owing to brucellosis is a very rare entity. Although rare, it is well known that *Brucella* can cause vasculitis of the cerebral vasculature with no predilection to size or location of vessels. Brucellosis can also cause deep venous thrombosis probably through an immune mechanism causing pseudotumor cerebri-like symptoms [1].

Ischemic stroke and transient ischemic attacks may be observed in CNS brucellosis. The pathogenesis may be caused by cerebral vasospasm, infectious vasculitis, or embolism. There are two types of cerebrovascular involvement in brucellosis, the first being mycotic aneurysm that can rupture with secondary subarachnoid hemorrhage. The second mechanism is inflammation of the vessels causing arteritis with subsequent infarcts, hemorrhage, or venous thrombosis. The mycotic aneurysm is most likely secondary to embolus from *Brucella* endocarditis [9].

CT scan may demonstrate intraparenchymal hemorrhage and perivascular enhancement after contrast material administration. MRI is superior in showing acute lacunar infarcts. FLAIR- and T2-weighted images reveal multiple hyperintense foci in the white matter compatible with vasculitis. Diffusion-weighted imaging is useful in acute ischemia where it shows restricted diffusion in acute infarct. The lacunar infarcts are mainly seen in the distribution of perforating vessels in the basal ganglia, brainstem, and the white matter of the brain. On the other hand, magnetic resonance angiography and digital subtraction angiography (DSA) may be normal, but DSA is superior in resolution and can demonstrate stenosis, occlusion of intracranial vessels, or vascular wall irregularities.

In patients with venous thrombosis, CT shows venous infarct as cortical and subcortical hypodensity in a venous territory with or without hemorrhage. On MRI, venous infarct appears as subcortical high T2 signal with mild mass effect. The diffusion is heterogeneous, most of the time not reduced. In some cases, there is small hemorrhage or hematoma. As a rule, MRI and CT venography are reliable techniques to make the diagnosis of venous sinus thrombosis. In the acute phase, the thrombus appears hyperdense on non-enhanced CT scan. In the subacute and acute phases, CT with contrast shows the filling defect within the sinus. On MRI, in the acute phase, the thrombus is hypointense on T2 and isointense on T1 and may be missed. Magnetic resonance venography 2D phase contrast can demonstrate the filling defect and make the diagnosis; when the thrombus is subacute, it appears hyperintense on T1 and T2 and it is easy to identify [4, 6, 10].

Conclusion

Neuroimaging findings of neurobrucellosis are variable, not specific and indistinguishable from other infectious or inflammatory conditions. The combination of neuroimaging, microbiological diagnostic tools, and neurophysiology is crucial for the diagnosis of neurobrucellosis. Contrast-enhanced MRI is the modality of choice, able to demonstrate meningeal and parenchymal lesions and involvement of cranial nerves.

References

1. Adaletli I, Albayram S, Gurses B, Ozer H, Yilmaz MH, Gulsen F, Sirikci A (2006) Vasculopathic changes in the cerebral arterial system with neurobrucellosis. AJNR Am J Neuroradiol 27:384–386
2. Al-Sous MW, Bohlega S, Al-Kawi MZ, Alwatban J, McLean DR (2004) Neurobrucellosis: clinical and neuroimaging correlation. AJNR Am J Neuroradiol 25:395–401
3. Alvis Miranda H, Castellar Leones SM, Elzain MA, Moscote Salazar LR (2013) Brain abscess: current management. J Neurosci Rural Pract 4:S67–S81
4. Budnik I, Fuchs I, Shelef I, Krymko H, Greenberg D (2012) Unusual presentations of pediatric neurobrucellosis. Am J Trop Med Hyg 86:258–260
5. Ceran N, Turkoglu R, Erdem I, Inan A, Engin D, Tireli H, Goktas P (2011) Neurobrucellosis: clinical, diagnostic, therapeutic features and outcome. Unusual clinical presentations in an endemic region. Braz J Infect Dis 15:52–59
6. Erdem G, Güngör S, Alkan A, Tabel Y (2014) Magnetic resonance imaging findings of pediatric neurobrucellosis. Med-Science 3:1732–1742
7. Feigin VL, Saadah M (2013) Abstracts of 3rd International Congress on Neurology and Epidemiology. Abu Dhabi, UAE, November 21–23, 2013. Neuroepidemiology 41:223–316
8. Habeeb YKR, Al-Najdi AKN, Sadek SAH, Al-Onaizi E (1998) Paediatric neurobrucellosis: case report and literature review. J Infect 37:59–62
9. Jabbour R, Khalifeh R, Al Kutoubi A, Atweh S (2003) Dissecting aneurysm of the basilar trunk in a young man. Arch Neurol 60:1016–1018
10. Kizilkilic O, Calli C (2011) Neurobrucellosis. Neuroimaging Clin N Am 21:927–937

11. Koussa S, Chemaly R (2003) Neurobrucellosis presenting with diffuse cerebral white matter lesions. Eur Neurol 50:121–123
12. Martınez-Chamorro E, Muñoz A, Esparza J, Muñoz MJ, Giangaspro E (2002) Focal cerebral involvement by neurobrucellosis: pathological and MRI findings. Eur J Radiol 43:28–30
13. Shakir RA, Al-Din ASN, Araj GF, Lulu AR, Mousa AR, Saadah MA (1987) Clinical categories of neurobrucellosis. Brain 110:213–223
14. Sharma BS, Khosla VK, Kak VK, Gupta VK, Tewari MK, Mathuriya SN, Pathak A (1995) Multiple pyogenic brain abscess. Acta Neurochir 133:36–43
15. Solaroglu I, Kaptanoglu E, Okutan O, Beskonakli E (2003) Solitary extra-axial posterior fossa abscess due to neurobrucellosis. J ClinNeurosci 10:710–712
16. World Organisation for Animal Health. Handistatus II: zoonoses (human cases): global cases of brucellosis in 2004. http://www.oie.int/hs2/gi_zoon_mald.asp?c_cont=6&c_mald=172&annee=2004
17. Yetkin MA, Bulut C, Erdinc FS, Oral B, Tulek N (2006) Evaluation of the clinical presentations in neurobrucellosis. Int J Infect Dis 10:446–452

Part III

Spinal Brucellosis

Brucellar Spondylitis as a Complication of Brucellosis

12

Mitra Ranjbar, Ahmet Tuncay Turgut, Marzieh Nojomi, and Mehmet Turgut

Contents

M. Ranjbar, MD (✉)
Department of Infectious Diseases,
Iran University of Medical Sciences, Tehran, Iran
e-mail: mitraranjbar@yahoo.com

A.T. Turgut, MD
Department of Radiology,
Hacettepe University School of Medicine,
Ankara, Turkey
e-mail: ahmettuncayturgut@yahoo.com

M. Nojomi, MD, MPH
Department of Community Medicine,
Iran University of Medical Sciences, Tehran, Iran
e-mail: mnojomi@gmail.com

M. Turgut, MD, PhD
Department of Neurosurgery,
Adnan Menderes University School of Medicine,
Aydın, Turkey
e-mail: drmturgut@yahoo.com

Abstract

Brucellosis, being a systemic disease, may affect many organ systems. The involvement of the musculoskeletal involvement is associated with 10–85 % of the focal complications. Spinal involvement is one of the most commonly encountered localized forms of human brucellosis. It is a destructive disease process requiring a correct and early diagnosis and an immediate treatment. Spinal brucellosis is more prevalent in older patients or in subjects with prolonged illness prior to treatment. The lumbar vertebrae are involved more frequently than the thoracic and cervical ones. Paravertebral, epidural, and psoas abscess can occur in the setting of brucellar spondylitis. Medical treatment for brucellar spondylitis should consist of two antibiotic agents for at least 12 weeks.

Keywords

Brucella • Brucellosis • Spondylitis

Abbreviations

CRP	C-reactive protein
CT	Computed tomography
ELISA	Immunocapture enzyme-linked immunosorbent assay

M. Turgut et al. (eds.), *Neurobrucellosis: Clinical, Diagnostic and Therapeutic Features*,
DOI 10.1007/978-3-319-24639-0_12

ESR	Erythrocyte sedimentation rate
HNP	Herniated nucleus pulposus
MRI	Magnetic resonance imaging
PET	Positron emission tomography
SUVmax	Maximum standardized uptake value
TMP/SMX	Trimethoprim/sulfamethoxazole

12.1 Introduction

Osteoarticular involvement is known to be the most commonly encountered complication of brucellosis (10–85 %). Anatomically, spinal brucellosis implies the involvement of the vertebral column, interspinal spaces, and/or paraspinal regions. Brucellar spondylitis was first described by Kulowski and Vinke in 1932, and it is one of the most serious complications of brucellosis [30, 33].

Spondylodiscitis is a serious complication because it may be associated with abscess formation [17]. Treatment of patients with brucellar spondylodiscitis is still problematic, because the most appropriate regimen and duration of treatment are not known. This complication may also require surgical intervention and may result in various functional sequelae [10, 17, 21].

Clinical diagnosis may be challenging owing to the fact that the associated symptoms and signs are variable and nonspecific. Therefore, it should be considered in the differential diagnosis of the patients presenting with back pain and spinal neurological disorders.

12.2 Incidence

The reported incidence of spinal brucellosis is quite variable (2–54 %), depending on the study population [9, 23, 32]. Spinal involvement was found in only 130 of 6300 (2 %) brucellosis patients from Malta [15]. According to Tekkök et al. [33], on the other hand, the incidence was 6 % in the report of Ariza et al. which included 331 patients, whereas 30 % of the patients with brucellosis was reported to have spinal involvement by Lifesso et al. Brucella causes vertebral osteomyelitis in endemic area. In a study on a total of 100 patients with vertebral osteomyelitis, 44 had pyogenic, 24 had brucellar, and 32 had tuberculous spondylodiscitis [22]. In a study in Turkey of 307 patients with brucellosis, 46 (15 %) were accompanied by spondylitis [37]. In another study in Turkey, 86 patients with brucellosis were diagnosed and mean age was 44.2 ± 17.7 years (range 16–79), and 33 (38 %) of the patients were female [5]. In this series, spondylitis was diagnosed in 26 (30 %) of the patients [5].

In another study, a total of 135 brucellosis spondylodiscitis were detected in 31 (23 %) patients [20]. In these series, the mean age of patients was 54 years (age range 24–74 years), with 52 % of males [20].

In a study in the west of Iran of 245 patients with brucellosis diagnosed between January 2004 and December 2005, sacroiliitis was the most common complication (75.7 %), followed by spondylitis (21.4 %) [16]. Spondylitis was the most common form of osteoarticular involvement encountered in the elderly (>60 years) and the second most common in other age groups [16].

In another study in Spain of 593 patients with brucellosis, of whom 58 (9.7 %) had spondylitis [8], the mean overall age of the patients with spondylitis was 48 ± 13 years [8]. In another study of 55 cases of spondylitis aged ranging between 25 and 79, 33 (59 %) were female [26]. The cases with tuberculous spondylodiscitis, pyogenic spondylodiscitis, and brucellar spondylodiscitis were found in 24 (%43), in 19 (34 %), and 12 (21 %) patients [26]. The 49 (88 %) patients had dorsalgia, whereas fever was present in only 16 (29 %) patients [26]. Increased erythrocyte sedimentation rate (ESR), increased C-reactive protein (CRP), and leukocytosis were present in 51 (91 %), 22 (39 %), and 8 (14 %) cases, respectively [26]. The number of the cases with history of previous surgery or trauma was 14 (25 %) [26].

In another study, the total number of reported spinal brucellosis cases from a total of 34 secondary or tertiary referral centers in Turkey published during the last century was reported to be 452 [35]. The clinical and radiological findings associated with spinal involvement of brucellosis were usually atypical leading to a diagnostic difficulty for this infectious disease because of its nonspecific nature and variability of the clinical presentation [35]. Therefore, it may easily result in misdiagnosis of herniated nucleus pulposus (HNP) or other spinal infections, and a high index of suspicion is required to diagnose this condition in endemic parts of the world [35]. In addition to serological tests, computed tomography (CT) and/or magnetic resonance imaging (MRI) techniques were found to be very helpful for the diagnosis and the follow-up, thanks to their capability for providing early detection of the lesions in the spine and more accurate localization of intraspinal and paraspinal infestation by means of multiplanar imaging [35].

12.3 Clinical Features

The initial clinical presentation in spinal brucellosis may be nonspecific due to the insidious nature of the disease. The most commonly encountered complaints are fever, malaise, sweating, back pain, and anorexia [14, 17]. The fever may be more prominent in its acute form, whereas constitutional symptoms such as myalgia, malaise, and anorexia are common findings in both subacute and chronic forms [8]. Nevertheless, localized symptoms like weakness in the lower extremities involving one or both legs, called monoparesis or paraparesis, paraesthesia, and reflex changes may be seen secondary to spinal cord or nerve root compression. Furthermore, neurobrucellosis with the clinical manifestations of meningitis or meningoencephalitis may develop as a complication of spinal brucellosis [4, 14]. On the other hand, physical examination reveals various findings compatible with brucellosis including hepatomegaly, splenomegaly which may be concomitant with back pain, a positive Lasegue test, and rarely signs of cauda equina syndrome or spinal cord syndrome composed of sensory and motor loss, areflexia/hyporeflexia, and loss of bladder function [13].

Brucellar spondylitis is frequently localized and affects continuous segments of the vertebral column. A case of simultaneous involvement of the cervical, thoracic, and lumbar spine in a patient with brucellar spondylodiscitis was described [12]. A 64-year-old male presented to the emergency department with a 2-month history of headaches, mainly localized in the occipital area, neck pain, and low back pain [12]. These were associated with fatigue and night sweats during the same interval but he denied having any fever [12]. He also reported falling twice at home with no apparent cause but because his legs suddenly felt "very weak" and he needed assistance to get up [12]. Spinal MRI disclosed abnormalities compatible with spondylodiscitis in the cervical, thoracic, and lumbar areas [12].

Spinal brucellosis usually starts from the vertebral body and then spreads to the intervertebral disk space. It is important to note that brucellar discitis without spondylitis is extremely rare. Recently, a 50-year-old man with brucellar discitis without spondylitis which resulted in HNP was reported [37]. Likewise, Turgut et al. [34] reported a case which presented with radicular pain and restricted mobility of spine due to localized muscle spasm, and patient had a complete recovery with antibrucellosis treatment.

Spondylodiscitis is a serious complication because it may be associated with abscess formation. In a study, abscesses occurred in about 60 % patients and were associated with low hemoglobin levels [20]. The duration of treatment was longer if an abscess was present [20]. Two female patients with abscesses required surgical intervention [20]. Both patients presented with fever, neurologic deficit, and high *Brucella* standard tube agglutination test titers [20].

Sponylodiscitis was complicated with epidural, paravertebral, prevertebral and psoas abscesses, or radiculitis. Brucellar sponylodiscitis should be considered particularly in elderly patients with back pain and debility in endemic areas. Radiologically, MRI is recommended in suspected cases for early diagnosis and for deciding the duration of treatment. Attention should be drawn to this disease given the need for prolonged duration of treatment particularly in complicated cases in order to avoid possible sequelae.

12.4 Diagnosis

Diagnosis of brucellosis requires the assessment of medical history, clinical evaluation, and routine laboratory and radiologic tests combined with culture, serology, or polymerase chain reaction assay. The routine laboratory tests are complete blood count, ESR, CRP, and liver function tests, although they are not specific for the diagnosis, and wide patient variability is known to exist. Median value of ESR was found to be 44.7 and significantly higher in patients with brucellar spondylodiscitis [1]. This finding may be helpful for diagnosis of brucellar spondylodiscitis together with other clinical and laboratory parameters; however, the absence of elevated ESR does not exclude the diagnosis. ESR was normal in 10 % of patients. Anemia was the most common hematological abnormality among patients with brucellosis and found to be significantly higher in the patients with brucellar spondylodiscitis related to older age and the nature of chronic disease [1]. Blood and bone marrow are the most suitable specimens used in the isolation of *Brucella*. In patients receiving antibiotics, as well as patients with a chronic form of brucellosis, bone marrow culture appears more sensitive. In addition, automated culture systems have improved the speed of brucella isolation, usually within 3 days. Numerous serologic methods are used in the diagnosis of brucellosis.

Although serum agglutination test is usually recognized as the reference technique, it is labor intensive and time consuming. The Coombs' antiglobulin test is used to detect nonagglutinating antibodies against *Brucella* cells. Serial dilutions up to high titers may be necessary to get beyond prozones with this process. Immunocapture enzyme-linked immunosorbent assay (ELISA, Brucellacapt) adds patient serum to a microwell, which is coated with antibodies against human IgM, IgG, and IgA. Stained killed *Brucella* cells are added, and agglutination is observed. This method is comparable to the Coombs' test. Likewise, ELISA may be comparable to conventional serologic tests in the diagnosis of the disease. Nevertheless, the center for disease control and prevention has warned that false-positive ELISA tests for brucellosis require that positive results should be confirmed by standard agglutination tests.

Negative serology does not exclude the diagnosis in brucellosis, and using more than one test is recommended in probable cases. In addition, *Brucella* antibodies can persist long after the patient's recovery, and thus it is not always possible to distinguish patients with active disease from those with past infection. In these cases, the IgG avidity test may be valuable, since high IgG avidity would suggest immune memory, not a new-onset disease. On the other hand, patients with titers lower than the diagnostic threshold and low avidity would suggest primary infection. Diagnosis of brucellosis was confirmed by blood culture and/or the presence of specific antibodies by tube agglutination (1:160 or higher) [17].

12.5 Radiologic Findings

Various findings which are consistent with vertebral osteomyelitis can be seen on MRI; namely, decreased signal intensity on T1-weighted image and increased signal intensity on T2-weighted image of the vertebral body, hyperintense signal on T2-weighted image of the disk, end plate degeneration, involvement of the epidural soft tissue, abscess formation, and contrast enhancement in the vertebral surfaces facing disk space, disk, and soft tissue following the administration of intravenous gadolinium diethylene triamine pentaacetic acid (Figs. 12.1, 12.2, 12.3, and 12.4) [35, 38]. A case of a patient with brucellar spondylodiscitis, affecting simultaneously the cervical, thoracic, and lumbar spine, had responded well to conservative management [12].

Bone scan is very sensitive in the early stage despite being nonspecific and also fails to demonstrate the extent of the lesion appropriately [6, 27]. At present, it is demonstrated that positron emission tomography (PET)-CT scan may provide useful information in the management of brucellar spondylodiscitis. In a recent review, the clinical impact of this technique in diagnosing spinal infections, with sensitivities ranging from 94 to 100 % and specificities ranging from 87 to 100 %, was emphasized [36]. In addition, PET-CT

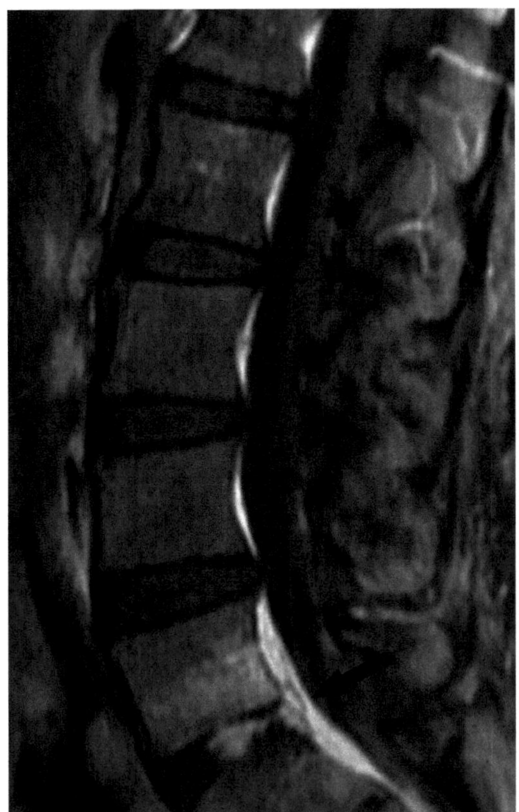

Fig. 12.1 Sagittal T1-weighted MRI shows posterior longitudinal ligament elevation (*arrow*) and marked enhancement of disk and vertebral end plate after gadolinium administration

was reported in a recent retrospective study to have a significant role in the clinical management of 52 % of patients with infectious spondylitis. However, the utility of PET-CT in monitoring the efficacy of treatment was less clear because only one patient had a negative PET-CT, whereas four patients had a negative MRI of the affected spine at the end of treatment [18]. Importantly, a significant decrease was detected in maximum standardized uptake value (SUVmax) by means of a successful treatment, whereas patients without any residual MRI findings had significantly lower SUVmax compared to those having residual MRI findings. Virtually negative indices of inflammation were detected in all patients after a successful treatment, as expected. In general, MRI should be the preferred imaging modality for the diagnosis of brucellar spondylodiscitis owing to its high sensitivity and specificity. Nevertheless, it should be kept in mind that it has several inherent technical limitations such as sensitivity to motion degradation implying that the patients with movement disorders may not be suitable candidates for the examination. Additionally, certain metallic implants are accepted to be a contraindication for this modality. Also, MRI cannot always help distinguish spondylitis from severe degenerative arthritis. Another challenge is that usually MRI scans only of the spinal region with the suspected target lesion are requested by the referring physicians. However, in a recently published series of patients with brucellar spondylodiscitis, a rate of 9 % of noncontiguous multifocal spinal involvement was detected which can be missed if only one spinal region is assessed. Therefore, in every case of suspected brucellar spondylitis, the entire spine should be evaluated with MRI, though this may be logistically challenging in the routine clinical practice [18].

12.6 Comparison of Tuberculous and Brucellar Spondylodiscitis

In a study with the purpose of comparison, the clinical, radiological, and prognostic features of spontaneous spondylodiscitis secondary to tuberculosis and brucellosis, some useful information was obtained [7]. According to the results of this study, the most important differential diagnosis is tuberculosis, in addition to the usual causes of vertebral osteomyelitis or septic arthritis [7]. This may have a significant impact on the therapeutic approach as well as the prognosis, given that several antimicrobial agents used to treat brucellosis are also used to treat tuberculosis. Septic arthritis in brucellosis starting with small pericapsular erosions progresses slowly. Anatomically, anterior erosions of the superior end plate in the vertebrae are typically the first features to become evident, with eventual involvement and sclerosis of the whole vertebra. Anterior osteophytes eventually develop, though vertebral destruction or impingement on the spinal cord is rare and usually suggestive of tuberculosis.

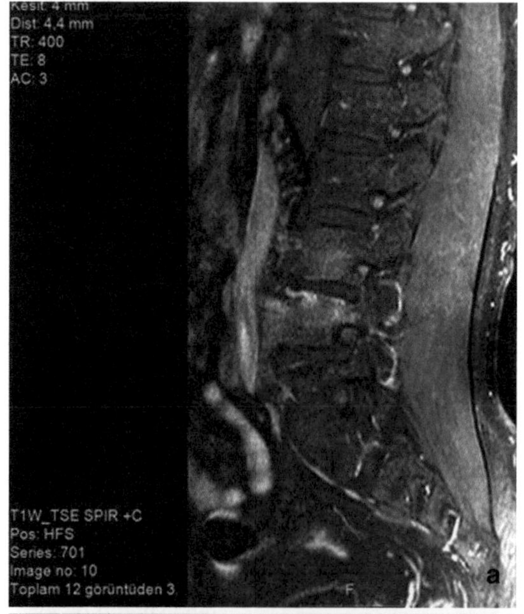

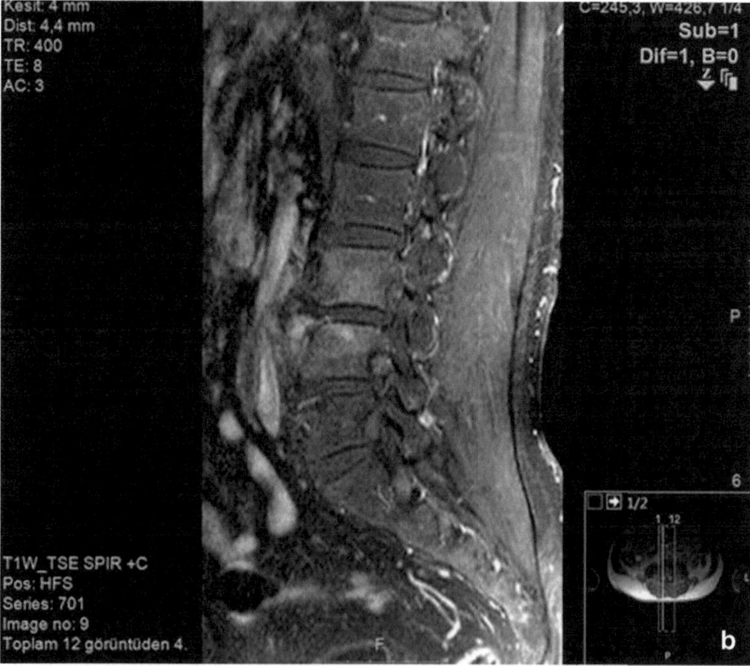

Fig. 12.2 (**a**, **b**) Sagittal T1-weighted MRI shows enhancement at the anterior surfaces of L3 and L4 vertebrae extending through the adjacent L3-4 disk space after gadolinium administration (Courtesy of O. Tuncyurek, M.D.)

12.7 Treatment of Spinal Brucellosis

Treatment for brucellar spondylitis should consist of two antibiotic agents for at least 12 weeks [2, 29]. Patients with brucellar spondylitis appear to respond better to doxycycline (100 mg orally twice daily for 12 weeks) plus streptomycin (1 g intramuscularly once daily for the first 14–21 days) than to doxycycline-rifampin [2]. Alternative choices include doxycycline (100 mg orally twice daily) plus rifampin (600–900 mg (15 mg/kg) once daily) for at least 12 weeks or ciprofloxacin (500 mg twice daily) plus rifampin for at least 12 weeks [2, 3, 29].

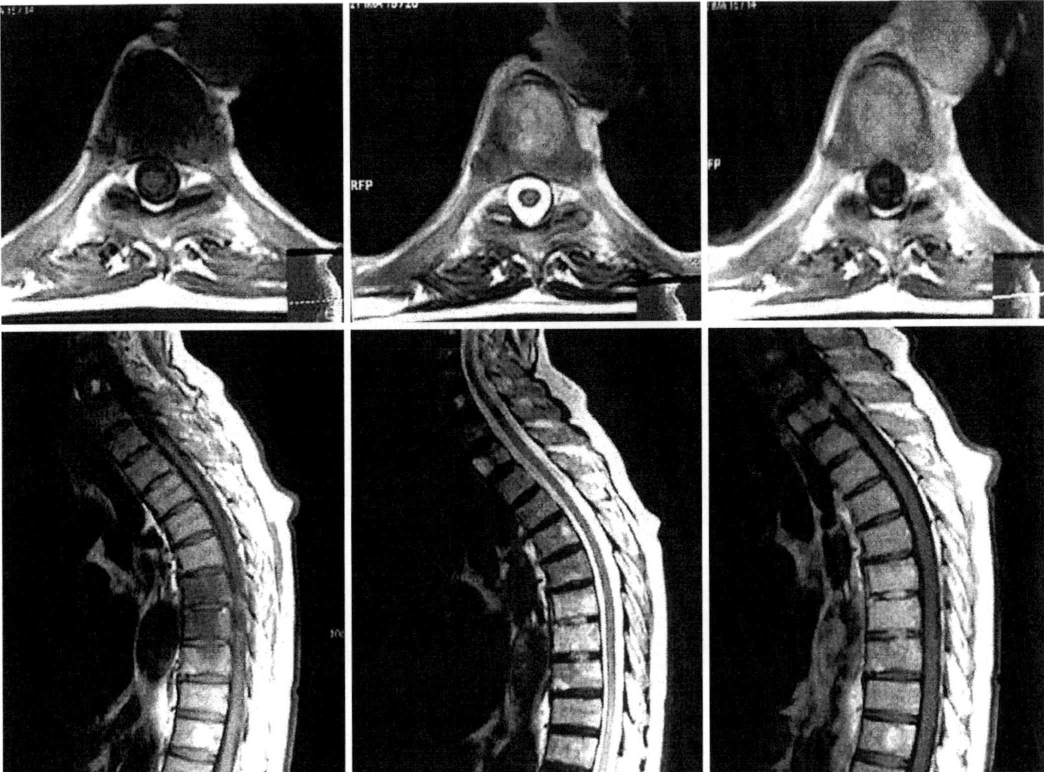

Fig. 12.3 MRI of a 77-year-old man with brucellar discitis and spondylitis, misdiagnosed as spinal metastasis with unknown origin. Axial and sagittal T1-and T2-weighted images demonstrate a contrast-enhanced infectious lesion involving the intervertebral spaces of T6-T7 and T7-T8, in addition to the vertebral bodies of T6 and T7 (From Turgut et al. [35], with permission)

The duration of therapy is at least as important as the choice of antimicrobial agents [25]. In one meta-analysis, the failure rate for patients treated less than 6 weeks was 43 %; the failure rate for patients treated more than 12 weeks was 17 % [25].

In a study in Greece, the standard treatment of brucellar spondylitis with a combination of two antibiotics for 6–12 weeks is associated with high rates of treatment failure and relapse [19]. A total of 18 patients with brucellar spondylitis were treated with a combination of at least three suitable antibiotics: doxycycline, rifampin, plus intramuscular streptomycin or trimethoprim/sulfamethoxazole (TMP/SMX, co-trimoxazole) or ciprofloxacin until the completion of at least 6 months of treatment [19]. If required, the treatment was continued with additional 6-month cycles, until resolution or significant improvement of clinical and radiological findings, or for a maximum of 18 months [19]. During the follow-up period with a mean of 36.5 months ranging from 1 to 96 months, no relapses were observed [19].

As a final management option, diagnostic or curative surgery can be performed in spinal brucellosis. Surgical intervention should be preferred when spinal instability, cord compression, radiculopathy, cauda equine syndrome, and severe weakness of the muscles due to extradural inflammatory mass or progressive collapse are present [11, 24, 31, 33].

Alternatively, percutaneous drainage or aspiration of epidural and paravertebral abscesses can be performed rather than surgery [33]. Nevertheless, abscess drainage is not always mandatory in the absence of neurological deterioration, and medical management can provide

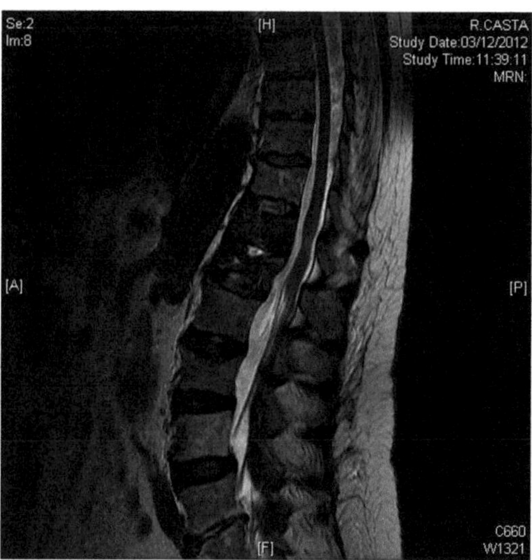

Fig. 12.4 MRI of a 69-year-old woman with brucellar spondylodiscitis. Midsagittal T2-weighted image reveals high signal intensity at T12 and L1 levels and medullar compression by the T12 pedicle (Courtesy of A. Cervan, M.D.)

cure as well. Furthermore, analgesics and immobilization with orthosis as supportive management tools can bc helpful to reduce the pain associated with spinal brucellosis [1, 27].

In spinal brucellosis, delayed convalescence after treatment is a well-known clinical sequela. Although the exact mechanism for this condition is not clearly understood, psychoneurosis exacerbated by the infection has been proposed as a causative factor for the delay. Clinically, this sequela is considered when pain, abnormal physical findings, or functional limitation persist for longer than 6 months in the posttreatment period. The severity of this clinical sequela may be mild, moderate, and severe depending on the patient's functional condition. Accordingly, the sequela is accepted as mild if no neurological deficits remain, but the patient suffers from pain during exercise which does not interfere with work. The sequela is considered as moderate if pain interferes with work or milder motor or sensorial deficits remain, whereas permanent and excruciating pain requiring rest and analgesics or remaining motor or sensorial deficits imply severe form of sequela. Anti-inflammatory drugs can be helpful for the treatment of mild clinical sequela, whereas the presence of moderate or severe sequelae may necessitate surgery [24, 31].

The early diagnosis, the administration of appropriate antimicrobial treatment, and the control of animal infection in endemic regions is crucial for the prevention of spinal brucellosis. Bone and joint involvement and epididymo-orchitis are considered the most frequently encountered complications of brucellosis [28]. Relapse of brucellosis is frequently detected owing to the fact that it is an intracellular organism.

Apparently, the diagnosis requires a high degree of clinical suspicion and thorough occupational and travel history. Nevertheless, a definitive diagnosis of the disease requires isolation of *Brucellae* spp. from blood cultures and bone marrow samples and demonstration of antigens and antibodies to *Brucella* by serological tests.

Importantly, brucellosis can be prevented mainly by increasing public awareness to safe livestock practices and mass vaccination of animals. Classically, the treatment recommended by the World Health Organization for acute brucellosis in adults is rifampicin 600–900 mg and doxycycline 100 mg twice daily for a minimum of 6 weeks [28]. Combined use of intramuscular streptomycin (1 g daily for 2–3 weeks) and an oral tetracycline (2 g daily for 6 weeks) results in fewer relapses [28]. Tetracycline monotherapy for a duration of 6 weeks may be considered as a good treatment option for patients with brucellosis with no focal disease, and a low risk of patients with focal disease, such as endocarditis or spondylitis, may require administration of extended courses of antibiotics [28]. Surgery should be preferred for patients with endocarditis and cerebral or hepatosplenic abscess that are antibiotic resistant [28].

Conclusion

Spinal involvement is still an important complication of brucellosis particularly in endemic areas of the world. The development of sequelae can usually be prevented by early diagnosis. Diagnostic tools with superior sensitivity such as CT or MRI should be used for early diagnosis as well as and for the evaluation of the treatment efficacy. Patients with brucellosis should be carefully evaluated for the localized form and spinal brucellosis in developing countries having limited resources. A combination of doxycycline (200 mg/day, for at least 12 weeks) with streptomycin (1 g/day, for 2 or 3 weeks) should still be the initial antimicrobial regimen in patients with spinal brucellosis. Alternatively, doxycycline plus rifampin or TMP/SMX plus rifampin or ciprofloxacin plus rifampin or ciprofloxacin plus streptomycin can be considered as in the presence of adverse reactions or contraindications (ototoxicity, nephrotoxicity, pregnancy, lactation, etc.). Antimicrobial therapy with optimal duration and surgical intervention when required can be helpful for preventing relapses and reducing the rate of occurrence of sequelae.

References

1. Abdi-Liae Z, Soudbakhsh A, Jafari S, Emadı H, Tomaj K (2007) Haematological manifestations of brucellosis. Acta Med Iran 45:145–148
2. Alp E, Doganay M (2008) Current therapeutic strategy in spinal brucellosis. Int J Infect Dis 12:573–577
3. Alp E, Koc RK, Durak AC, Yildiz O, Aygen B, Sumerkan B, Doganay M (2006) Doxycycline plus streptomycin versus ciprofloxacin plus rifampicin in spinal brucellosis. BMC Infect Dis 6:72
4. Aygen B, Doganay M, Sümerkan B, Yildiz O, Kayabas Ü (2002) Clinical manifestations, complications and treatment of brucellosis: a retrospective evaluation of 480 patients. Med Mal Infect 32:485–493
5. Bodur H, Erbay A, Colpan A, Akinci E (2004) Brucellar spondylitis. Rheumatol Int 24:221–226
6. Bruschwein DA, Brown ML, McLeod RA (1980) Gallium scintigraphy in the evaluation of disc-space infections: concise communication. J Nucl Med 21:925–927
7. Celik AK, Aypak A, Aypak C (2011) Comparative analysis of tuberculous and brucellar spondylodiscitis. Trop Doct 41:172–174
8. Colmenero JD, Cisneros JM, Orjuela DL, Pachón J, Garcia-Portales R, Rodriguez-Sampedro F, Juarez C (1992) Clinical course and prognosis of Brucella spondylitis. Infection 20:38–42
9. Colmenero JD, Reguera JM, Fernández-Nebro A, Cabrera-Franquelo F (1991) Osteoarticular complications of brucellosis. Ann Rheum Dis 50:23–26
10. Colmenero JD, Ruiz-Mesa JD, Plata A, Bermúdez P, Martín-Rico P, Queipo-Ortuño MI, Reguera JM (2008) Clinical findings, therapeutic approach, and outcome of brucellar vertebral osteomyelitis. Clin Infect Dis 46:426–433
11. Colmenero JD, Reguera JM, Martos F, Sánchez-De-Mora D, Delgado M, Causse M, Martín-Farfán A, Juárez C (1996) Complications associated with Brucella melitensis infection: a study of 530 cases. Medicine (Baltimore) 75:195–211
12. Charalambides C, Papademetriou K, Sgouros S, Sakas D (2010) Brucellosis of the spine affecting multiple non-contiguous levels. Br J Neurosurg 24:589–591
13. Daglioglu E, Bayazit N, Okay O, Dalgic A, Hatipoglu HG, Ergungor F (2009) Lumbar epidural abscess caused by brucella species: report of two cases. Neurocirugia (Astur) 20:159–162
14. Doganay M, Aygen B (2003) Human brucellosis: an overview. Int J Infect Dis 7:173–182
15. Ganado W, Craig AJ (1958) Brucellosis myopathy. J Bone Joint Surg Am 40:1380–1387
16. Hashemi SH, Keramat F, Ranjbar M, Mamani M, Farzam A, Jamal-Omidi S (2007) Osteoarticular complications of brucellosis in Hamedan, an endemic area in the west of Iran. Int J Infect Dis 11:496–500
17. Gul HC, Erdem H (2015) Brucella species. In: Mandell douglas, and Bennett's principles and practice of infectious diseases, 8th edn. Elsevier Inc, Philadelphia
18. Ioannou S, Chatziioannou S, Pneumaticos SG, Zormpala A, Sipsas NV (2013) Fluorine-18 fluoro -2-deoxy-D-glucose positron emission tomography/computed tomography scan contributes to the diagnosis and management of brucellar spondylodiscitis. BMC Infect Dis 13:73
19. Ioannou S, Karadima D, Pneumaticos S, Athanasiou H, Pontikis J, Zormpala A, Sipsas NV (2011) Efficacy of prolonged antimicrobial chemotherapy for brucellar spondylodiscitis. Clin Microbiol Infect 17:756–762
20. Kaptan F, Gulduren HM, Sarsilmaz A, Sucu HK, Ural S, Vardar I, Coskun NA (2013) Brucellar spondylodiscitis: comparison of patients with and without abscesses. Rheumatol Int 33:985–992
21. Luzzati R, Giacomazzi D, Danzi MC, Tacconi L, Concia E, Vento S (2009) Diagnosis, management and outcome of clinically-suspected spinal infection. J Infect 58:259–265
22. Mete B, Kurt C, Yilmaz MH, Ertan G, Ozaras R, Mert A, Tabak F, Ozturk R (2012) Vertebral osteomyelitis: eight years' experience of 100 cases. Rheumatol Int 32:3591–3597
23. Mousa A, Muhtaseb SA, Almudallal DS, Khodeir SM, Marafie AA (1987) Osteoarticular complications of brucellosis: a study of 169 cases. Rev Infect Dis 9:531–543
24. Nas K, Gür A, Kemaloğlu MS, Geyik MF, Cevik R, Büke Y, Ceviz A, Saraç AJ, Aksu Y (2001) Management of spinal brucellosis and outcome of rehabilitation. Spinal Cord 39:223–227
25. Pappas G, Seitaridis S, Akritidis N, Tsianos E (2004) Treatment of brucella spondylitis: lessons from an impossible meta-analysis and initial report of efficacy of a fluoroquinolone-containing regimen. Int J Antimicrob Agents 24:502–507

26. Pehlivanoglu F, Cicek G, Sengoz G (2012) The evaluation of the clinical, laboratory and the radiological findings of the fifty-five cases diagnosed with tuberculous, brucellar and pyogenic spondylodiscitis. J Neurosci Rural Pract 3:17–20
27. Pourbagher A, Pourbagher MA, Savas L, Turunc T, Demiroglu YZ, Erol I, Yalcintas D (2006) Epidemiologic, clinical, and imaging findings in brucellosis patients with osteoarticular involvement. AJR Am J Roentgenol 187:873–880
28. Rahil AI, Othman M, Ibrahim W, Mohamed MY (2014) Brucellosis in Qatar: a retrospective cohort study. Qatar Med J 2014:25–30
29. Smailnejad Gangi SM, Hasanjani Roushan MR, Janmohammadi N, Mehraeen R, Soleimani Amiri MJ, Khalilian E (2012) Outcomes of treatment in 50 cases with spinal brucellosis in Babol, Northern Iran. J Infect Dev Ctries 6:654–659
30. Solera J, Lozano E, Martínez-Alfaro E, Espinosa A, Castillejos ML, Abad L (1999) Brucellar spondylitis: review of 35 cases and literature survey. Clin Infect Dis 29:1440–1449
31. Solera J, Martínez-Alfaro E, Espinosa A (1997) Recognition and optimum treatment of brucellosis. Drugs 53:245–256
32. Tasova Y, Saltoĝlu N, Sahin G, Aksu HS (1999) Osteoarticular involvement of brucellosis in Turkey. Clin Rheumatol 18:214–219
33. Tekkök IH, Berker M, Ozcan OE, Ozgen T, Akalin E (1993) Brucellosis of the spine. Neurosurgery 33:838–844
34. Turgut M, Sendur OF, Gurel M (2003) Brucellar spondylodiscitis in the lumbar region-case report. Neurol Med Chir (Tokyo) 43:210–212
35. Turgut M, Turgut AT, Koşar U (2006) Spinal brucellosis: Turkish experience based on 452 cases published during the last century. Acta Neurochir (Wien) 148:1033–1044
36. Van der Bruggen W, Bleeker-Rovers CP, Boerman OC, Gotthardt M, Oyen WJ (2010) PET and SPECT in osteomyelitis and prosthetic bone and joint infections: a systematic review. Semin Nucl Med 40:3–15
37. Yilmaz C, Akar A, Civelek E, Köksay B, Kabatas S, Cansever T, Caner H (2010) Brucellar discitis as a cause of lumbar disc herniation: a case report. Neurol Neurochir Polska 44:516–519
38. Yilmaz E, Parlak M, Akalin H, Heper Y, Ozakin C, Mistik R, Oral B, Helvaci S, Töre O (2004) Brucellar spondylitis. Review of 25 cases. J Clin Rheumatol 10:300–307

13 Clinical Presentation of Vertebral Brucellosis

Oreste de Divitiis, Michelangelo de Angelis, and Andrea Elefante

Contents

O. de Divitiis, MD (✉) • M. de Angelis, MD
Department of Neurosciences, Reproduction and Odontostomatological Sciences, School of Medicine and Surgery, University of Naples Federico II, Naples, Italy
e-mail: oreste.dedivitiis@unina.it

A. Elefante, MD
Department of Advanced Biomedical Sciences, School of Medicine and Surgery, University of Naples Federico II, Naples, Italy
e-mail: andrea.elefante@unina.it

Abstract

In this chapter, the vertebral involvement of brucellosis will be discussed. Within the bone infection of brucellosis, spinal localization is the most frequent and is an important proper management of this complication. The diagnosis of spinal brucellosis with laboratory tests and imaging and the medical and the surgical treatment are described in the following paragraphs.

Keywords

Drainage • Neurobrucellosis • Paravertebral abscess • Spinal brucellosis • Spine fusion

Abbreviations

CSF Cerebrospinal fluid
CT Computed tomography
MRI Magnetic resonance imaging

13.1 Introduction

The most frequent complication of brucellosis is bone involvement that is observed in about 25 % of cases. Within the bony infection, spinal involvement represents the most frequent one,

M. Turgut et al. (eds.), *Neurobrucellosis: Clinical, Diagnostic and Therapeutic Features*, DOI 10.1007/978-3-319-24639-0_13

accounting for about 50 % of the cases of osteo-articular extension with a vertebral infection rate of 6–12 % of cases of brucellosis [2, 6, 22, 27].

Chronic brucellosis should be considered in the differential diagnosis of every destructive spinal lesion, especially in the countries where it is endemic.

13.2 Physiopathology

First described by Kulowski and Vinke in 1932, the involvement of the spine in brucellosis most commonly affects the lumbosacral region while the thoracic and cervical spines are rarely involved. In some cases, the destruction may be extensive involving different regions at the same time especially in those for which the institution of a specific treatment comes too late because of a delay in the diagnosis.

An accompanying proliferative sclerotic reaction to a destructive process involving the articular structures of the vertebral body is the main pathological finding in spinal involvement which slowly develops into ankylosis of the involved area during a long period as months or years [20, 24].

The superior endplate, with its rich blood supply, usually represents the first area to be involved in spinal brucellosis, but infrequently, the inferior endplate may also be affected. The size of the initial inoculum, the virulence of the organism, and the immunity of the host are crucial parameters for the progression of the infection that may either regress to heal completely or progress to involve the entire vertebral body, intervertebral disc space, and then neighbouring vertebrae [28–31].

Spinal brucellosis is frequently caused by *B. melitensis*, the most virulent and invasive ones among the different *Brucella* species, but also by *B. suis*. The extent of spinal damage may be severe. In accord with Madkour and Sharif classification of spinal brucellosis [23], we can classify it as early and advanced stages. In the early form, where the organism is localized in the ventral aspect of a superior cartilage endplate, with a small area of osseous destruction, the disease continues with the formation of an osteophyte called "parrot's beak". In the advanced form, the entire vertebral body is involved with a chronic inflammation composed of plasma cells, lymphocytes, histiocytes, and polymorphonuclear cells; at times or randomly or infrequently, granulomatous tissue may develop. As a general rule, there is no necrosis or central caseation [9–11].

13.3 Clinical Signs

Although vertebral involvement in brucellosis can occur at any level, the disease was commonly reported to settle in the lumbar spine, in particular at the level of L4–L5. In only 9 % of all cases, multiple levels are involved.

A constant symptom is pain, relieved by rest, lasting late into the convalescent period and localized to the diseased region of the spine. This stage is usually not identified as brucellosis usually occurring before radiographic findings have appeared. In more than one-half of the cases, a girdle pain radiating into the extremities is present with muscle spasm, restriction of movement, tenderness, and signs of involvement of nerve root. Paravertebral abscess and extradural compression may also occur especially in severe infections [13, 14].

13.4 Diagnosis

Both cellular and humoral mechanisms work to get immunity following active infection with *Brucella* spp. The IgM antibodies are the first to increase after the *Brucella* infection and may persist for several years. Following the progression of the disease, IgM declines and IgG increases, but the IgG level decreases gradually and gets lost within 6–18 months after adequate treatment. By using the 2-mercaptoethanol extracts, determination of IgG is possible without any difficulty and elevated IgG level signifies an active disease process, suggesting the need for medical treatment. It is important to keep in the mind that false-positive reactions can be seen owing to cross-reacting antibodies during certain infections including

Yersinia enterocolitica, *Salmonella* strains, and *Francisella tularensis* and following cholera vaccine [1, 18, 26].

A small number of organisms make the microscopic diagnosis harder in specimens obtained by biopsy or surgical intervention and they can therefore be identified by culture. Regarding the blood culture in many cases, the test may fail. The causes can be the no-bacteremic state and the prolonged time required by the test (up to 6 weeks) to become positive. The use of antibiotics before the confirmation of the diagnosis is an important topic in the case of negative *Brucella* culture result. Also, patients with spinal brucellosis have a positive blood culture less frequently than patients with systemic brucellosis [16, 17].

Radiologic imaging has a critical role in the evaluation of these lesions to provide information about the disease process, to guide biopsy procedure with/without drainage, and to guide the selection of appropriate treatment method, medical and/or surgical, and the monitoring of treatment response [34]. Magnetic resonance imaging (MRI) with gadolinium enhancement has become the gold standard approach for assessing the neural structures with high-resolution images [12]. Also, radiographs of the spine and computed tomography (CT) may provide some information. From these, CT imaging is useful in making image-guided biopsies of the vertebral body or aspiration of the paravertebral abscesses, although it is less sensitive than MRI. In particular, CT scan is invaluable in the differential diagnosis of *Brucella* involving the spine from other spinal diseases [8].

13.5 Differential Diagnosis

Tuberculosis of the spine, pyogenic osteomyelitis due to other bacteria, herniated disc, and metastatic lesion have to be considered in the differential diagnosis. While in tuberculosis the changes appear relatively early and in osteoporosis the changes are more marked and the destruction more severe, in the healing stage of brucellosis, the proliferative changes are not seen in tuberculosis. Paravertebral abscesses and vertebral collapses are more common in tuberculosis. In a pyogenic infection due to other bacteria, the onset is usually more rapid and the disease is more acute with early destruction of the bone. A herniated disc does not show the severe bone destruction observed in untreated brucellosis. Metastatic deposits do not usually involve two neighbouring vertebral bodies and the intervening intervertebral disc is usually spared [32, 36, 38, 40–42].

13.6 Treatment

Most of the cases with spinal brucellosis need no surgical intervention and could be controlled with medical treatment. Today, the treatment of choice is conservative approach with immobilization of the affected region and long-term antibiotic treatment. In most of the cases, antimicrobial therapy is effective, with a high cure rate as 90 % in patients with spinal brucellosis, although there is some evidence that bone infection may be more resistant to the treatment. A large number of antibiotics in certain combinations have been used to treat osteomyelitis due to *Brucella* spp., including tetracyclines, trimethoprim-sulfamethoxazole (TMP/SMZ, co-trimoxazole), and aminoglycosides, but currently, the most effective combination is doxycycline and rifampin [3–5]. In general, at least 6 months of therapy would be beneficial to prevent recurrence and it should be continued until MRI demonstrates the changes of the signal intensity due to the regression of the inflammatory process or serological examination is negative.

Importantly, urgent operative exploration should be considered in patients with acute neurological deficits or progressive worsening, as did in cases with cervical brucellar epidural abscess [7, 35]. Other indications for surgical intervention are the presence of vertebral body destruction with segmental instability and failure of medical treatment. As a general rule, these patients must be treated with a combination of antibiotic treatment and surgery including removal of involved intervertebral disc, debridement of spinal infection, and surgical drainage of epidural abscess, with/without stabilization and fusion procedure. A CT-guided needle biopsy before surgical intervention could be performed in some cases of epidural/paravertebral abscess formation [15, 21, 25, 33, 37]. Currently, there is an agreement regarding the optimal treatment approach, spinal instrumentation, and fusion with an autogenous iliac strut bone graft.

There is no standard method for determining whether or not brucellosis has resolved. Usually, the resolution of infection is indicated by the improvement of clinical symptoms, negative blood culture, decrease in inflammatory markers (C-reactive protein and erythrocyte sedimentation rate), seroconversion, and the disappearance of the imaging findings [19, 39, 40].

Conclusion

- The most common complication of brucellosis is bone involvement that is observed in about 25 % of cases.
- Pain is the most common symptom.
- MRI with gadolinium is the gold standard to detect the spinal involvement of brucellosis.
- The treatment of choice is conservative approach with immobilization of the affected region and long-term antibiotic treatment.
- Main indication for surgery is the quick worsening of the neurological symptoms.
- Drainage of the abscess and stabilization of the involved segment of the spine are the options of choice.
- Improvement of clinical symptoms, seroconversion, negative blood culture, decrease in inflammatory markers, and imaging finding confirm the resolution of the disease.

References

1. Araj GF (2010) Update on laboratory diagnosis of human brucellosis. Int J Antimicrob Agents 36(Suppl 1): S12–S17
2. Ariza J, Gudiol F, Valverde J, Pallares R, Fernandez-Viladrich P, Rufi G, Espadaler L, Fernandez-Nogues F (1985) Brucella spondylitis. A detailed analysis based on current findings. Rev Infect Dis 7:656–664
3. Baykal M, Akalin HE, Firat M, Serin A (1989) In vitro activity and clinical efficacy of ofloxacin in infections due to Brucella melitensis. Rev Infect Dis 11:S993–S994
4. Bingol A, Yucemen N, Meco O (1999) Medically treated intraspinal "Brucella" granuloma-MR imaging. Surg Neurol 52:570–576
5. Bodur H, Erbay A, Colpan A, Akinci E (2004) Brucellar spondylitis. Rheumatol Int 24:221–226
6. ChelliBouaziz M, Ladeb MF, Chakroun M, Chaabane S (2008) Spinal brucellosis: a review. Skeletal Radiol 37:785–790
7. deDivitiis O, Elefante A (2012) Cervical spinal brucellosis: a diagnostic and surgical challenge. World Neurosurg 78:257–259
8. Demirci M, Tan E, Durguner M, Zileli T, Eryilmaz M (1989) Spinal brucellosis. A case with "cauliflower" appearance on CT. Neuroradiology 31:282–283
9. Ganado W, Craig AJ (1958) Brucellosis myelopathy. J Bone Joint Surg Am 40:1380–1388
10. Glasgow MMS (1976) Brucellosis of the spine. Br J Surg 63:283–288
11. Goodhart GL, Zakem JF, Collins WC, Meyer JD (1987) Brucellosis of the spine. Report of a patient with bilateral paraspinal abscesses. Spine 12:414–416
12. Harman M, Unal O, Onbas KT, Kýymaz N, Arslan H (2001) Brucellar spondylodiscitis: MRI diagnosis. J Clin Imaging 25:421–427
13. Horasan ES, Colak M, Erzōz G, Uḡuz M, Kaya A (2012) Clinical findings of vertebral osteomyelitis: Brucella spp. versus other etiologic agents. Rheumatol Int 32:3449–3453
14. Jaffe H (1972) Metabolic, degenerative and inflammatory disease in bones and joints. Lea & Febiger, Philadelphia
15. Katonis P, Tzermiadianos M, Gikas A, Papagelopoulos P, Hadjipavlou A (2006) Surgical treatment of spinal brucellosis. Clin Orthop Relat Res 444:66–72
16. Keenan JD, Metz CW Jr (1972) Brucella spondylitis. A brief review and case report. Clin Orthop 82:87–91
17. Kelly PJ, Martin WJ, Schirger A, Weed LA (1960) Brucellosis of the bones and joints. Experience with thirty-six patients. JAMA 174:347–353
18. Klein GC, Behan KA (1981) Determination of Brucella immunoglobulin G agglutinating antibody titer with dithiothreitol. J Clin Microbiol 14:24–25
19. Koubaa M, Maaloul I, Marrakchi C, Lahiani D, Hammami B, Mnif Z, Ben Mahfoudh K, Hammami A, Ben Jemaa M (2014) Spinal brucellosis in South of Tunisia: review of 32 cases. Spine J 14:1538–1544
20. Kulowski J, Vinke TH (1932) Undulant (Malta) fever spondylitis. Report of a case due to Brucella melitensis bovine variety, surgically treated. JAMA 99:1656–1659
21. Lifeso RM, Harder E, McCorkell SJ (1985) Spinal brucellosis. J Bone Joint Surg Br 67:345–351
22. Madkour MM, Gargani G (1989) Epidemiological aspects. In: Madkour MM (ed) Brucellosis. Butterworths, London, pp 11–28

23. Madkour MM, Sharif H (1989) Bone and joint imaging. In: Madkour MM (ed) Brucellosis. Butterworths, London, pp 105–114
24. Meltzer E, Sidi Y, Smolen G, Banai M, Bardenstein S, Schwartz E (2010) Sexually transmitted brucellosis in humans. Clin Infect Dis 51:e12–e15
25. Mousa AM, Bahar RH, Araj GF, Koshy TS, Muhtaseb SA, Al-Mudallal DS, Marafie AA (1990) Neurological complications of Brucella spondylitis. Acta Neurol Scand 81:16–23
26. Namiduru M, Karaoglan I, Gursoy S, Bayazit N, Sirikci A (2004) Brucellosis of the spine: evaluation of the clinical, laboratory, and radiological findings of 14 patients. Rheumatol Int 24:125–129
27. Pappas G, Papadimitriou P, Akritidis N, Christou L, Tsianos EV (2006) The new global map of human brucellosis. Lancet Infect Dis 6:91–99
28. Paul B, Gopakumar TS, Vasu CK (1999) Brucellar spondylitis. J Assoc Physicians India 47:451–453
29. Rajapakse CNA, Al-Aska KA, Al-Orainey I, Halim K, Arabi K (1987) Spinal brucellosis. Br J Rheumatol 26:28–31
30. Raptopoulou A, Karantanas AH, Poumboulidis K, Grollios G, Raptopoulou-Gigi M, Garyfallos A (2006) Brucellar spondylodiscitis: noncontiguous multifocal involvement of the cervical, thoracic, and lumbar spine. Clin Imaging 30:214–217
31. Samra Y, Hertz M, Shaked Y, Zwas S, Altman G (1982) Brucellosis of the spine. A report of 3 cases. J Bone Joint Surg Br 64:429–431
32. Scully RE, Mark EJ, Mc Neely BU (1986) Case records of the MGH. N Engl J Med 315:748–753
33. Sgouros S, Sakas D (2010) Brucellosis of the spine affecting multiple non-contiguous levels. Br J Neurosurg 24:589–591
34. Solé-Llenas J, Rotés-Querol J, Dalmau-Ciria M (1966) Radiologic aspects of spinal brucellosis. Acta Radiol Diagn 5:1132–1139
35. Song KJ, Yoon SJ, Lee KB (2012) Cervical spinal brucellosis with epidural abscess causing neurologic deficit with negative serologic tests. A case report. World Neurosurg 78(375):e15–e19
36. Spink WW (1981) Brucella. In: Braude AI (ed) International textbook of medicine, vol 2, Medical microbiology and infectious diseases. WB Saunders, Philadelphia, pp 374–379
37. Tekkok IH, Berker M, Ozcan OE, Ozgen T, Akalin E (1993) Brucellosis of the spine. Neurosurgery 33:838–844
38. Torres-Rojas J, Taddonio RF, Sanders CV (1979) Spondylitis caused by Brucella abortus. South Med J 72:1166–1169
39. Turgut M, Turgut AT, Koşar U (2006) Spinal brucellosis: Turkish experience based on 452 cases published during the last century. Acta Neurochir Wien 148:1033–1044
40. Ugarriza LF, Porras LF, Lorenzana LM, Rodriguez-Sanchez JA, Garcia-Yagie LM, Cabezudo JM (2005) Brucellar spinal epidural abscesses. Analysis of eleven cases. Br J Neurosurg 19:235–240
41. Wu P-C, Khin M-M, Pang S-W (1985) Salmonella osteomyelitis. An important differential diagnosis of granulomatous osteomyelitis. Am J Surg Pathol 9:531–537
42. Young EJ (1983) Human brucellosis. Rev Infect Dis 5:821–842

Imaging of Vertebral Brucellosis

14

Ahmet Tuncay Turgut, Recep Brohi, Pelin Demir, and Andrea Elefante

Contents

A.T. Turgut, MD (✉)
Department of Radiology,
Hacettepe University School of Medicine,
Ankara, Turkey
e-mail: ahmettuncayturgut@yahoo.com

R. Brohi, MD
Department of Neurosurgery, Ankara Training and Research Hospital,
Ankara, Turkey
e-mail: recepbrohi@yahoo.com

P. Demir, MD
Department of Radiology,
Numune Training and Research Hospital,
Ankara, Turkey
e-mail: drrpelindemir6@hotmail.com

A. Elefante, MD
Department of Advanced Biomedical Sciences,
"Federico II" University,
Via S.Pansini, 5, Naples 80131, Italy
e-mail: aelefant@unina.it

Abstract

Brucellosis is a zoonotic disease, with sheep, goat, camel, livestock animals, etc., as the primary hosts and human beings as the secondary host. It is a member of the specie brucella with melitensis, abortus, suis, and canis subgroups being a Gram-negative short rodlike bacteria which are intracellular. This infection is endemic in some parts of the world, in particular in the Mediterranean basin. Involvement of the nervous system by the organism is seen in about 5–10 % of cases which may involve the central nervous system or may involve the spinal system, the latter being the subject of this chapter. The diagnosis is done by clinical and laboratory findings such as blood agglutinin levels, isolation of the species from blood flow, or other specimens. Along with the laboratory findings, plain X-rays, CT, MRI, and radionuclide studies are of importance. The treatment options are antibiotics as the first step in case of lack of neurologic deterioration. If neurologic deterioration occurs, surgical procedures can be carried by an anterior, posterior, or combined approach. Brucellosis is an infection which causes socioeconomic problems, so its diagnoses and treatment should be done carefully. Recent investigations and developments in medications and invasive techniques provide the chance to treat it thoroughly.

M. Turgut et al. (eds.), *Neurobrucellosis: Clinical, Diagnostic and Therapeutic Features*,
DOI 10.1007/978-3-319-24639-0_14

Keywords

Spine • Brucella • Neurobrucellosis • Neuroimaging

Abbreviations

CT Computed tomography
MRI Magnetic resonance imaging
PET Positron emission tomography

14.1 Introduction

A zoonotic infectious disease caused by brucella species in human which is not common in the western world including the United States as well as Central and Northern Europe, this pathogenous group is a common and significant health issue in many underdeveloped regions of the world and also in partly developed countries. Central and South America, Middle East, and Mediterranean regions are geographic areas where these species are still endemic and causing severe public health and socioeconomic problems. Contact with livestock and products such as unpasteurized milk and untanned hides which are products related to livestock may lead to the infection. Person-to-person transmission is very unusual with only few cases being reported [1]. Outbreak of disease is possible when a common source of food is involved such as cheese [2]. Brucellosis can occur by different means, occupational, recreational, and foodborne, or may be linked to travel and even to bioterrorism [3].

Human brucellosis (Malta fever, Mediterranean fever, Gibraltar fever, undulant fever, typhomalarial fever, or Cyprus fever) may involve any organ of the body, and it may show a generalized or localized pattern; the latter, being the osteoarticular form, is also the most common localized form [4, 5]. If involvement of a specific organ far outweighs, the disease is meant as localized or focal [6]. Osteoarticular form of the disease is the most common complication of its chronic form and ranges from 5 to 85 % [6–9]. Spondylitis caused by brucella is one of the most serious forms of osteoarticular involvement including epidural abscesses, myelitis/radiculoneuritis, or demyelinating neuropathy [10, 11].

The infection affects the disc and causes discitis as many other infectious agents do. When the vertebral body is affected by brucella species, the form of the infection is named spondylitis. Brucella spondylitis influences the cauda equina and spinal nerves and mobility problems. Spinal cord and cauda equina compression is a major reason for the main complaints in spinal brucellosis. There is a lack of specific clinical manifestations with nocturnal fever, malaise, polyarthromyalgia, headache, profuse sweating, and weight loss [12, 13]. This lack of specific manifestations may lead to misdiagnose with other infectious entities such as spinal tuberculosis and also mistreatment.

14.2 Clinical Diagnosis for Spinal Brucellosis

Different authors group the infection into acute, subacute, and chronic phases with periods, respectively, being less than 2–3 months, 2 to 3–12 months, and more than 12 months [9, 14–16]. Being in close contact with animals and all sorts of livestock products causes a predominancy of males over females especially young adults. Osteoarticular symptoms and manifestations are more frequent in the chronic form [16]. Due to the involvement of osteoarticular structures, there is a high amount of morbidity presenting with different clinical pictures. The level of the affected spine determines the complications and clinical presentation [17]. The lumbar spine is the most frequently involved spine segment followed by the thoracic and cervical spine segments [5, 18]. L4–L5 involvement tops the lumbar spondylitis followed by the L5–S1 level [8, 12, 14].

Laboratory tests should be used for serologic confirmation. Red bengal plate agglutination test is a test for this purpose. If it is negative, further tests, like compliment fixation tests and brucellosis antihuman immunoglobulin tests (Coombs test), should be determined.

Plain radiographs and computed tomography (CT) are not very helpful in the differential diagnoses of this entity. It can be misdiagnosed as lumbar disc herniation because this may compress the spinal root(s) [19].

14.3 Radiologic Imaging Specificities of Spinal Brucellosis

14.3.1 Radiography

On plain X-rays, brucellar involvement of the bone and end plate is visualized as four different stages: (1) localized area of bone erosion at the discovertebral junction, (2) active bone sclerosis, (3) peripheral vacuum phenomenon entrapped between the intervertebral disc and the cartilage end plate of the vertebra, and (4) a parrot's beak (anterior osteophyte formation) [20]. The anterior erosion is quite similar to the one seen at Schmorl nodes.

On plain X-rays, the spine gap is narrow, and there may be an increase in bone density. The vertebral edges can be destroyed with a feature like worm eaten, and the vertebral edges may have sclerosis and bone hyperplasia which is called osteophyte (beaklike). There could be facet destruction causing instability resulting in spondylolisthesis.

14.3.2 Computed Tomography

Especially in case of diffuse brucellar spondylitis, CT scans show bone sclerosis which is associated with bone destruction and paraspinal tissue edema which leads to obliteration of the paraspinal muscle-fat plane. About 25–30 % of cases may show disc gas (vacuum phenomenon). Usually there is no Gibbus deformity because the vertebral body morphology is almost totally preserved. Such features and absence of paraspinal soft tissue abscesses are differential diagnostic tools from tuberculosis spondylosis. But the exact and clear proof of the infection and differential diagnosis depends on isolation of the organism. High and increasing titer of brucella organisms with or without isolation of the organism and prompt response to antibrucellar treatment regimens are diagnostic findings.

CT scans can show articular surface hyperplasia and sclerosis at the end plate, central bone destruction, and round and hypodense hairlike bone lesions [13]. Similar changes can also be seen on facet joints. The periosteum of the vertebral edge may be hypertrophied and calcified.

14.3.3 Magnetic Resonance Imaging

Since its introduction to the medical science, this modality is the choice of imaging for detecting spinal brucellosis along with serologic confirmation tests for the last two to three decades. MRI can detect the histopathologic changes earlier than other imaging modalities.

Radiologically, T1-weighted images demonstrate decreased signal intensity (hypointense), T2-weighted images reveal increased signal intensity (hyperintense), and, if gadolinium-like contrast media is given, T1-weighted images will reveal a high contrast enhancement (Figs. 14.1, 14.2, 14.3, and 14.4). Narrowing of the intervertebral disc space can be visualized in all types of MRI sequences, and the intervertebral disc appears to be hypointense [21]. Diagnostic MRI features of brucellar spondylitis such as signal changes in the vertebral bone and cartilaginous end plate without morphologic alterations and enhancement of the adjacent facet joints following administration of gadolinium contrast material have been described. Fat-saturated sequence with contrast medium is one of the sequences that is helpful to see vertebral involvement by brucella.

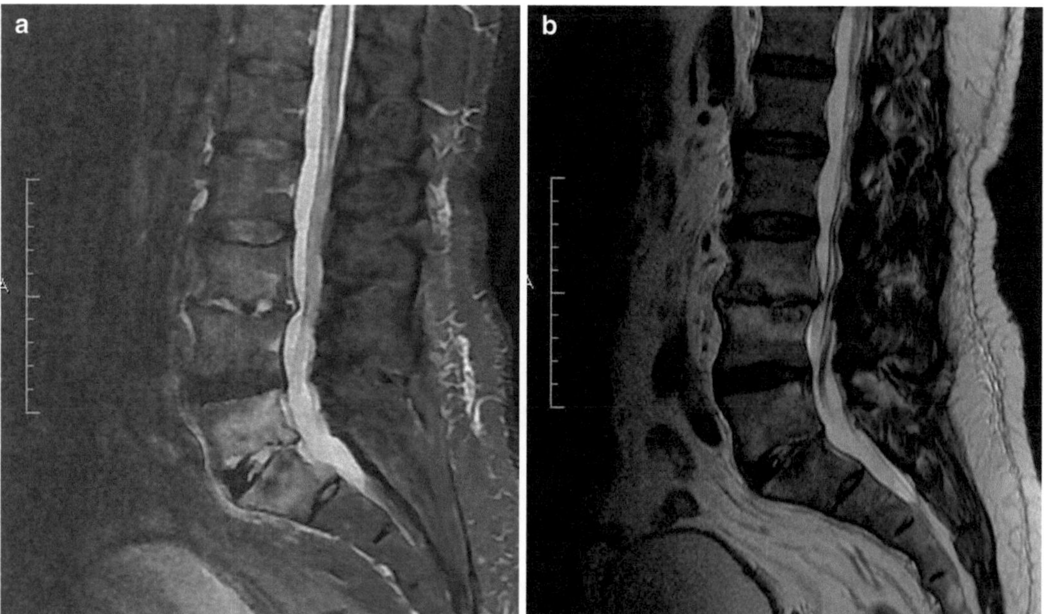

Fig. 14.1 (**a**) Sagittal STIR FAST image of a male patient showing involvement of two segments. (**b**) Sagittal T2-weighted image of the same patient. Note the different stages of the disease for each segment

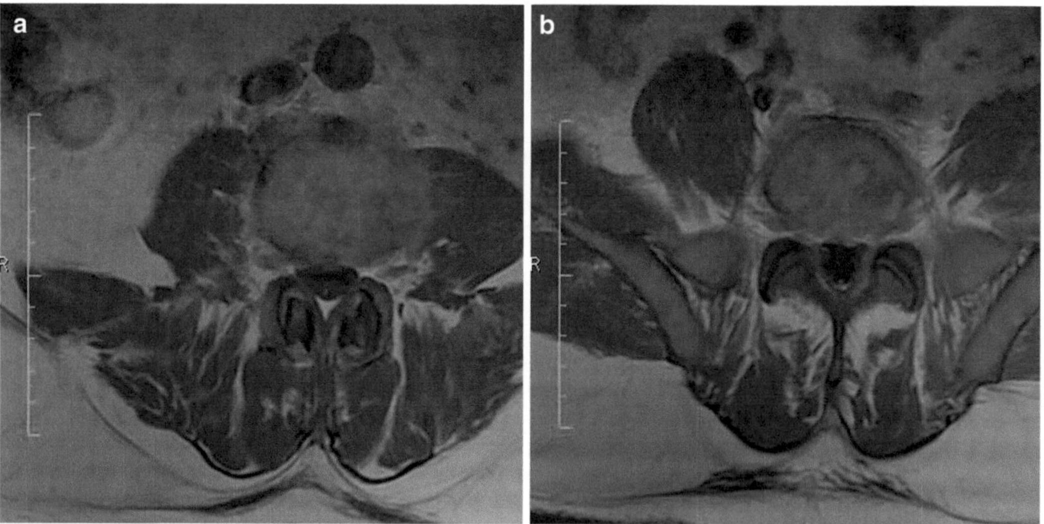

Fig. 14.2 (**a**) Contrast-enhanced MRI images of the same patient with same level, axial L3–L4. (**b**) Contrast-enhanced MRI images of the same patient with same level, axial L5–S1

14.3.4 Scintigraphy

Radionuclide bone scintigraphy is also an important diagnostic study for detecting spinal infections including brucellosis. The authors who first mentioned the role and importance of nuclear medicine were Bahar and Madkour [22, 23]. Scintigrams may show focal or diffuse increased uptake in the vertebral bodies. The entire vertebral body may be involved, or there may be the caries sign (focal and marked uptake at the intersection region of the upper and lateral margins of

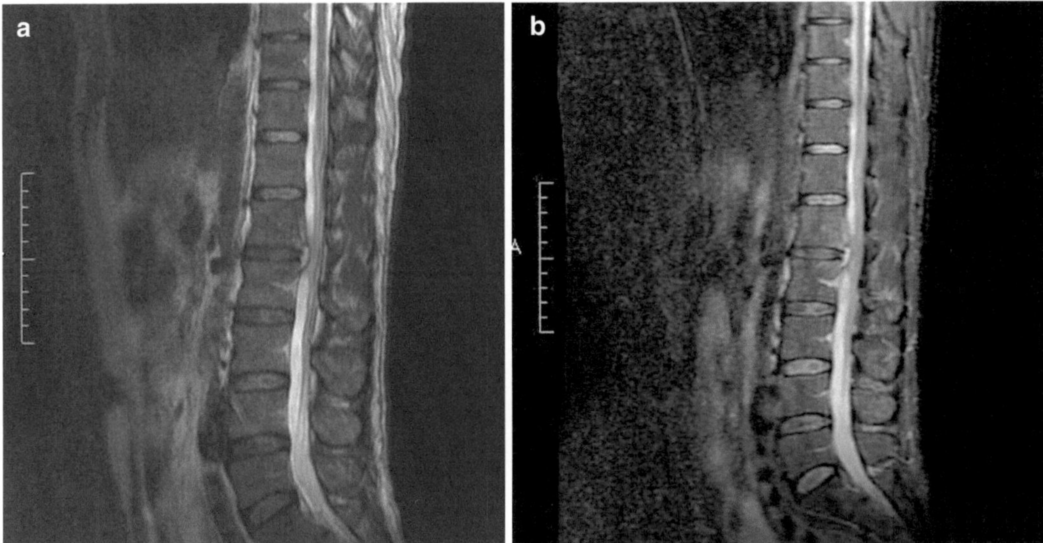

Fig. 14.3 (**a**) A patient with spinal brucellosis, note the posterior beaklike protrusion, sagittal T2-weighted image, L1–L2. (**b**) STIR sagittal-weighted image of the same level of the same patient on (**a**)

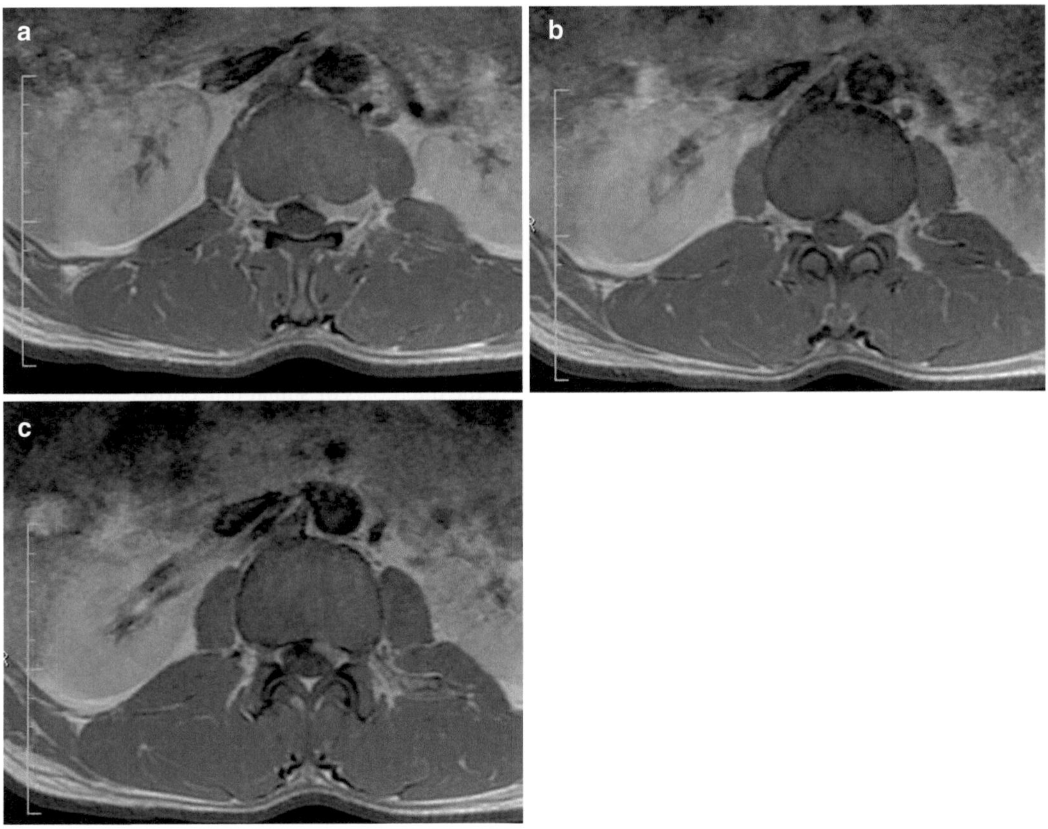

Fig. 14.4 Axial contrast-enhanced images of L1–L2 level with three different axial levels, respectively, lower end plate of L1 (**a**), mid-level between L1–L2 disc (**b**), and upper end plate of L2 (**c**)

the vertebra). Scintigraphy may show involvement of focal long bones, costovertebral joints, and costochondral junction. Sacro-ileitis may also be present and can be seen on radionuclide imaging. Nevertheless, MRI is the choice imaging for spinal brucella.

As mentioned by a recent article and investigation [24], positron emission tomography (PET) can show lesions which are and may not be visualized on MRI. PET/CT combination with metabolites such as fluorine-18 fluoro-deoxy-D-glucose may reveal additional lesions of the spine and paravertebral tissues too.

14.4 Treatment

The first step in the treatment of spinal brucellosis is medication which includes antibiotics effective in intracellular organisms of the brucella genus. As the infection is intracellular, a long medication period is required and close follow-up is needed. One important issue which should be taken into consideration is a sudden neurologic deterioration, in case medical treatment with antibiotics is the initial regimen of therapy. Surgery may be needed in case of neurologic deterioration. In such a case, anterior, posterior, or combined surgeries may be performed.

Involvement of the cervical column is infrequent compared to the lumbar or thoracic region but is more susceptible to severe complications. Epidural mass and spinal cord compression may cause serious neurologic deficits. The anterior surgical approach is the first choice in this region.

Conclusion

The brucella organism can affect all the nervous system regardless of location with manifestations of spinal or central nervous involvement all together named as neurobrucellosis. Laboratory tests and imaging modalities such as MRI, PET, and scintigraphy are used to diagnose this entity.

Although brucella is a systemic infection, local manifestation such as brucellar involvement of the spinal column is a treatable disease and has a good outcome in most cases. Usually, it may cause different complications in the nervous system such as meningitis, granuloma and abscess development, and spondylitis depending on its location, and sometimes all of these manifestations can be seen in one case [25].

Treatment of the infection is mainly conservative with medications unless it has formed an abscess or granuloma. The medications should include drugs acting on intracellular organisms. If antibiotic drugs are administered, blood serum agglutinin levels can be used for the progression of the treatment. Surgery should be kept on hand as an option in case of failure of medical treatment and especially in case of abscesses and neurologic deterioration. In case of surgery, not the only one but the most critical prognostic factor in recovery from the infection is the preoperative neurologic condition.

As a standard manner of diagnostic algorithm, a stepwise imaging modality of choice could be done for the diagnosis of spinal brucellosis, starting from plain X-rays and going through CT and MRI. Plain X-ray is a cheap and easy to access technique for imaging spinal brucellosis, but the overmentioned signs for the disease has a disadvantage; as details may be easily passed over. But along with laboratory tests and with a careful eye, this easy and cheap imaging modality can lead to the diagnosis of spinal brucellosis.

CT, the more precise imaging modality than plain X-ray, comes as the second stage, but recently MRI is almost always the choice as the first step of imaging for spinal brucellosis and all other manifestations of the disease. MRI reveals an early diagnosis of vertebral involvement of spinal brucellosis and has the advantage of avoidance of X-rays of CT. With enhancement of contrast media, it provides a precise diagnosis. Recently additional nuclear medicine imaging techniques such as scintigraphy may help in the diagnosis of the disease earlier than MRI, especially that PET has this advantage. But as MRI has widespread accessibility and advantage of protection from ionizing radiation, it can be used as the diagnostic study of choice for spinal brucellosis.

References

1. Rubin B, Band JD, Wong P, Colville J (1991) Person-to-person transmission of Brucella melitensis. Lancet 1:14–15
2. Hines PD, Overturf GD, Hatch D, Kim J (1986) Brucellosis in a California family. Pediatr Infect Dis 5:579–582
3. Godfroid J, Cloeckaert A, Liautard JP, Kohler S, Fretin D, Walravens K, Garin-Bastuji B, Letesson JJ (2005) From the discovery of the Malta fever's agent to the discovery of a marine mammal reservoir, brucellosis has continuously been a re-emerging zoonosis. Vet Res 36:313–326
4. Bosilkovski M, Krteva L, Caparoska S, Dimzova M (2004) Osteoarticular involvement in brucellosis: study of 196 cases in the Republic of Macedonia. CMJ 45:727–733
5. Turgut M, Turgut AT, Koşar U (2006) Spinal brucellosis: the Turkish experience based on 452 cases published during the last century. Acta Neurochir (Wien) 148:1033–1044
6. Young EJ (2000) Brucella species. In: Mandell GL, Bennet JE, Dolin R (eds) Principles and practice of infectious diseases, 5th edn. Churchill Livingstone, New York, pp 2386–2393
7. Tekkök IH, Berker M, Özcan OE, Özgen T, Akalın E (1993) Brucellosis of the spine. Neurosurgery 33: 838–844
8. Özaksoy D, Yücesoy K, Yücesoy M, Kovanlıkaya I, Yüce A, Naderi S (2001) Brucellar spondylitis: MRI findings. Eur Spine J 10:529–533
9. Gur A, Geyik MF, Dikici B, Nas K, Çevik R, Sarac AJ, Hosoglu S (2003) Complications of brucellosis in different age groups in Southeastern Anatolia of Turkey: a study of 283 cases. Yonsei Med J 44:33–44
10. Ariza J, Gudiol F, Valvarde R, Pallares R, Fernandez-Viladrich P, Rufi G, Espalder L, Fernandez-Nogues F (1985) Brucella spondylitis: a detailed analysis based on current findings. Rev Infect Dis 7:656–664
11. Bodur H, Erbay A, Çolpan A, Akıncı E (2004) Brucellar spondylitis. Rheumatol Int 24:221–226
12. Yang XM, Wang YY, Shi W, Zhang Y, Zhang P, Ren YX (2014) Imaging classification and clinical significance of brucellosis spondylitis. J Spine 3:172
13. Turgut M, Şendur ÖF, Gürel M (2003) Brucellar spondylitis in the lumbar region. Neurol Med Chir (Tokyo) 43:210–212
14. Gotuzzo W, Seas C, Guera JG, Carillo C, Bocanegra TS, Calvo A, Castaneda O, Alarcon GS (1987) Brucella arthritis: a study of 39 peruvian families. Ann Rheum Dis 46:506–509
15. Yıldırım RC, Afşar OZ, Eker L (1997) Brucellosis in the World and Turkey (in Turkish). Sürekli Tıp Eğitimi Dergisi 6:189–192
16. Pourbagher A, Pourbagher MA, Savaş L, Turunç T, Demiroğlu YZ, Erol İ, Yalçıntaş D (2006) Epidemiologic, clinical, and imaging findings in brucellosis in patients with osteoarticular involvement. AJR Am J Roentgenol 187:873–880
17. Özgeçmen S, Ardıçoğlu Ö (1999) Osteoarticular brucellosis. J Rheumatol 3:322–325
18. Naderi S, Yücesoy K, Mertol T, Arda MN (2000) Epidural brucella abscess. Report of a spinal brucellosis manifesting itself with epidural abscess. Neuro-orthopedics 28:11–15
19. Demirci I (2003) Brucella discitis mimicking herniation without spondylitis: MRI findings. Zentralbl Neurochir 64:178–181
20. Sharif HS, Aediyan OA, Clark DC, Madkour MM, Aebed MY, Mattsson TA, al-Deeb SM, Moutaer KR (1989) Brucella and tuberculous spondylitis: comparative imaging features. Radiology 171: 419–425
21. Turgut M, Çullu E, Şendur ÖF, Gürer G (2004) Brucella spine infection: four case reports. Neurol Med Chir (Tokyo) 44:562–567
22. Madkour MM, Sharif HS, Abed MY, Al-Fayez MA (1988) Osteoarticular brucellosis: results of bone scintigraphy in 140 patients. AJR Am J Roentgenol 150:1101–1105
23. Bahar RH, Al-Suhaili AR, Mousa AM, Nawaz MK, Kaddah N, Abdel Dayem HM (1988) Brucellosis: appearance on skeletal imaging. Clin Nucl Med 13:102–106
24. Savvas I, Chatziioannou S, Pneumaticos SG, Zormpala A, Sipsas NV (2013) Fluorine-18 fluoro-2-deoxy-D-glucose positron emission tomography/computed scan contributes to the diagnosis and management of brucellar spondylodiskitis. BMC Infect Dis 13:73
25. Goktepe AS, Alaca R, Mohur H, Coskun U (2003) Neurobrucellosis and a demonstration of its involvement in spinal roots via magnetic resonance imaging. Spinal Cord 41:574–576

15 Epidural and Subdural Spinal Brucellosis

Ebru Kursun, Ahmet Tuncay Turgut, Naime Altınkaya Tokmak, and Mehmet Turgut

Contents

E. Kursun, MD (✉)
Department of Infectious Diseases and Clinical Microbiology, Baskent University School of Medicine, Ankara, Turkey
e-mail: ebru.kursun@hotmail.com

A.T. Turgut, MD
Department of Radiology, Hacettepe University School of Medicine, Ankara, Turkey
e-mail: ahmettuncayturgut@yahoo.com

N.A. Tokmak, MD
Department of Radiology, Baskent University School of Medicine, Ankara, Turkey
e-mail: naimeto@yahoo.com

M. Turgut, MD, PhD
Department of Neurosurgery, Adnan Menderes University School of Medicine, Aydın, Turkey
e-mail: drmturgut@yahoo.com

Abstract

The present paper discusses the characteristics, diagnosis, and treatment of epidural and subdural spinal abscesses, which are the rare complications of brucellosis. Epidural and subdural spinal abscesses have high mortality and their prognosis is quite good with early diagnosis and treatment. There is no standard practice concerning treatment; long-term combined antibiotic therapy, with additional surgical therapy in those having neurological deficit, is required. Attention should be paid particularly for epidural and subdural spinal involvement in the places where brucellosis is endemic.

Keywords

Epidural spinal abscess • Neurobrucellosis • Spinal brucellosis • Spinal subdural abscess

Abbreviations

CT	Computed tomography
MRI	Magnetic resonance imaging
TMP/SMX	Trimethoprim-sulfamethoxazole

M. Turgut et al. (eds.), *Neurobrucellosis: Clinical, Diagnostic and Therapeutic Features*, DOI 10.1007/978-3-319-24639-0_15

15.1 Introduction

Brucellosis is a zoonosis caused by a type of bacteria called *Brucella* and is still widespread all around the world (Fig. 15.1). It is a disease that has the ability of disease in involving humans and animals, resulting in serious health problems. Brucellosis is still endemic in India, Mexico, the Middle East, the Caribbean Islands, Eastern Europe, the Middle and South American countries, and the Mediterranean basin (Turkey, Portugal, Spain, Italy, Greece, South France, North Africa) [37]. While the main mode of transmission of the disease is the consumption of unpasteurized products like milk, ice cream, butter, and cheeses in the developing countries, it is most commonly the occupational exposure in the developed countries [13, 44]. Brucellosis is a systemic infectious disease that could manifest with different clinical pictures; signs and symptoms in the clinical picture are usually not specific to the disease. Clinically, arthralgia, high fever, weakness, perspiration, and low back pain are the most common symptoms [7].

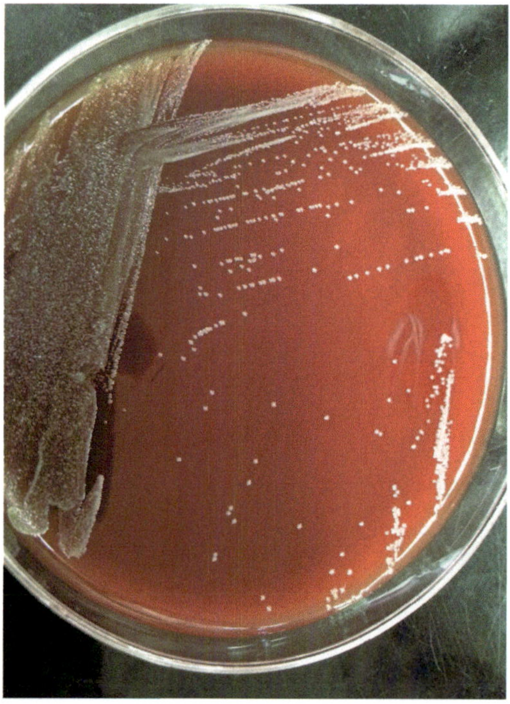

Fig. 15.1 *Brucella* colonies recovered on blood agar from blood culture of a patient with brucellosis (Courtesy of G.F. Araj, M.D.)

Brucellosis-associated central nervous system involvement is called neurobrucellosis, and while the incidence of neurological involvement changes from 3 to 25 % in various studies, it is reported to be 3–5 % in average [1, 32, 45]. Neurobrucellosis manifests with different neurological pictures as encephalitis, meningitis, myelitis, radiculoneuritis, demyelination, epidural abscess, brain abscess, spinal abscess, and granuloma [37]. Pathogenesis of central nervous system involvement is unclear, although several mechanisms have been suggested. As the bacterium *Brucella* lives intracellular, it avoids phagocytosis and accordingly survives for a long time. The bacteria that get rid of phagocytosis reproduce by suppression of the immunity of the host involve the central nervous system either directly or indirectly via endotoxins.

Brucellosis involves many tissues and organs, primarily the osteoarticular system, which is seen in 5–85 % of the cases [39]. The spine is the most commonly involved of bony brucellosis [26]. Brucellar spondylodiscitis begins at the upper end plates, which are rich in vascularization, depending on the virulence and inoculum of the bacteria and the immune status of the host, and may spread to the vertebral body, intervertebral disk space, and adjacent vertebra [20].

15.2 Epidural Spinal Brucellosis

Brucellar epidural abscess is encountered most frequently due to direct invasion of spondylitis, whereas it rarely develops via direct hematogeneous route without spondylitis [35]. Although brucellosis-associated spinal epidural abscesses are rarely encountered and are found in the literature usually as case reports [20, 37], their prevalence rates are reported to be 10–22 % in many studies on brucellosis [24, 26, 39, 42]. The lumbar vertebra is the most common location of involvement followed by the thoracic and the cervical vertebrae [19, 35]. Koubaa et al. [26] investigated the patients with spinal brucellar epidural abscess and demonstrated that the lumbar region is the most common location of involvement by 84.2 %.

Clinical symptoms of epidural abscess include significant spinal pain, local tenderness, and fever; however, fever may not be present in half and pain may not be present in 10–15 % of the patients [26]. Diagnosis is sometimes delayed until the appearance of neurological symptoms. Neurological complications of brucellar epidural spinal abscess are seen in 1.5 % of the cases and are usually accompanied by spondylitis [22]. Neurological complication of epidural abscess occurs due to spinal cord injury caused by direct compression effect, thrombosis, and thrombophlebitis in the adjacent veins, interruption of arterial blood flow, or the inflammation that occurs due to bacterial toxins and mediators [18]. Depending on the nerve root involved, epidural abscess leads to typical neurological symptoms such as nerve root pain defined as shooting or electric shock, motor weakness, sensorial alterations, bladder or intestinal dysfunction, and paralysis [11].

15.2.1 Diagnosis

The diagnosis of epidural spinal brucellosis is made using the combination of clinical, laboratory, and imaging methods. Brucellosis-associated epidural abscess must be considered in patients with arthralgia, high fever, perspiration, and weight loss together with epidemiological history (consumption of unpasteurized dairy products, involvement in livestock farming and veterinarian, history of past brucellosis), as well as with spinal pain, local tenderness and motor weakness, sensorial alterations, bladder and intestinal dysfunction, and paralysis. Definite diagnosis of brucellosis is made by isolating the agent from blood flow, bone marrow, or a number of other tissues. Positivity of the culture for *Brucella* was reported to be 41.1 % by Aygen et al. [4], 68.8 % by Colmenero et al. [9], 43 % by Kursun et al. [24], 22.6 % by Demirdağ et al. [12], 21 % by Kurtaran et al. [25], and 11.4 % by Buzgan et al. [7]. Sensitivity of blood culture ranges from 17 to 85 % depending on previous antibiotic use and duration of the disease [8, 33].

15.2.1.1 Laboratory Tests

The rose Bengal test for brucellosis is an important screening test and positive results should be verified by serum agglutination test. Quantitative standard tube agglutination test is the most common serological method used for the diagnosis of brucellosis. Detecting >160 titers in the presence of clinical findings or fourfold increase in serum antibody level in the serum samples obtained at 2–3-week intervals is diagnostic. Failing to detect seropositivity in the patients with strong clinical suspicion should suggest presence of blocking antibodies, prozone phenomenon (absence of agglutination due to excessive antibody in the patient's serum), or early period of infection [2].

15.2.1.2 Radiological Studies

Plain X-ray, ultrasonography, computed tomography (CT), magnetic resonance imaging (MRI), and bone scintigraphy are used in the radiological diagnosis of brucellosis involving musculoskeletal system. Typical signs of brucellar spondylitis on radiography appear 3–5 weeks following the beginning of the infection [8]. The focal destructions involving the superior or inferior vertebral body angle, known as brucellar epiphysitis, are the pathognomonic signs of brucellosis. Focal anterior or diffuse disk collapse is quite common [8]. Bone erosion is less common compared to tuberculous spondylitis (also called tuberculosis of the spine). Perilesional bone formation and osteophyte formations in the anterior vertebral end plates are typical and productive osseous changes appear earlier period compared to tuberculous spondylitis. It may be difficult to radiographically distinguish it from degenerative diseases because of slow bone remodeling.

Involvement of intervertebral disk in the early period is seen as small hypodense area in the disk on CT. Flattening of disk and destruction of cartilage end plate, which cannot be detected on plain radiography in the early period, are seen on CT [31]. After administering contrast agent, paravertebral abscess and psoas involvement are easily determined. Displacement of intraspinal enlargement of epidural abscess in the posterior aspect of dural sac after contrast agent administration can be seen on CT; however, this change is identified better on MRI [30]. Sample can be obtained from disko-vertebral area by needle biopsy under the guidance of tomography. Although it is not specific, histopathological examination helps in diagnosing the brucellosis.

MRI is a scanning method used in the diagnosis and monitoring of response to medical treatment in brucellar spondylitis. In a previous study, the veteran authors of this chapter reported that MRI has high sensitivity in detecting the disease at early stage and in detecting enlargement in the epidural and paravertebral areas [39]. MRI findings in the brucellosis-associated spinal involvement show differences between acute and chronic phases. Intervertebral disk and adjacent vertebrae appear to be hypointense on T1-weighted sequences and hyperintense on T2-weighted sequences in acute brucellosis, whereas nonhomogeneous signal intensity is seen in vertebral corpus on T1-weighted images in chronic brucellosis (Fig. 15.2). Spinal involvement and paravertebral and epidural abscesses are observed as hyperintense areas due to contrast agent uptake on T1-weighted images obtained following the administration of intravenous contrast agent (gadolinium) (Fig. 15.3). Therefore, using contrast agent is critical in demonstrating spinal involvement and abscess [30, 36]. Figure 15.4 is showing spondylodiscitis (arrow) complicated with epidural abscess at the T11–T12 level.

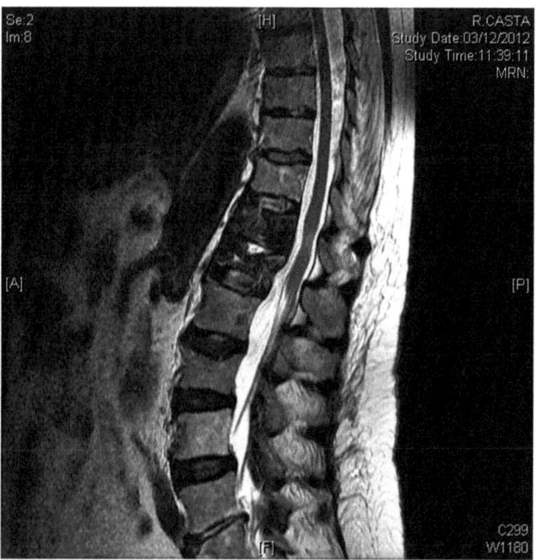

Fig. 15.2 Sagittal T2-weighted MRI reveals high signal intensity at T12 and L1, consistent with *Brucella* spondylodiscitis (Courtesy of M. Rodriguez, M.D.)

Bone scintigraphy is a sensitive method in detecting brucellosis-related bone involvement and is routinely recommended in the patients with musculoskeletal system symptoms [3, 15]. Bone scintigraphy allows early diagnosis of all osteoarticular involvements of the disease with a high sensitivity ranging from 69 to 91 % [3, 8]. In particular, an increased uptake limited to the anterior vertebral body angle strongly suggests presence of brucellosis [27].

15.2.2 Treatment

Eradication of microorganism forms the basis of treatment; however, there is no consensus on choice and duration of antibiotic therapy and surgical therapy. Antibiotic therapy for epidural spinal abscess is recommended for a long time ranging from 6 weeks to 1 year [20, 26, 29, 37, 40]. Antibiotics in the combinations used for the treatment of disease include tetracycline, rifampicin, aminoglycosides, trimethoprim-sulfamethoxazole (TMP/SMX or co-trimoxazole), and quinolones. Dual or triple antibiotic combinations are recommended in treatment. While neurological complications have initially been considered as indications for surgical intervention, surprisingly better responses to the medical therapy achieved in the recent times have made surgery to be considered as the last option [6]. Nevertheless, nerve root, spinal cord and dural compression, wide vertebral involvement, anterior abscess larger than 2.5 cm, and instability remain as the indications for early surgery [16, 21, 23].

Solera et al. [35] reported that they were successful with combined antibiotic therapy without surgical intervention in several cervical epidural abscess cases, which had the symptoms of spinal

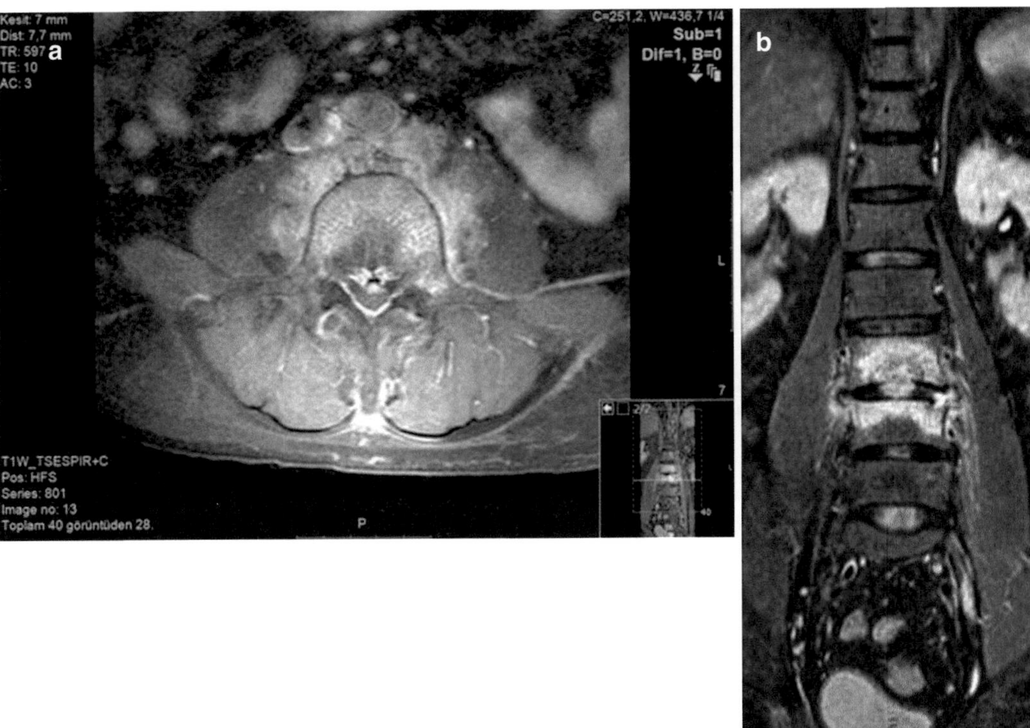

Fig. 15.3 MRI of a patient with brucellar spondylodiscitis. Axial postcontrast T1-weighted MRI (**a**) and coronal fat suppression fast spin-echo image (**b**) reveal the presence of brucellar spondylitis with involvement of neighboring disk space (Courtesy of Y. Ozsunar, M.D.)

cord compression. Pina et al. [26] reported that they achieved cure with surgical treatment performed together with antibiotherapy due to neurological worsening in 3 of 4 patients with cervical epidural abscess. Kubaao et al. [26] investigated 19 patients with epidural abscess and reported that nine cases received dual (doxycycline and rifampicin) antibiotic combination and 10 received triple (doxycycline and rifampicin and TMP/SMX or doxycycline and rifampicin and ofloxacine) antibiotic combination for a period of 4–14 months and that none of the patients required surgical intervention and end-treatment responses were good. Faria et al. [17], Özateş et al. [28], and Ugarizza et al. [41] reported that some of the patients (36 %–89 %) required surgical treatment. Reviewing the literature, it is observed that some authors initially obtained response with medical therapy, whereas some authors obtained response with surgical intervention in addition to medical therapy. Therefore, therapy choice and duration of treatment should base on the opinions of neurosurgeons, infectious disease specialists, and radiologists depending actually on the clinical condition of the patient. The patients should be closely monitored for potential adverse drug reactions and neurological complications.

Laminectomy, hemilaminectomy, inferior laminectomy, and interlaminar fenestration methods can be preferred for decompression and drainage in the patients with lumbar epidural abscess, for whom surgery is considered [14]. In thoracic epidural abscess, anterior (decompression and fusion) or posterior (decompression and instrumentation) approach can be considered according to the involvement of posterior element. In cervical epidural abscess, decompression or fusion and debridement are preferred together with anterior or posterior approach depending on the localization of abscess [21].

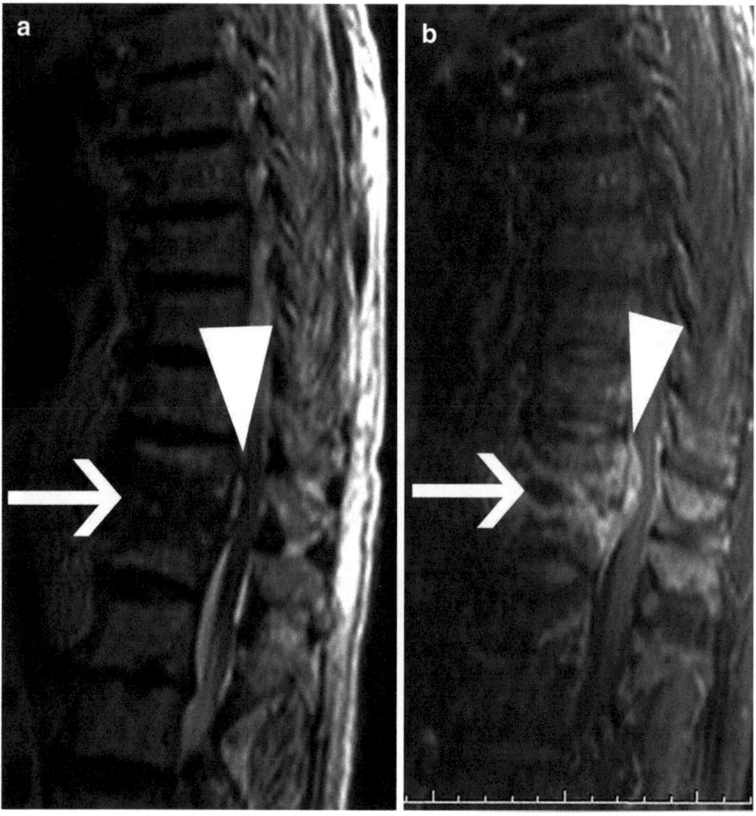

Fig. 15.4 T2-weighted sagittal MRI (**a**) and T1-weighted fat-saturated sagittal MRI after intravenous gadolinium (**b**), showing *Brucella* spondylodiscitis (*arrow*) associated with epidural abscess at the T11–T12 level (*arrowheads*)

15.3 Subdural Spinal Brucellosis

Spinal subdural abscesses are rarely encountered. Although their prevalence is unclear, there are a few cases reported in the literature. It is defined as the infection in the area between dura and arachnoid. It results from underlying immunosuppressing conditions such as alcoholism, diabetes mellitus, tumors, renal insufficiency, hemodialysis, and infectious diseases such as human immunodeficiency virus infection, as well as anatomic changes in the vertebra and spinal cord such as degenerative joint diseases, trauma, and surgery. Although its involvement is unclear, it is thought that the disease spreads by contiguity directly from the epidural space or via the blood circulation [10, 46]. Brucellosis-related subdural involvement is quite rarely seen and it is usually in the form of a case reports. Shoshan et al. [34] reported a neurobrucellosis case presenting with chronic subdural empyema. Tuncer et al. [38] also reported neurobrucellosis-related subdural hemorrhage.

15.3.1 Diagnosis

The diagnosis is made based upon the clinical, radiological, and laboratory findings together. Spinal subdural abscess clinically manifests with fever, back pain, para/tetraparesis, bladder dysfunction, loss of rectal tonus, and alterations in conscious [42]. Demonstrating the presence of *Brucella* bacterium by serological and/or culture methods is necessary. CT and MRI are used as radiological methods. Contrast-enhanced MRI is a superior scanning method in localization of the abscess as well as the spinal cord compression [43].

15.3.2 Treatment

Since brucellosis-associated subdural abscesses have been introduced as case reports, there is no consensus on its treatment. Nevertheless, surgical drainage of the abscess and long-term combined antibiotic therapy establish the basis of treatment.

Treatment should be started promptly as the disease has a high mortality and morbidity. Dual or triple medications that have antibrucellar efficacy should be used in the treatment. Surgical treatment includes laminectomy and debridement depending on the site of involvement in the cases with neurological deficit [5, 43].

Conclusion

- Brucellosis-associated epidural abscesses are rarely encountered and have high morbidity and mortality unless treated early.
- Diagnosis of epidural spinal brucellosis is made using clinical, laboratory, and radiological methods together.
- Epidural spinal abscess should necessarily be considered in newly developed neurological events with back pain in patients living in endemic regions and who have systemic symptoms of brucellosis.
- Epidural spinal abscess shows good prognosis with early diagnosis and treatment.
- Although there is response to antibiotic therapy, surgical therapy should urgently be considered in patients with signs of spinal cord compression.
- Dual or triple antibiotic combinations should be used in the medical treatment of epidural spinal abscess and the duration of antibiotic therapy should be from 6 months to 1 year.
- Brucellosis-associated subdural spinal abscesses are quite rare and have a high mortality unless treated promptly.
- The diagnosis of subdural spinal brucellosis is made on clinical, laboratory, and radiological evidence.
- Subdural spinal abscess should necessarily be considered in the presence of fever, para/tetraparesis, bladder dysfunction, loss of rectal tonus, and altered consciousness in patients living in an endemic region or having systemic symptoms of brucellosis.
- Despite the response to antibiotic therapy, surgical intervention should necessarily be considered in patients who still show signs of spinal cord compression.
- Medical treatment of subdural spinal abscess should include long-term usage of dual or triple antibiotic combination.

References

1. Al Deeb SM, Yaqub BA, Sharif HS, Phadke JG (1989) Neurobrucellosis: clinical characteristics, diagnosis, and outcome. Neurology 39:489–501
2. Alişkan H (2008) The value of culture and serological methods in the diagnosis of human brucellosis. Mikrobiyol Bul 42:185–195
3. Aydin M, Fuat Yapar A, Savas L, Reyhan M, Pourbagher A, Turunc TY, Ziya Demiroglu Y, Yologlu NA, Aktas A (2005) Scintigraphic findings in osteoarticular brucellosis. Nucl Med Commun 26:639–647
4. Aygen B, Doğanay M, Sümerkan B, Yıldız O, Kayabaş Ü (2002) Clinical manifestations, complications and treatment of brucellosis: a retrospective evaluation of 480 patients. Med Mal Infect 32:485–493
5. Bartels RH, de Jong TR, Grotenhuis JA (1992) Spinal subdural abscess. Case report. J Neurosurg 76:307–311
6. Bingöl A, Yücemen N, Meço O (1999) Medically treated intraspinal "Brucella" granuloma. Surg Neurol 52:570–576
7. Buzgan T, Karahocagil MK, Irmak H, Baran AI, Karsen H, Evirgen O, Akdeniz H (2010) Clinical manifestations and complications in 1028 cases of brucellosis: a retrospective evaluation and review of the literature. Int J Infect Dis 14:469–478
8. Chelli Bouaziz M, Ladeb MF, Chakroun M, Chaabane S (2008) Spinal brucellosis: a review. Skeletal Radiol 37:785–790
9. Colmenero JD, Reguera JM, Martos F, Sanchez-De-Mora D, Delgado M, Causse M, Martin-Farfan A, Juarez C (1996) Complications associated with Brucella melitensis infection: a study of 530 cases. Medicine (Baltimore) 75:195–211
10. Coumans JV, Walcott BP (2011) Rapidly progressive lumbar subdural empyema following acromial bursa injection. J Clin Neurosci 18:1562–1563
11. Darouiche RO, Hamill RJ, Greeberg SB, Weathers SW, Musher DM (1992) Bacterial spinal epidural abscess. Review of 43 cases and literature survey. Medicine (Baltimore) 71:369–385
12. Demirağ K, Özden M, Kalkan A, Çelik I, Kılıç SS (2002) Brucellosis: retrospective evaluation of 146 cases. Flora 7:120–125
13. Doğanay M, Meşe Alp E (2008) Brucellosis. In: Topçu AW, Söyletir G, Doğanay M (eds) Infection diseases and microbiology (in Turkish), 3rd edn. Nobel Tıp Kitabevleri, İstanbul, pp 897–909
14. Erdem M, Namiduru M, Karaoglan I, Kecik VB, Aydin A, Tanriverdi M (2012) Unusual presentation of neurobrucellosis: a solitary intracranial mass lesion

mimicking a cerebral tumor: a case of encephalitis caused by Brucella melitensis. J Infect Chemother 18:767–770

15. el-Desouki M (1991) Skeletal brucellosis: assessment with bone scintigraphy. Radiology 181:415–418
16. Tezer M, Ozturk C, Aydogan M, Camurdan K, Ertuer E, Hamzaoglu A (2006) Noncontiguous dual segment thoracic brucellosis with neurological deficit. Spine J 6:321–324
17. Faria F, Viegas F (1999) Spinal brucellosis: a personal experience of nine patients and a review of literature. Paraplegia 33:294–295
18. Gelin BG, Weiengarten K, Gamache FW Jr, Hartman BJ (1997) Epidural abscess. In: Scheld WM, Whitely RJ, Durack DT (eds) Infection of the central nervous system, 2nd edn. Lippincott-Raven Publishers, Philadelphia, pp 507–522
19. Gonzâlez-Gay MA, Garcia-Porrua C, Ibañez D, Garcia-Pais MJ (1999) Osteoarticular complications of brucellosis in an Atlantic area of Spain. J Rheumatol 26:141–145
20. Görgülü A, Albayrak BS, Görgülü E, Tural O, Karaaslan T, Oyar O, Yilmaz M (2006) Spinal epidural abscess due to Brucella. Surg Neurol 66:141–146
21. Guerado E, Cervăn AM (2012) Surgical treatment of spondylodiscitis, an update. Int Orthop 36:413–420
22. İzyi Y (2005) Lumbosacral spinal epidural abscess caused by Brucella mellitensis. Acta Neurochir (Wien) 147:1207–1209
23. Karikari IO, Powers CJ, Reynolds RM, Mehta AI, Isaac RE (2009) Management of spontaneous spinal epidural abscess: a single center 10-year experience. Neurosurgery 65:919–923
24. Kursun E, Turunc T, Demiroglu Y, Arslan H (2013) Evaluation of four hundred and forty seven brucellosis cases. Intern Med 52:745–750
25. Kurtaran B, Candevir A, Inal AS, Kõmür S, Akyıldız O, Saltoglu N, Aksu HSZ, Taşova Y (2012) Clinical appearance of brucellosis in adults: fourteen years of experience. Turk J Med Sci 42:497–505
26. Koubâa M, Mâaloul I, Marrakchi C, Lahiani D, Znazen A, Hammami B, Haddar S, Mnif Z, Hammami A, Ben Jemaa M (2013) Brucellar spinal epidural abscesses. Single center experience of nineteen patients and review of literature. Egypt Rheumatologist 35:15–20
27. Madkour MM, Sharif HS, Abed MY, Al-Fayez MA (1988) Osteoarticular brucellosis: results of bone scintigraphy in 140 patients. AJR Am J Roentgenol 150:1101–1105
28. Ozateş M, Ozkan U, Bukte Y, Ceviz A, Sari I, Simsek M (1999) Lumbar epidural brucellar abscess causing nerve root compression. Spinal Cord 37:448–449
29. Pina M, Modrego PJ, Uroz JJ, Cobeta JC, Lerin FJ, Baiges JJ (2001) Brucellar spinal epidural abscess of cervical location: report of four cases. Eur Neurol 45:249–253
30. Pourbagher A, Pourbagher MA, Savas L, Turunc T, Demiroglu YZ, Erol I, Yalcıntas D (2006) Epidemiologic, clinical, and imaging findings in brucellosis patients with osteoarticular involvement. Am J Roentgenol 187:873–880
31. Raininko RK, Aho AJ, Laine MO (1985) Computed tomography in spondylitis. CT versus other radiographic methods. Acta Orthop Scand 56:372–377
32. Shakir RA, Al-Din AS, Araj GF, Lulu AR, Mousa AR, Saadah MA (1987) Clinical categories of neurobrucellosis. A report of 19 cases. Brain 110:213–223
33. Sharif HS, Aideyan OA, Clark DC, Madkour MM, Aabed MY, Mattsson TA, al-Deeb SM, Moutaery KR (1989) Brucellar and tuberculous spondylitis: comparative imaging features. Radiology 171:419–425
34. Shoshan Y, Maayan S, Gomori MJ, Israel Z (1996) Chronic subdural empyema: a new presentation of neurobrucellosis. Clin Infect Dis 23:400–401
35. Solera J, Lozano E, Martinez-Alfaro E, Espinosa A, Castilejos ML (2000) Brucellar spondylitis: review of 35 cases and literature survey. Clin Infect Dis 29:1440–1449
36. Talı ET, Koc AM, Oner AY (2015) Spinal brucellosis. Neuroimaging Clin N Am 25:233–245
37. Tufan K, Aydemir F, Sarica FB, Kursun E, Kardes Ö, Cekinmez M, Caner H (2014) A extremely rare case of cervical intramedullary granuloma due to Brucella accompanied by Chiari Type-1 malformation. Asian J Neurosurg 9:173–176
38. Tuncer Ertem G, Tülek N, Yetkin MA (2004) Case report: subdural hemorrhage in neurobrucellosis. Mikrobiyol Bul 38:253–256
39. Turgut M, Turgut AT, Kosar U (2006) Spinal brucellosis: Turkish experience based on 452 cases published during the last century. Acta Neurochir (Wien) 148:1033–1044
40. Turgut M, Cullu E, Sendur OF, Gürer G (2004) Brucellar spine infection four case reports. Neurol Med Chir 44:562–567
41. Ugarizza LF, Porras LF, Lorenzana LM, Rodriquez-Sănchez JA, Garcia-Yagüe LM, Cabezudo JM (2005) Brucellar spinal epidural abscesses. Analysis of eleven cases. Br J Neurosurg 19:235–240
42. Ulu-Kilic A, Karakas A, Erdem H, Turker T, Inal AS, Ak O, Turan H, Kazak E, Inan A, Duygu F, Demiraslan H, Kader C, Sener A, Dayan S, Deveci O, Tekin R, Saltoglu N, Aydın M, Horasan ES, Gul HC, Ceylan B, Kadanalı A, Karabay O, Karagoz G, Kayabas U, Turhan V, Engin D, Gulsun S, Elaldı N, Alabay S (2014) Update on treatment options for spinal brucellosis. Clin Microbiol Infect 20:75–82
43. Usoltseva N, Medina-Flores R, Rehman A, Samji S, D'Costa M (2014) Spinal subdural abscess: a rare complication of decubitus ulcer. Clin Med Res 12:68–72
44. Young EJ (2005) Brucella species. In: Mandell GL, Bennet JE, Dolin R (eds) Principles and practice of infectious diseases, 6th edn. Churchill Livingstone, Philadelphia, pp 2669–2674
45. Vajramani GV, Nagmoti MB, Patil CS (2005) Neurobrucellosis presenting as an intra-medullary spinal cord abscess. Ann Clin Microbiol Antimicrob 4:14–18
46. Wu AS, Griebel RW, Meguro K, Fourney DR (2004) Spinal subdural empyema after a dural tear. Case report. Neurosurg Focus 17:1–4

16 Intramedullary Brucellosis

Erdal Kalkan, Fatih Erdi, Ahmet Tuncay Turgut, and Bülent Kaya

Contents

E. Kalkan, MD (✉) • F. Erdi, MD • B. Kaya, MD
Department of Neurosurgery,
Necmettin Erbakan University,
Meram Faculty of Medicine,
Konya, Turkey
e-mail: erdalkalkan62@yahoo.com;
mfatiherdi@hotmail.com;
drbulentkaya1977@gmail.com

A.T. Turgut, MD
Department of Radiology,
Hacettepe University School of Medicine,
Ankara, Turkey
e-mail: ahmettuncayturgut@yahoo.com

Abstract

Human neurobrucellosis has a broad spectrum of clinical manifestations depending on the stage of the infection and affected part of the nervous system. Neurobrucellosis is the second most common and severely debilitating complication of the systemic brucellosis and may occur at any stage, even years after and without the sytemic symptoms. Clinically, neurobrucellosis can present in an acute form as meningitis, meningoencephalitis, myelopathy, or neuropathy; in chronic form as granuloma, demyelinization, or degeneration; or in any combination of these. In this chapter, we analyze the etiology, physiopathology, clinical picture, diagnosis, and management of intramedullary brucellosis in detail.

Keywords

Abscess • Brucella • Granuloma • Intramedullary • Neurobrucellosis

Abbreviations

CSF	Cerebrospinal fluid
CT	Computed tomography
MRI	Magnetic resonance imaging
PET/CT	Positron emission tomography combined with computed tomography

M. Turgut et al. (eds.), *Neurobrucellosis: Clinical, Diagnostic and Therapeutic Features*,
DOI 10.1007/978-3-319-24639-0_16

16.1 Introduction

The exact pathogenesis of neurobrucellosis is not well enlightened and has some controversies. *Brucella* have some direct or indirect effects by its endotoxins on the central nervous system [7]. Spinal cord or nerve root may secondarily be affected due to spondylitis, vasculitis, or arachnoiditis [3]. Primary intramedullary brucellosis is exceptionally infrequent and includes intramedullary abscesses and granulomas [1].

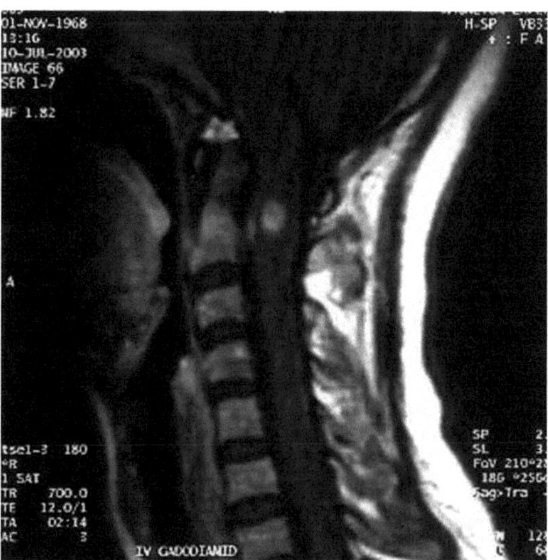

Fig. 16.1 T1-weighted sagittal cervical MRI shows homogenously contrast-enhanced intramedullary lesion with regular shape at the C2 level (From Nas et al. [10], with permission)

16.2 Diagnosis

Regardless of their etiology, intramedullary spinal cord abscesses and granulomas are rare but potentially harmful lesions. They can lead to undesirable, sometimes irreversible neurological problems. While they have no specific symptomatology or clinical findings, the only way for accurate and early diagnosis is a high index of suspicion [6, 10].

Plain radiographs, computed tomography (CT), scintigraphic techniques, and magnetic resonance imaging (MRI) can all be used in the diagnosis. Plain radiographic evaluation generally provides little information. CT and/or MRI can provide useful anatomic and topographic confirmation of lesions involving the spine and more accurate localization of intraspinal intramedullary and paraspinal infestation by means of multiplanar images as well as planning of medical and surgical treatment of brucellosis [13, 14, 18].

Advances in the imaging field have produced successful results in the diagnosis of brucellosis. Improved CT (such as diffusion/perfusion studies) and MRI (such as fluid-attenuated inversion recovery modalities) have enabled improved sensitivity in detecting both bone and soft tissue lesions [4].

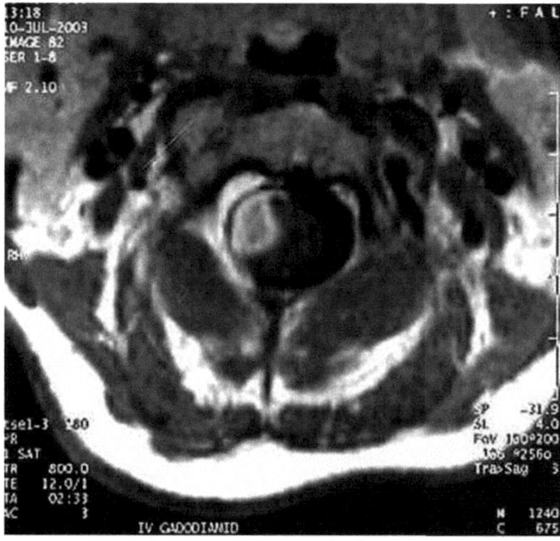

Fig. 16.2 T1-weighted axial MRI scan shows the same lesion which was located on the right side of spinal cord intramedullary and extending to epidural space (From Nas et al. [10], with permission)

Radiologically, MRI findings may differ in a wide spectrum from mild/diffuse edema and swelling with mild or no contrast enhancement to marked edema and abscess formation with diffuse, patchy, or ring enhancement consistent with the stage of the infection (Figs. 16.1 and 16.2) [10, 14]. Intramedullary high signal intensities, expansion of the cord, and necrotic center are well seen on T2-weighted images. The MRI findings of granulomatous myelitis are similar to intracranial tuberculomas [14]. Focal spinal cord swelling, high-signal edema, and low-signal nodular lesion ("tuberculoma") on T2-weighted images and nodular contrast enhancement on T1-weighted images are among the frequently detected radiological findings. Intramedullary tumors may simulate spinal cord granulomas. The fusiform dilatation of the cord and the pattern of enhancement are the shared imaging characteristics among these entities [13]. MRI with gadolinium contrast (Figs. 16.1 and 16.2) seems to be the modality of choice [10, 14]. Sensitivity of MRI varies between 91 and 100 % [5, 13, 14].

Positron emission tomography combined with computed tomography (PET/CT) scan can provide additional information on the spread of brucellar spondylitis. The efficacy of treatment and the need for further antimicrobial chemotherapy could be assessed with PET/CT [8].

16.3 Incidence

Previously reported available cases of intramedullary brucellosis in the English literature are summarized in Table 16.1. As shown in Table 16.1, systemic brucellosis was present in all cases suffering from intramedullary involvement [1, 2, 6, 7, 9–11, 14, 15, 19]. The reported lesions were generally abscesses except three cases [1, 14, 15]. The most common site for involvement was the thoracic and upper cervical spinal cord. Keihani-Douste et al. [9] reported a case of multilevel cervicothoracic spinal cord lesion with concurrent multiple brain abscesses. Isolated cervical intramedullary involvement was reported by Nas et al. [10], Hendam et al. [7], Tufan et al. [15], and Talı et al. [14]. *Brucella abortus* and *B. melitensis* were the identified pathogens in all the available cases. Blood serology was positive in all cases except the cases of Cokca et al. [2] and Talı et al. [14].

16.4 Treatment

In some cases with intramedullary brucellosis, the symptoms of neurobrucellosis may resolve spontaneously in the ordinary course of the

Table 16.1 Previously reported cases of intramedullary neurobrucellosis

Authors/year	Patient age/sex	Type/location of the lesion	Pus culture	Blood culture	Serology	Treatment	Systemic disease
Cokca et al. [2], 1994	17/M	Abscess/ T11–L2	*B abortus*	*B. abortus*	?	Surgical + medical	Present
Bingol et al. [1],1999	40/F	Granuloma/T5	Not done	No growth	+	Medical	Present
Novati et al. [11], 2002	24/M	Abscess/T3	Not done	*B. melitensis*	+	Medical	Present
Helvaci et al. [6], 2002	15/F	Abscess/ T11–T12	No growth	No growth	+	Surgical + medical	Present
Vajramani et al. [18], 2005	40/F	Abscess/conus medullaris	*B. melitensis*	*B. melitensis*	+	Surgical + medical	Present
Keihani-Douste et al. [9], 2006	12/M	Abscess/C1–L4	Not done	?	+	Surgical + medical	Present
Nas et al. [10], 2007	45/F	Abscess/ C1-2	Not done	Not done	+	Medical	Present
Hendam et al. [7], 2014	57/F	Abscess/C4–C5	Not done	Not done	+	Medical	Present
Tufan et al. [15], 2014	19/M	Granuloma/C2	Not done	Not done	+	Medical	Present
Talı et al. [14], 2015	NS	Granuloma/C4	NS	NS	NS	NS	NS

NS not stated

disease. Nevertheless, there is no guarantee that spontaneous resolution will occur, and it may take a long period of time [1].

In the current literature, the management strategies of intramedullary brucellosis vary. Bingöl et al. [1], Novati et al. [11], Nas et al. [10], and Hendam et al. [7] were treated and followed their cases with medical treatment. Bingöl et al. [1] indicated the suprisingly well response of *Brucella* abscess to antibiotics. The duration of antibiotherapy is variable and it depends mainly on the type of lesion ("granuloma" or "abscess") or presence of surgical drainage and the patient's response to treatment. On the other hand, the reported time ranges vary from 3 months to a few years.

High relapsing rate is the most important issue for short-length antibiotic usage. In the literature, relapse rate of brucellar spondylitis varies between 4 and 55 % [12]. While there is no study investigating the relapsing rate and outcomes of intramedullary brucellosis, complete resolution or clinically stabilization of related symptoms with biochemical and cellular normalization of the cerebrospinal fluid (CSF) content and lowering of the CSF antibody levels could be accepted as the criteria for stopping therapy. Extending the therapy from 18 to 24 months was advocated previously [1]. The optimal duration of treatment remains a controversial issue. Serology and imaging are not always helpful, as residual MRI findings are present long after successful treatment [5, 13].

Ioannou et al. [8] reported a significant decrease in maximum standardized uptake values in successfully treated brucellar spondylodiscitis cases. Thus, they stated that PET/CT scan may be a complementary method to MRI for determining the efficacy of treatment and the need for further antimicrobial chemotherapy [8].

Antibiotics such as doxycycline, rifampicin, and trimethoprim-sulfamethoxazole have been advocated for their good blood-brain barrier penetrance and synergistic actions [15–19]. Streptomycin and ceftriaxone could be added to this regimen [6, 19].

Surgical drainage by myelotomy after laminectomy could be reserved for intramedullary abscess rather than granuloma formation. Progressive neurological impairment, inadequate response to antibiotics with evident spinal cord edema, and an absolute indication for the obtention of tissue sampling were reported as surgical indications [12, 19].

Importantly, the location of the lesion and the general medical status of the patient are crucial factors for considering to operate an intramedullary abscess, like all other neurosurgical interventions [17].

As most of these patients have systemic brucellosis as well, they should undergo an antibiotherapy postoperatively, especially in the initial stages. It should be noted that appropriate surgical intervention has an additional benefit, namely, reducing the duration of antibiotic usage [19].

According to some authors, the operation for intramedullary brucellar abscess may be a last resort decision due to the surprisingly good response of the disease to antibiotics. Bingöl et al. [1] believe that almost half of the abscesses are asymptomatic and will resolve with antibiotics. Nevertheless, there are some who are against this point of view. Vajramani et al. [19] concluded that neurosurgical drainage with antibiotics usually results in resolution of the infection. Based on their experience, early intervention could prevent the neurological disability and improve functional outcome [19]. The authors of this chapter advise to act depending on each individual cases.

As a rule, corticosteroid usage should be considered in these cases initially, especially if edema is present in radiological studies [19]. It is speculated that corticosteroids seem to have effects on tissue protection from bacterial toxins and antigenic stimulations and reduces long-term complications [6]. Lastly, it is important to know that prolonged follow-up is necessary in all patients with spinal brucellosis including intramedullary ones [16].

Conclusion

- Intramedullary brucellosis is a rare, but severe infection of the spinal cord.
- A high index of suspicion is crucial for early diagnosis and to prevent significant

morbidity and mortality associated with this disease.

- Expeditious diagnosis and appropriate medical and surgical treatment can lead to a satisfactory outcome in these patients.
- Intramedullary brucellosis must be considered in the differential diagnosis of spinal lesions, particularly in endemic countries.
- It is important to know that an early correct intervention could prevent the harmful effects of neurobrucellosis involving the spinal cord and the neurological disability due to its complications.

References

1. Bingöl A, Yücemen N, Meço O (1999) Medically treated intraspinal "Brucella" granuloma. Surg Neurol 52:570–576
2. Cokça F, Meço O, Arasil E, Unlu A (1994) An intramedullary dermoid cyst abscess due to Brucella abortus biotype 3 at T11-L2 spinal levels. Infection 22:359–360
3. al Deeb SM, Yaqub BA, Sharif HS, Phadke JC (1989) Neurobrucellosis: clinical characteristics, diagnosis, and outcome. Neurology 39:498–501
4. Franco MP, Mulder M, Gilman RH, Smits HL (2007) Human brucellosis. Lancet Infect Dis 7:775–786
5. Harman M, Unal O, Onbaşi KT, Kiymaz N, Arslan H (2001) Brucellar spondylodiscitis: MRI diagnosis. Clin Imaging 25:421–427
6. Helvaci M, Kasirga E, Cetin N, Yaprak I (2002) Intramedullary spinal cord abscess suspected of Brucella infection. Pediatr Int 44:446–448
7. Hendam AT, Barayan SS, Anazi AH Al (2014) Cervical intramedullary brucellosis: a case report. Neurosurg Q 24:203–206
8. Ioannou S, Chatziioannou S, Pneumaticos SG, Zormpala A, Sipsas NV (2013) Fluorine-18 fluoro-2-deoxy-D-glucose positron emission tomography/computed tomography scan contributes to the diagnosis and management of brucellar spondylodiskitis. BMC Infect Dis 13:73
9. Keihani-Douste Z, Daneshjou K, Ghasemi M (2006) A quadriplegic child with multiple brain abscesses: case report of neurobrucellosis. Med Sci Monit 12:119–122
10. Nas K, Tasdemir N, Cakmak E, Kemaloglu MS, Bukte Y, Geyik MF (2007) Cervical intramedullary granuloma of Brucella: a case report and review of the literature. Eur Spine J 16(Suppl 3):2559
11. Novati R, Viganò MG, de Bona A, Nocita B, Finazzi R, Lazzarin A (2002) Neurobrucellosis with spinal cord abscess of the dorsal tract: a case report. Int J Infect Dis 6:149–150
12. Solera J, Lozano E, Martinez-Alfaro E, Espinosa A, Castillejos ML, Abad L (1999) Brucellar spondylitis: review of 35 cases and literature survey. Clin Infect Dis 29:1440–1449
13. Tali ET, Gültekin S (2005) Spinal infections. Eur Radiol 15:599–607
14. Talı ET, Koc AM, Oner AY (2015) Spinal brucellosis. Neuroimaging Clin N Am 25:233–245
15. Tufan K, Aydemir F, Sarica FB, Kursun E, Kardes Ö, Cekinmez M, Caner H (2014) A extremely rare case of cervical intramedullary granuloma due to Brucella accompanied by Chiari type 1 malformation. Asian J Neurosurg 9:173–176
16. Turgut M, Cullu E, Sendur OF, Güyrer G (2004) Brucellar spine infection-four case reports. Neurol Med Chir (Tokyo) 44:562–567
17. Turgut M, Sendur OF, Gürel M (2003) Brucellar spondylodiscitis in the lumbar region. Neurol Med Chir (Tokyo) 43:210–212
18. Turgut M, Turgut AT, Koşar U (2006) Spinal brucellosis: Turkish experience based on 452 cases published during the last century. Acta Neurochir (Wien) 148:1033–1044
19. Vajramani GV, Nagmoti MB, Patil CS (2005) Neurobrucellosis presenting as an intra-medullary spinal cord abscess. Ann Clin Microbiol Antimicrob 4:14

Part IV

Peripheral and Cranial Nerves

Brucella Polyradiculoneuritis

17

Farhad Abbasi, Soolmaz Korooni,
and Ahmet Tuncay Turgut

Contents

Abstract

Brucella polyradiculopathy is a rare manifestation of neurobrucellosis. Polyradiculopathy usually gradually progress and cause numbness and muscle weakness in extremities. Patients may present with pain, sensory abnormality, weakness of the extremities, and gate abnormality. Neurobrucellosis is diagnosed according to signs and symptoms, using laboratory tests including serology and imaging. Magnetic resonance imaging with gadolinium injection usually shows enhancement of lumbar nerve roots in *Brucella* polyradiculopathy. For confirmation of polyradiculopathy, nerve conduction studies and electromyography examination are used. Treatment of *Brucella* polyradiculopathy is not different from that of neurobrucellosis. The most common medications used for the treatment are rifampicin, trimethoprim-sulfamethoxazole, doxycycline, ceftriaxone, ciprofloxacin, and streptomycin. Clinical features of the patients guide the physician for duration of treatment. Prompt diagnosis without delay in treatment is associated with fewer sequelae and excellent prognosis.

Keywords

Brucellosis • Neurobrucellosis • Polyradiculopathy • Polyradiculoneuritis

F. Abbasi, MD (✉)
Department of Infectious Diseases,
Bushehr University of Medical Sciences,
Bushehr, Iran
e-mail: f_abbasi55@yahoo.com

S. Korooni, MD
Department of Internal Medicine,
Bushehr University of Medical Sciences,
Bushehr, Iran
e-mail: s_korooni62@yahoo.com

A.T. Turgut, MD
Department of Radiology,
Hacettepe University School of Medicine,
Ankara, Turkey
e-mail: ahmettuncayturgut@yahoo.com

M. Turgut et al. (eds.), *Neurobrucellosis: Clinical, Diagnostic and Therapeutic Features*,
DOI 10.1007/978-3-319-24639-0_17

Abbreviations

CNS	Central nervous system
CSF	Cerebrospinal fluid
EMG	Electromyography
MRI	Magnetic resonance imaging
NCV	Nerve conduction velocity
PNS	Peripheral nervous system

17.1 Introduction

Brucella infection rarely involves the central nervous system (CNS) with different clinical manifestations [2, 16, 21, 30]. Presentation may be with depression, encephalitis, meningitis, brain abscess, convulsion, cranial nerve palsy, subarachnoid hemorrhage, and decreased level of consciousness [19]. Brucellosis may affect the peripheral nervous system (PNS) with a variety of signs and symptoms [27]. Neurologic involvement due to brucellosis was reported in 1.7–10 % of the patients with brucellosis [8, 11, 25].

Complications of neurobrucellosis may be due to the acute-febrile phase of the diseases or may be due to the toxic-febrile phase, i.e., those related to primary involvement of CNS or PNS by the *Brucella* bacteria. Involvement of the CNS is commonly acute and presents as meningitis or encephalitis. Involvement of the PNS mainly present as polyradiculoneuritis [6]. Neurobrucellosis may affect any part of the CNS and PNS and present as any neurological disease [18]. Neurobrucellosis presentations are myelitis, myelopathy, paraplegia, radiculoneuritis, intracerebral abscess, epidural abscess, intradural abscess, demyelination, Guillain-Barré syndrome, polyneuritis, and cranial nerve palsy [7, 8, 10, 11, 16, 30]. Shehata et al. [26] demonstrated that CNS involvement was detected in 33 % of patients and PNS involvement was seen in 22 % of patients. In some cases, however, combined involvement of both CNS and PNS may occur simultaneously [4].

17.2 Clinical Manifestations

Clinical manifestations of neurobrucellosis are categorized as central and peripheral involvement. Peripheral involvements include neuropathy or radiculopathy. Central involvements include meningitis, cranial nerve palsy, and encephalitis [24].

Clinical manifestation of neurobrucellosis may be due to direct effect of microorganism on the nervous system or may be due to indirect effect with immune mechanisms that eventually lead to neuropathy. In animal model, anti-GM1 ganglioside antibodies are found to be produced in the response to ganglioside-like molecules of *Brucella*. These antibodies can cause flaccid weakness and ataxia-like symptoms.

Neurobrucellosis may present as meningoencephalitis, polyradiculoneuropathy, or both. The main presentation of the peripheral form is polyradiculoneuropathy and the main presentation of the central form is meningoencephalitis [17]. *Brucella* involvement of the spine has no specific manifestation. It may be due to an abscess or granuloma with compression effect on the spinal cord [24]. Polyradiculopathy is one of the rare clinical manifestations of brucellosis.

Brucellosis may affect the CNS and PNS via direct effects of microorganisms or indirect effect by toxin or cytokines. So the presentation may differ ranging from acute illness to chronic form [13]. Polyradiculopathy usually gradually progress and cause sensory and motor weakness in upper and lower limbs [20]. Patients may present with pain, sensory loss and weakness of the limbs, and difficulty of walking [13] but usually present with weakness of the lower extremities [5]. Spinal root involvement presents as lower motor neuron diseases [3]. Magnetic resonance imaging (MRI) is a useful imaging modality for the diagnosis of spinal root involvement. Spinal root involvement and subsequence polyradiculopathy are similar to other neurological diseases [17]. Radiculopathy is probably due to inflammation of the meninges and the intrathecal portion of the roots. The pathogenesis of myelopathy may involve demyelination as spasticity persists or worsens after radiculopathy improves [5]. Neurobrucellosis may present as Guillain-Barré-like syndrome with bilateral polyradiculopathy without sensory involvement [3]. Neurobrucellosis may be manifest as recurrent transverse myelitis. Immune system response and recurrent transverse myelitis due to neurobrucellosis has been reported. Krishnan et al. [22] reported a patient with four episodes of transverse myelitis that lead to quadriplegia.

Brucella antibody was detected from his cerebrospinal fluid (CSF). High level of interleukin-6, IL-8, and macrophage chemoattractant protein-1 in CSF was detected. The patient responded to intravenous cyclophosphamide and plasma exchange [22]. Neurobrucellosis symptoms may last 8 weeks before diagnosis, ranging from 1 week to 4 months [6]. The recovery from neurobrucellosis may be accompanied by some sequelae. Paraparesis, dementia, sphincter dysfunction, and peripheral facial paralysis may occur [10].

17.3 Diagnosis

Brucellosis polyradiculopathy is often diagnosed by its neurological manifestations, laboratory tests, and imaging [9]. Neurobrucellosis is a treatable disease. Most of the diagnostic methods may reveal negative results. That is why high index of suspicion is necessary for the diagnosis of neurobrucellosis especially in endemic areas [1]. Clinical suspicion and accurate evaluation of patients with polyradiculoneuritis is the most important clue in diagnosis and treatment [14]. Early diagnosis is essential to prevent severe and permanent complications and sequelae of nerve roots [2, 8, 24]. *Brucella* tube agglutination with Coombs test is sensitive and specific. Enzyme-linked immunosorbent assay is considered superior to the agglutination tests [9]. Blood culture is not a useful laboratory test for diagnosis of *Brucella* polyradiculopathy. It takes a long time for results; moreover the results are usually negative [28]. In Erdem et al.'s study [12], blood culture was positive for brucellosis in 37 % by automated method and CSF culture was positive in 25 % and 9 % by automated and conventional CSF culture, respectively. Clinical and radiologic correlations are necessary. It may have a range from a normal imaging of a patient with severe clinical manifestation to imaging abnormality with or without significant clinical finding (Figs. 17.1 and 17.2) [4]. MRI of the spine may reveal swelling of the nerve root that may be enhanced by the use of gadolinium [20]. Diagnosis of *Brucella* polyradiculopathy or polyradiculoneuritis can be achieved by CSF analysis, laboratory tests including serology, electromyography (EMG) and nerve conduction velocity (NCV) examinations, and correlation with clinical manifestations [13]. MRI with gadolinium injection usually shows enhancement of the lumbar nerve root [5]. For confirmation of polyradiculopathy, NCV studies and EMG

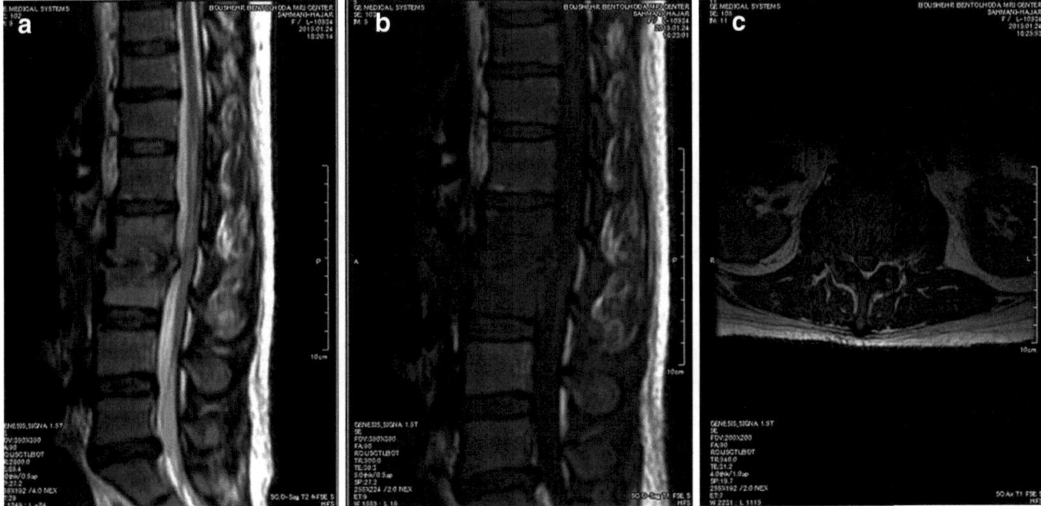

Fig. 17.1 A 35-year-old woman with numbness of lower extremity. (**a**) Sagittal T2-weighted MRI scan shows loss of low signal intensity of the cortical end plates and high signal in disk space and herniated disk. (**b**) T1-weighted MRI depicts loss of low signal intensity of the cortical end plates, destruction of the intervertebral disk space and end plates and decreased signal intensity in L1–L2 vertebral bodies. (**c**) Axial T1-weighted MRI shows end plates with decreased signal intensity and high signal intensity in paravertebral soft tissues

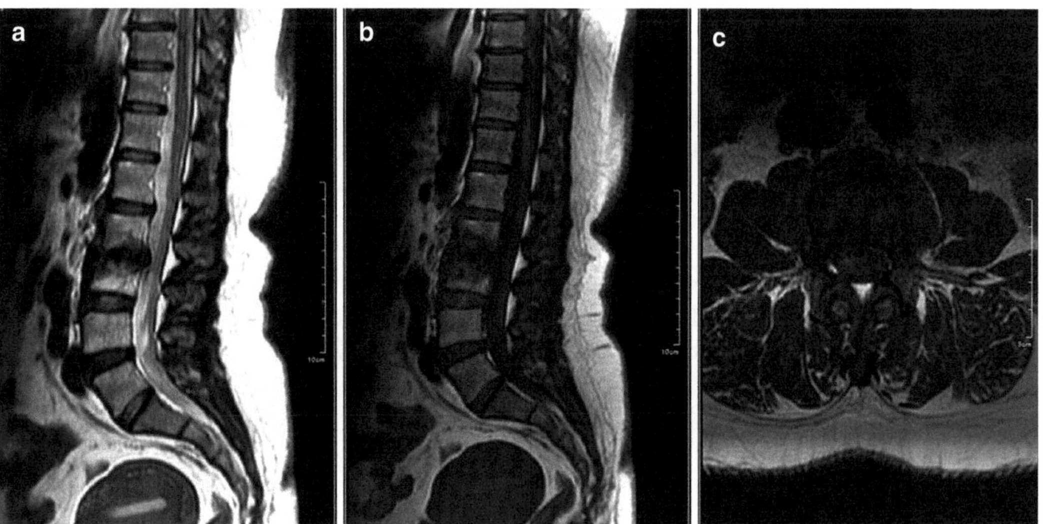

Fig. 17.2 A 41-year-old woman with pain and weakness of lower extremity. (**a**) Sagittal T2-weighted MRI shows intervertebral disk with decreased signal intensity. (**b**) T1-weighted MRI reveals destruction of the intervertebral disk space and end plates and decreased signal intensity in L2–L3 vertebral bodies. (**c**) Axial T1-weighted MRI depicts end plates with decreased signal intensity

examination are used. Prolonged F waves, decreased NCVs and amplitude, and paraspinal muscle denervation potentials may be seen by NCV and EMG study [13].

17.4 Treatment

As polyradiculoneuritis is one manifestation of neurobrucellosis, the treatment is the same as neurobrucellosis. Polyradiculoneuritis should be diagnosed and managed promptly. It may cause permanent and irreversible sequelae with diagnosis or treatment delay [29]. Treatment of polyradiculoneuritis may be a combination of doxycycline, rifampicin, trimethoprim/sulfamethoxazole, ciprofloxacin, ceftriaxone, and streptomycin. Duration of therapy varies in different studies, most of them recommend at least 3 months treatment [5, 23]. Duration of treatment ranging from several weeks to several months depends on patient's condition; it may be shortened to 12 weeks if rapid improvement occurs. According to Gül et al.'s study [18], duration of therapy is 6 months with combination antibiotic therapy, in spite of the fact that the therapy should be individualized. In contrast in Asadipouya et al.'s study from Iran [6], duration of treatment was as short as 8 weeks in about half of the patients. Corticosteroids are not proven to be useful on localized brucellosis [13]. Moreover, rehabilitation should also be a part of the treatment in brucellosis polyradiculopathy [15].

Conclusion

Diagnosis of *Brucella* polyradiculoneuritis needs a high index of suspicion [9]. In patients with polyradiculoneuritis, brucellosis should be considered in the differential diagnosis especially in endemic areas. That may lead to early diagnosis and treatment [13], and in this situation the prognosis will be excellent. Some items will correlate closely with prognosis that includes duration of illness, *Brucella* spp. virulence, timing between diagnosis and starting antibiotic, and duration of antibiotic therapy [6].

References

1. Adeva-Bartolomé MT, Montes-Martínez I, Castellanos-Pinedo F, Zurdo-Hernández JM, de Castro-García FJ (2005) Neurobrucellosis: four case reports. Rev Neurol 41:664–666

2. Ahmed R, Patil BS (2009) Neurobrucellosis: a rare cause for spastic paraparesis. Braz J Infect Dis 13:245
3. Alshareef AA (2009) Case report of polyradiclopathy, hearing loss, and ataxia as presentation of neurobrucellosis. JKAU Med Sci 16:85–92
4. Al-Sous MW, Bohlega S, Al-Kawi MZ, Alwatban J, McLean DR (2004) Neurobrucellosis: clinical and neuroimaging correlation. AJNR Am J Neuroradiol 25:395–401
5. Al-Sous MW, Bohlega SA, Al-Kawi MZ, McLean DR, Ghaus SN (2003) Polyradiculopathy. A rare complication of neurobrucellosis. Neurosciences (Riyadh) 8:46–49
6. Asadipooya K, Dehghanian A, Omrani GH, Abbasi F (2011) Short-course treatment in neurobrucellosis: a study in Iran. Neurol India 59:101–103
7. Babamahmoodi F, Babamahmoodi A (2011) Brucellosis, presenting with Guillain-Barré syndrome. J Glob Infect Dis 3:390–392
8. Baykal T, Baygutalp F, Senel K, Levent A, Erdal A, Ugur M, Ozgocmen S (2012) Spastic paraparesis and sensorineural hearing loss in a patient with neurobrucellosis. J Back Musculoskelet Rehabil 25: 157–159
9. Budnik I, Fuchs I, Shelef I, Krymko H, Greenberg D (2012) Unusual presentations of pediatric neurobrucellosis. Am J Trop Med Hyg 86:258–260
10. Demiroğlu YZ, Turunç T, Karaca S, Arlıer Z, Alışkan H, Colakoğlu S, Arslan H (2011) Neurological involvement in brucellosis; clinical classification, treatment and results. Mikrobiyol Bul 45:401–410
11. Elzein FE, Mursi M (2014) Case report: Brucella induced Guillain-Barré syndrome. Am J Trop Med Hyg 91:1179–1180
12. Erdem H, Kilic S, Sener B, Acikel C, Alp E, Karahocagil M, Yetkin F, Inan A, Kecik Bosnak V, Gul HC, Tekin-Koruk S, Ceran N, Demirdal T, Yilmaz G, Ulu-Kilic A, Ceylan B, Dogan-Celik A, Nayman-Alpat S, Tekin R, Yalci A, Turhan V, Karaoglan I, Yilmaz H, Mete B, Batirel A, Ulcay A, Dayan S, Seza Inal A, Ahmed SS, Tufan ZK, Karakas A, Teker B, Namiduru M, Savasci U, Pappas G (2013) Diagnosis of chronic brucellar meningitis and meningoencephalitis: the results of the Istanbul-2 study. Clin Microbiol Infect 19:E80–E86
13. Ertem G, Kutlu G, Hatipoglu ÇA, Bulut C, Demirz AP (2012) A rare presentation of brucellosis: polyradiculopathy and peripheral neuritis. Turk J Med Sci 42:359–364
14. Faraji F, Didgar F, Talaie-Zanjani A, Mohammadbeigi A (2013) Uncontrolled seizures resulting from cerebral venous sinus thrombosis complicating neurobrucellosis. J Neurosci Rural Pract 4:313–316
15. Goktepe AS, Alaca R, Mohur H, Coskun U (2003) Neurobrucellosis and a demonstration of its involvement in spinal roots via magnetic resonance imaging. Spinal Cord 41:574–576
16. Guenifi W, Rais M, Gasmi A, Ouyahia A, Boukhrissa H, Mechakra S, Houari M, Nouasria B, Lacheheb A (2010) Neurobrucellosis: description of 5 cases in Setif Hospital Algeria. Med Trop 70:309–310
17. Gul HC, Erdem H, Bek S (2009) Overview of neurobrucellosis: a pooled analysis of 187 cases. Int J Infect Dis 13:e339–e343
18. Gul HC, Erdem H, Gorenek L, Ozdag MF, Kalpakci Y, Avci IY, Besirbellioglu BA, Eyigun CP (2008) Management of neurobrucellosis: an assessment of 11 cases. Intern Med 47:995–1001
19. Hadda V, Khilnani GC, Kedia S (2009) Brucellosis presenting as pyrexia of unknown origin in an international traveller: a case report. Cases J 2:7969
20. Ishibashi M, Kimura N, Takahashi Y, Kimura Y, Hazama Y, Kumamoto T (2011) A case of neurosarcoidosis with swelling and gadolinium enhancement of spinal nerve roots on magnetic resonance imaging. Rinsho Shinkeigaku 51:483–486
21. Kanik-Yüksek S, Gülhan B, Ozkaya-Parlakay A, Tezer H (2014) A case of childhood brucellosis with neurological involvement and epididymo-orchitis. J Infect Dev Ctries 8:1636–1638
22. Krishnan C, Kaplin AI, Graber JS, Darman JS, Kerr DA (2005) Recurrent transverse myelitis following neurobrucellosis: immunologic features and beneficial response to immunosuppression. J Neurovirol 11:225–231
23. Koussa S, Tohmé A, Ghayad E, Nasnas R, El Kallab K, Chemaly R (2003) Neurobrucellosis: clinical features and therapeutic responses in 15 patients. Rev Neurol (Paris) 159:1148–1155
24. Nas K, Tasdemir N, Cakmak E, Kemaloglu MS, Bukte Y, Geyik MF (2007) Cervical intramedullary granuloma of Brucella: a case report and review of the literature. Eur Spine J 16(Suppl 3):S255–S259
25. Ozkavukcu E, Tuncay Z, Selçuk F, Erden I (2009) An unusual case of neurobrucellosis presenting with unilateral abducens nerve palsy: clinical and MRI findings. Diagn Interv Radiol 15:236–238
26. Shehata GA, Abdel-Baky L, Rashed H, Elamin H (2010) Neuropsychiatric evaluation of patients with brucellosis. J Neurovirol 16:48–55
27. Tajdini M, Akbarloo S, Hosseini SM, Parvizi B, Baghani S, Aghamollaii V, Tafakhori A (2014) From a simple chronic headache to neurobrucellosis: a case report. Med J Islam Repub Iran 28:12
28. Trifiletti RR, Restivo DA, Pavone P, Giuffrida S, Parano E (2000) Diabetes insipidus in neurobrucellosis. Clin Neurol Neurosurg 102:163–165
29. Ulu-Kilic A, Karakas A, Erdem H, Turker T, Inal AS, Ak O, Turan H, Kazak E, Inan A, Duygu F, Demiraslan H, Kader C, Sener A, Dayan S, Deveci O, Tekin R, Saltoglu N, Aydın M, Horasan ES, Gul HC, Ceylan B, Kadanalı A, Karabay O, Karagoz G, Kayabas U, Turhan V, Engin D, Gulsun S, Elaldı N, Alabay S (2014) Update on treatment options for spinal brucellosis. Clin Microbiol Infect 20:75–82
30. Vajramani GV, Nagmoti MB, Patil CS (2005) Neurobrucellosis presenting as an intramedullary spinal cord abscess. Ann Clin Microbiol Antimicrob 4:14

Cranial Nerve Involvement in Brucellosis

18

Hakim Irfan Showkat, Basharat Mujtaba Jan, Arif Hussain Sarmast, Sadaf Anwar, Rouf Asimi, and Gull Mohammad Bhat

Contents

Abstract

Brucellosis is one of the common zoonotic infectious diseases in the world. It may involve all organs and systems. However, the central nervous system is unusually rarely involved. Meningitis is most frequently observed in neurobrucellosis and is associated with many complications like cranial nerve (CN) paralysis, meningoencephalitis, myelitis, radiculopathy, and neuropathy. Because of basal meningitis, one or more CN involvement is seen in more than 50 % of the patients with neurobrucellosis. Besides neurobrucellosis, causes of CN palsies in cases of brucellosis are pseudotumor cerebri and adverse reactions of tetracyclines which are used in the treatment of brucellosis.

Keywords

Brucellosis • Cranial nerve • Meningitis • Palsy • Radiculopathy

Abbreviations

CN	Cranial nerve
CNS	Central nervous system
CSF	Cerebrospinal fluid
ELISA	Enzyme-linked immunosorbent assay
PCR	Polymerase chain reaction

H.I. Showkat, MBBCh, MD, DNB (✉)
S. Anwar, MBBCh, PGDCC
Department of Cardiology, National Heart Institute New Delhi, New Delhi 110065, India
e-mail: docirfanshahi512@gmail.com; dr.sadaf4u@gmail.com

B.M. Jan, MS • A.H. Sarmast, MS
Department of Neurosurgery, SKIMS Kashmir, Kashmir 190001, India
e-mail: shahqul@yahoo.com; arifhsarmast@gmail.com

R. Asimi, MD, DM
Department of Neurology, SKIMS Kashmir, Kashmir 190001, India
e-mail: ravoufasimi@yahoo.co.in

G.M. Bhat, MD, DM
Department of Medical Oncology, SKIMS Kashmir, Kashmir 190001, India
e-mail: gmbhat@gmail.com

M. Turgut et al. (eds.), *Neurobrucellosis: Clinical, Diagnostic and Therapeutic Features*,
DOI 10.1007/978-3-319-24639-0_18

18.1 Introduction

Brucellosis is a chronic disease with varied clinical features [2, 9, 16, 30]. Neurobrucellosis occurs in 4–13 % of cases of brucellosis and involves the central (CNS) or peripheral nervous system [24, 25]. Neurological involvement may be the only presentation of focal chronic brucellosis [18]. The presence of neurobrucellosis in the acute stage may be due to direct harmful effects of bacteria invading the nervous tissues, with the existence of circulating endotoxins, or inflammatory and immunologic reactions of the host within the nervous system of the body.

Diffuse neurological syndrome of brucellosis, myelitis presents with backache, spastic paraparesis, and demyelination at any part in the CNS, including the spinal cord and cerebral white matter, as well as cerebellar dysfunction. Furthermore, mycotic aneurysms, ischemic strokes, and subarachnoid hemorrhage, intracerebral hemorrhage, subthalamic hemorrhage, and cerebral venous thrombosis are seen as meningovascular complications of neurobrucellosis [3, 6, 18, 23]. Moreover, it may present with Guillain-Barre syndrome [20], intracranial hypertension [22, 29], posterior fossa abscess [28], diabetes insipidus [31], subdural hemorrhage [32], pituitary abscess [11], and cerebral venous thrombosis [33].

Brucellosis in the acute may be associated with cranial nerve (CN) involvement that may resolve fully with the use of antibiotic treatment, while those with neurological infection usually have sequel neurologic deficits. They are best divided into (1) those seen with radiculopathy or peripheral neuropathy and (2) those seen with more diffuse CNS involvement with myelitis, with CN involvement and a syndrome of parenchymatous dysfunction [9, 18]. Symptoms of the radiculopathy and peripheral neuropathy are usually consist of back pain, loss of reflex activity, and paraparesis with proximal nerve radicular involvement.

18.2 Cranial Nerve Involvement

Neurobrucellosis may have CN involvement and are diagnosed based on laboratory parameters, especially serological ones. The diagnosis of neurobrucellosis may be positive even when tests are negative for serology and cerebrospinal fluid (CSF) culture [7] and is mainly on clinical response and response of CSF tests if abnormal with anti-*Brucella* treatment.

Around 50 % of cases with *Brucella* meningitis may show signs of meningeal irritation [18]. How the bacteria enters the CNS is not clear, but it has been postulated that bacteria may reach the reticuloendothelial system and then may enter the circulation and lodge into the meninges where it may cause meningitis or meningoencephalitis, and then the bacterial endotoxins lead to arteritis in the endothelium of the cerebral blood vessels, resulting in cerebral ischemia and infarct.

CN involvement in brucellosis may present with different signs depending on the cranial nerve involved. First CN (olfactory nerve) involvement has not been reported till now as per the searched literature, though reports of upper cervical spine nerve involvement (C_2 level) in neurobrucellosis has been reported and can involve the spinal root of the spinal accessory ncrvc [21].

Interestingly, optic neuritis due to neurobrucellosis in children has also been reported [17]. Therefore, in the presence of optic neuritis in endemic countries, like the Mediterranean Basin and the Middle East, neurobrucellosis must be investigated because brucellosis is a reversible and treatable cause.

Oculomotor nerve involvement is an extremely rare complication, though several adult cases are present in the literature. In *Brucella* meningoencephalitis, CN III, IV, or VI involvement may cause papilledema, neuritis, papillitis, total/subtotal ophthalmoplegia, and optic atrophy [5, 9, 14, 19, 30]. Sensory symptoms like paresthesias and gait apraxia may be the presentation in many cases. CNs VI, VII, or VIII involvement is a relatively usual involvement finding in neurobrucellosis. CN VIII involvement has been reported as very characteristic of *Brucella* meningitis. There is a predilection for the vestibulocochlear nerve [2, 25, 30], which can lead to sensorineural hearing loss. CN VII if involved will present as facial nerve palsy which may be a permanent feature of neurobrucellosis.

Lower CN involvement is rare and we have reported a case with involvement of the CN VIII with sensorineural bilateral hearing loss with left>right (on audiometry) and CNs IX, X, and XI also involved on the left side with impaired gag reflex and paresis of the uvula and soft palate on the same side; even then such presentation is unusual [26]. Nevertheless, brucellosis must always be kept in mind in the presence of multiple CN involvement.

18.3 Diagnosis

Investigations like serum agglutination test are to be used for screening, while complement fixation and Coombs' test are the confirmatory tests for brucellosis. Enzyme-linked immunosorbent assay (ELISA) for *Brucella*, more sensitive and specific than many other serological tests, can be used in place of other serological tests. Antibodies can form against *Brucella* in serum and CSF which can be detected by ELISA. Serological markers may be negative in the CSF and serum. The common abnormality in CSF is usually lymphocytic pleocytosis and elevated proteins. Blood culture is not useful test for the diagnosis of neurobrucellosis, as it is usually negative and also takes a long time [15]. In CSF (<20 %) *Brucella* can be grown in culture and the serological tests for antibodies in CSF are specific for the diagnosis of neurobrucellosis [4, 12]. PCR can be used when CSF culture is negative and it may be used as an alternative for the diagnosis of neurobrucellosis [27].

Definite diagnosis of neurobrucellosis can be obtained only in the presence of: (1) CSF tests with high protein and lymphocytic pleocytosis, (2) neurological dysfunction that cannot be explained by another neurologic disease, (3) response of CSF to the antibiotics with a significant drop in the CSF lymphocyte count and protein levels, and (4) CSF culture with growth of *Brucella* or positive *Brucella* IgG agglutination titers in serum [10].

Contrast-enhanced magnetic resonance imaging may show hyperintense lesions [26] or nodule in the cortex which may be surrounded by vasogenic edema but it is a feature of chronic meningitis and is not specific for brucellosis (Figs. 18.1 and 18.2).

18.4 Treatment

The intracellular location of the bacteria may pose problems in the treatment of brucellosis. The optimal regimen is not uniformly accepted. Adequate

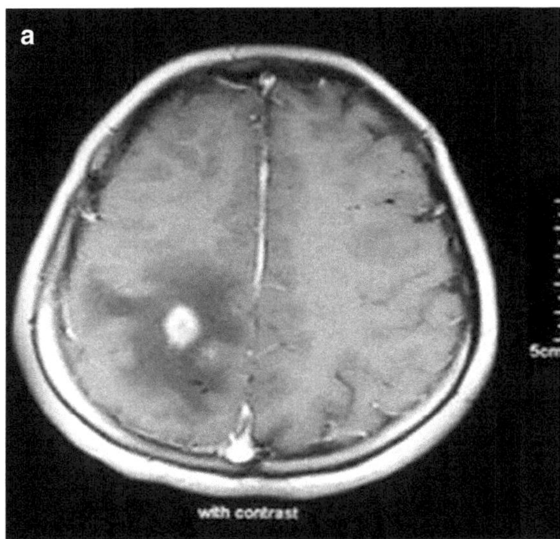

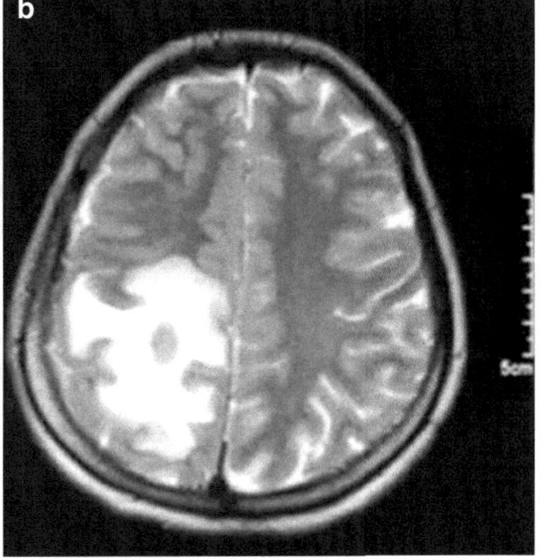

Fig. 18.1 (**a**) Axial T1-weighted gadolinium-enhanced MRI showing the presence of a solid nodule with a diameter of 1.5 cm in the right parietal cortex with vasogenic edema. (**b**) Axial T2-weighted image demonstrating the presence of marked vasogenic edema surrounding a hypointense central nodule (From Erdem et al. [8])

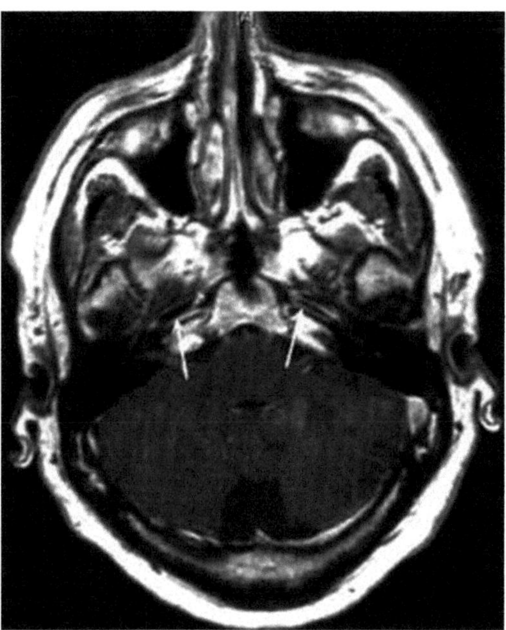

Fig. 18.2 Contrast-enhanced axial T1-weighted MRI in a 56-year-old man with cranial nerve neuritis. Note the presence of bilateral enhancement of the CN VIII after gadolinium administration (*arrowhead*) (From Jochum et al. [13])

CSF levels may not be achieved for tetracycline and aminoglycosides. The recommended dose of doxycycline accepted by most authorities is 100 mg orally twice a day combined with two or more other drugs (rifampin 600–900 mg orally once a day/streptomycin 1 g intramuscular once a day) and treatment has to be continued for a few weeks as per the response of the patient. Doxycycline crosses the blood-brain barrier better than generic tetracycline, and with trimethoprim-sulfamethoxazole and rifampin, better and more successful response has been seen for *Brucella* meningitis. Other drugs like 3rd-generation cephalosporins have high penetration to CSF but sensitivity and response of *Brucella* spp. is variable, and in vitro sensitivity should be ensured before using it. Antibiotic treatment has to be given for 1–19 months and CSF should be cleared. Steroids are to be used and are recommended for neurobrucellosis treatment, but the efficacy has not been proved in the absence of controlled studies. All patients are to be kept under review for 1 year after the completion of antibiotic treatment and the serum agglutinins has to fall to normal levels [1].

18.5 Prognosis

Meningitis caused by *Brucella* differs from other chronic meningitis as it has a better prognosis. Mortality in brucellosis is low for unknown reasons, and death has not been always clearly related to brucellosis. There has been high incidence for minor sequelae and only a few cases have suffered important limitations in their daily activity due to various motor, sensory, or intellectual deficits.

In cases of neurobrucellosis, the CNs usually remain affected permanently to some extent. Treatment usually does not cure the damage to the CNs, although little improvement may be seen after completion of treatment; however, in a few cases, complete resolution has been reported where diagnosis was made early and treatment was started early. This complete resolution has been reported in cases with involvement of CN VIII or VI and even in involvement of other CNs [14].

Conclusion

The most frequently observed complication in neurobrucellosis is meningitis yet it has many complications which may be in the form of meningoencephalitis, myelitis, CN paralyses, radiculopathy, and neuropathy. Basal meningitis may involve one or more CNs and this may be noted in more than half of the patients with neurobrucellosis. Tests which may be like serum agglutination are often used for screening but the confirmatory tests are complement fixation and Coombs' test. The more sensitive and specific test for *Brucella* is ELISA. Treatment is needed for a long period of time and early diagnosis with early treatment may prevent many long-term complications.

References

1. Akdeniz H, Irmak H, Anlar O, Demiroz AP (1998) Central nervous system brucellosis: presentation, diagnosis, and treatment. J Infect 36:297–301
2. Al Deeb SM, Yaqub BA, Sharif HS, Phadke JG (1989) Neurobrucellosis: clinical characteristics, diagnosis and outcome. Neurology 39:498–501
3. Al-Sous MW, Bohlega S, Al-Kawi MZ, Alwatban J, McLean DR (2004) Neurobrucellosis: clinical and

neuroimaging correlation. AJNR Am J Neuroradiol 25:395–401
4. Baldi PC, Araj GF, Racaro GC, Wallach JC, Fossati CA (1999) Detection of antibodies to Brucella cytoplasmic proteins in the cerebrospinal fluid of patients with neurobrucellosis. Clin Diagn Lab Immunol 6:756–759
5. Bashir R, Al-Kawi MZ, Harder EJ, Jinkins J (1985) Nervous system brucellosis: diagnosis and treatment. Neurology 35:1576–1581
6. Bouza E, Garcia de la Torre M, Parras F, Guerrero A, Rogríguez-Créixems M, Gobernado J (1987) Brucellar meningitis. Rev Infect Dis 9:810–822
7. Drevets DA, Leenen PJM, Greenfield RA (2004) Invasion of the central nervous system by intracellular bacteria. Clin Microbiol Rev 17:323–347
8. Erdem M, Namiduru M, Karaoglan I, Kecik VB, Aydin A, Tanriverdi M (2012) Unusual presentation of neurobrucellosis: a solitary intracranial mass lesion mimicking a cerebral tumor: a case of encephalitis caused by Brucella melitensis. J Infect Chemother 18:767–770
9. Finham RW, Sahs AL, Joynt RJ (1963) Protean manifestation of nervous system brucellosis: case histories of a wide variety of clinical forms. JAMA 184:269–275
10. Ghosh D, Gupta P, Prabhakar S (1999) Systemic brucellosis with chronic meningitis: a case report. Neurol India 47:58–60
11. Guven MB, Cirak B, Kutluhan A, Ugras S (1999) Pituitary abscess secondary to neurobrucellosis. Case illustration. J Neurosurg 90:1142
12. Izadi S (2001) Neurobrucellosis. Shiraz E-Medical J 2:2–6
13. Jochum T, Kliesch U, Both R, Leonhardi J, Bär KJ (2008) Neurobrucellosis with thalamic infarction: a case report. Neurol Sci 29:481–483
14. Karakurum GB, Yerdelen D, Karatas M, Pelit A, Demiroglu YZ, Kizilkilic O, Tan M, Toygar O (2006) Abducens nerve palsy and optic neuritis as initial manifestation in brucellosis. Scand J Infect Dis 38:721–725
15. Kochar DK, Agarwal N, Jain N, Sharma BV, Rastogi A, Meena CB (2000) Clinical profile of neurobrucellosis-a report on 12 cases from Bikaner (North-West India). J Assoc Physicians India 48:376–380
16. Lulu AR, Araj GF, Khateeb MI, Mustafa MY, Yusuf AR, Fenech FF (1988) Human brucellosis in Kuwait-a prospective study of 400 cases. Q J Med 66:39–54
17. Marques R, Martins C, Machado I, Monteiro JP, Campos N, Calhau P (2011) Unilateral optic neuritis as a presentation of neurobrucellosis. Pediatr Rep 3:e11
18. McLean DR, Russell N, Khan MY (1992) Neurobrucellosis: clinical and therapeutic features. Clin Infect Dis 15:582–590
19. Mousa AR, Koshy TS, Araj GF, Marafie AA, Muhtaseb SA, Al-Mudallal DS, Busharetulla MS (1986) Brucella meningitis: presentation, diagnosis and treatment. A prospective study of ten cases. Q J Med 60:873–885
20. Namiduru M, Karaoglan I, Yilmaz M (2003) Guillain-Barre syndrome associated with acute neurobrucellosis. Int J Clin Pract 57:919–920
21. Nas K, Tasdemir N, Cakmak E, Kemaloglu MS, Bukte Y, Geyik MF (2007) Cervical intramedullary granuloma of Brucella: a case report and review of the literature. Eur Spine J 16:255–259
22. Ozisik HI, Ersoy Y, Refik-Tevfik M, Kizkin S, Ozcan C (2004) Isolated intracranial hypertension: a rare presentation of neurobrucellosis. Microbes Infect 6:861–863
23. Pascual J, Combarros O, Polo JM, Berciano J (1988) Localized CNS brucellosis: report of 7 cases. Acta Neurol Scand 78:282–289
24. Ranjabar M, Razaiee AA, Hashemi SH, Mehdipour S (2009) Neurobrucellosis: report of a rare disease in 20 Iranian patients referred to a tertiary hospital. East Mediterr Health J 15:143–148
25. Shakir RA, Al-Din AS, Araj GF, Lulu AR, Mousa AR, Saadah MA (1987) Clinical categories of neurobrucellosis: a report of 19 cases. Brain 110:213–223
26. Showkat HI, Asimi R, Sarmast AH, Lone R, Hussain I, Kotwal S (2012) Neurobrucellosis with bilateral sensorineural hearing loss and ataxia A case report. Schweiz Arch Neurol Psychiatr 163:226–227
27. Sinopidis X, Kaleyias J, Mitropoulou K, Triga M, Kothare SV, Mantagos S (2012) An uncommon case of pediatric neurobrucellosis associated with intracranial hypertension. Case Rep Infect Dis Article ID 492467. doi:10.1155/2012/492467
28. Solaroglu I, Kaptanoglu E, Okutan O, Beskonakli E (2003) Solitary extra-axial posterior fossa abscess due to neurobrucellosis. J Clin Neurosci 10:710–712
29. Tekeli O, Tomac S, Gursel E, Hasiripi H (1999) Divergence paralysis and intracranial hypertension due to neurobrucellosis. A case report. Binocul Vis Strabismus Q 14:117–118
30. Thomas R, Kameswaran M, Murugan V, Okafor BC (1993) Clinical records. Sensorineural hearing loss in neurobrucellosis. J Laryngol Otol 107:1034–1036
31. Trifiletti RR, Restivo DA, Pavone P, Giuffrida S, Parano E (2000) Diabetes insipidus in neurobrucellosis. Clin Neurol Neurosurg 102:163–165
32. Tuncer-Ertem G, Tülek N, Yetkin MA (2004) Case report: subdural hemorrhage in neurobrucellosis. Mikrobiyol Bul 38:253–256
33. Zaidan R, Al Tahan AR (1999) Cerebral venous thrombosis: a new manifestation of neurobrucellosis. Clin Infect Dis 28:399–400

Part V

Laboratory Studies in Neuro-Brucellosis

Standard and New Laboratory Procedures in Neurobrucellosis

19

George F. Araj

Contents

Abstract

The nonspecific and protean presentation of brucellosis and what it can entail from a wide range of differential diagnosis necessitate the resort to *Brucella*-specific laboratory tests to help in reaching an accurate diagnosis. For this purpose, several test formats are available including culture, agglutination, ELISA, and molecular tests. Knowledge is necessary for the understanding of the usefulness and limitations of the laboratory tests for accurate interpretation of their results as correlates with the clinical stage of the disease. The simultaneous use of test combination that detects agglutinating and non-agglutinating antibodies is recommended to definitively exclude *Brucella* spp. infection especially in complicated, focal, or chronic presentation. As will be discussed in this chapter, the *Brucella-specific* laboratory tests are crucial for the diagnosis of brucellosis in humans.

Keywords

Agglutination tests • Brucellosis • Laboratory diagnosis • Molecular tests

Abbreviations

CNS	Central nervous system
CSF	Cerebrospinal fluid
ELISA	Enzyme-linked immunosorbent assay
IgA	Immunoglobulin A

G.F. Araj, PhD, D(ABMM), FAAM
Department of Pathology and Laboratory Medicine, American University of Beirut Medical Center, PO Box 11-0236, Beirut 1107-2020, Lebanon
e-mail: garaj@aub.edu.lb

M. Turgut et al. (eds.), *Neurobrucellosis: Clinical, Diagnostic and Therapeutic Features*,
DOI 10.1007/978-3-319-24639-0_19

IgG	Immunoglobulin G
IgM	Immunoglobulin M
PCR	Polymerase chain reaction
(RT)-PCR	Real-time PCR
SAT	Serum agglutination test

19.1 Introduction

Brucellosis is one of the major zoonotic diseases worldwide, responsible for a wide range of medical, public health, and economic problems, especially in those countries where this disease is endemic such as in the Mediterranean region and Arabian Peninsula [14].

The clinical diagnosis of brucellosis with its variations (systemic, complicated, localized, or neurobrucellosis) is challenging since clinical symptoms and signs can overlap with a wide range of infectious and noninfectious diseases (see Chap. 2 in this book). The *Brucella*-specific laboratory tests are crucial for the diagnosis, as will be discussed in this chapter.

19.2 Any Help from Routine Hematological and Chemical Tests?

The routine hematology and biochemical profiles in patients with brucellosis are usually within normal limits, with some elevation in erythrocyte sedimentation rate and liver function tests. The cerebrospinal fluid (CSF) analysis, in both adults and children, is nonspecific and can overlap with other central nervous system (CNS) diseases such as mycobacterial, viral, syphilitic, or fungal infections or with noninfectious diseases such as mental and psychiatric illnesses, multiple sclerosis, and cancer [17, 18, 21, 25].

19.3 *Brucella*-Specific Tests Are Needed for Reaching a Diagnosis

To reach an accurate diagnosis, the physician should be aware of this disease and its suggestive clinical signs and symptoms and must resort to specific *Brucella* tests. So far, the most practical, helpful, and useful laboratory diagnostic tests for the diagnosis of systemic or complicated cases of brucellosis, including the CNS involvement, are the standard culture and serologic tests. In order to reach the accurate diagnosis, the order for serologic investigation should include a combination of tests: the serum agglutination test (SAT) and the Brucella indirect Coombs test, SAT and Brucellacapt, or SAT and the enzyme-linked immunosorbent assay (ELISA), to be simultaneously tested on blood and CSF specimens [2]. Other tests such as the in-house-developed molecular tests have to be standardized before adopting and incorporating them in routine clinical use [1, 2, 22]. More detailed information on these laboratory tests is discussed below.

19.4 Molecular Tests for Direct Detection

The in-house-developed conventional polymerase chain reaction (PCR) and real-time (RT) PCR assays are being attempted to directly detect *Brucella* from clinical specimens, using *Brucella*-specific gene targets including: BCS P31 (encodes a 31-kDa cell surface protein), BP26 (encodes a 26-kDa periplasmic protein), 16S rRNA, and the insertion sequence rRNA. However, the sensitivities of these assays are quite variable, ranging from 50 to 100 %. Still, molecular assays have promising potential and can constitute a prominent role in the diagnosis but remain in need of further optimization, standardization, and improvement before their routine incorporation in the diagnosis of human brucellosis [20, 26, 28, 31].

19.5 Culture

Requesting to perform a culture (considered gold standard) of blood, CSF, and other specimen sources, when suspected, is essential for recovering *Brucella* spp. or other pathogens that can be considered in the differential diagnosis. Recovery of isolates can also be helpful for epidemiologic tracing and antimicrobial susceptibility testing.

Though *Brucella* spp. can easily grow on a wide range of culture media, the yield is generally variable, being higher among patients with acute brucellosis (40–90 %) than in patients in the chronic, focal, and complicated stages (5–20 %). The yield in CSF *Brucella* culture is also low (5–30 %) [4, 15, 25]. Its growth in culture is slow (7 days to 6 weeks) when using the conventional biphasic Ruiz-Castañeda bottle. The automated, continuously monitored blood culture systems like BacT/ALERT (bioMérieux, Durham, NC) and BACTEC (BD Diagnostics, Sparks, MD) show higher *Brucella* yields and earlier recovery (majority within 1 week) than the conventional culture method [2, 9, 29].

Once recovered in culture, the *Brucella* genus can be easily and rapidly identified using a couple of conventional tests (gram stain, catalase, oxidase, and specific agglutinating antisera). Most recently, the matrix-assisted laser desorption/ionization time-of-flight mass spectrometry which has been used in many laboratories for routine determination of microorganisms can be helpful in identification of the *Brucella* species [19].

However, when definitive identification, speciation, and characterization are required, *Brucella* isolates should be referred to specialized laboratories geared for handling and characterizing this and other highly infectious pathogens, by specific biochemical and molecular methods, under well-structured safe facilities.

19.6 Serologic Tests

Because of the above noted technical limitations, *Brucella* serologic assays are usually relied upon in the laboratory diagnosis of systemic, focal, and complicated brucellosis especially neurobrucellosis. Comprehensive information on the different *Brucella*-specific serologic tests used in the diagnosis of human brucellosis was detailed by Araj [2] and will be summarized below.

In order to have an accurate assessment, serologic results should be interpreted in the context of the evolution of antibody responses after infection with *Brucella* spp. IgM first appears, followed by the appearance of IgG, IgA, and other immunoglobulins within 10–14 days. Their evolution will depend on several factors, for example, the clinical category, response to treatment, and relapse. It is of interest to note that in this disease and after treatment and cure, *Brucella-specific* IgG and some IgM can persist for a very prolonged time (months and sometime years) in 15–20 % of asymptomatic patients, and the explanation for this remains elusive [14, 22].

A wide range of serologic tests have been used for diagnosis of patients with brucellosis. Currently, five tests are the most important and widely used for the diagnosis of brucellosis in humans and will be emphasized [2].

19.6.1 Serum Agglutination Test

The SAT is a widely used direct agglutination test in tubes (also known as Wright test). It is labor intensive, takes time to set up, and can only be read after 24 h.

19.6.2 Rose Bengal Test

The Rose Bengal test is a simple and rapid (10 min) slide agglutination test. Both of the aforementioned agglutination-based tests are relatively good methods in diagnosing acute cases, show high rates of false-negative results in chronic and complicated cases, and are liable to cross-react with a couple of other bacteria (i.e., false-positive result). Furthermore, neither can differentiate the types of antibodies involved.

19.6.3 Indirect Coombs Test

The indirect Coombs test is an extension of SAT, is cumbersome to perform, takes an additional 24 h to read (i.e., turnaround time is around 48 h), detects non-agglutinating or incomplete antibodies, and is good for chronic and complicated cases.

19.6.4 Brucellacapt Test (Vircell, Granada, Spain)

The Brucellacapt test is based on an immunocapture technique to detect, in a single step, the non-agglutinating IgG and IgA antibodies, as well as the agglutinating antibodies. Its performance is similar to that of Coombs test, but it is more rapid (18–24 h) and easier to carry out.

19.6.5 Enzyme-Linked Immunosorbent Assay

ELISA can detect immunoglobulin classes and subclasses and is the test of choice for complicated cases, especially neurobrucellosis, and chronic cases when other laboratory tests are negative. It is rapid, highly sensitive, and reveals total and individual specific immunoglobulins (IgM, IgG, and IgA) [2–6, 8]. Commercial ELISAs detecting *Brucella* IgG and IgM with a high degree of sensitivity and specificity have been available for a number of years [10].

Several other tests have also been available or being newly developed but may not be practical or commonly used or are still undergoing assessment to determine reliability for clinical laboratory diagnosis of brucellosis. These include indirect fluorescence antibody test, lateral flow test, and different formats of molecular tests [1, 2].

19.7 Evaluation, Interpretation, and Reporting of Results

An accurate assessment of the medical history and final condition of patients is mandatory for the management and the interpretation of serologic test and is necessary for the understanding of the usefulness and limitations of the laboratory tests [2, 22, 30]. Positive cutoff titers in the *Brucella* agglutination test for diagnosis have generally been considered to be ≥160 in symptomatic patients. Nevertheless, much lower titers with the SAT have been reported for patients with active disease [2]. Moreover, when brucellosis is suspected and negative serology is encountered, it is important to be careful since there are some subclasses such as *B. canis*, which can be missed by serologic assays using *B. abortus* or *B. melitensis* antigen. In addition, in very early disease presentation, slide test or SAT used alone can give a false-negative response, and so it is crucial to repeat these tests after 1–2 weeks [12]. A combination of agglutinating and non-agglutinating tests is recommended to definitively exclude *Brucella* spp. infection.

In an attempt to look for differential markers between acute and chronic brucellosis, *Brucella-specific* immunoglobulin classes and subclasses must be tested. In acute brucellosis, elevation in *Brucella*-specific IgM, IgG, IgA, IgE, IgG1, and IgG3 is shown, while in those patients with chronic brucellosis, elevations in IgA, IgG, IgE, IgG1, and IgG4 are usually seen [4, 7, 8, 11, 15, 22]. Monitoring the treatment response requires a close monitoring for patients with serologic titers. A decline means good prognosis, persistently high titers necessitate sequential follow-up, and a resurgence in antibody titers usually indicates relapse or reinfection. Slide and SAT titers fall faster than with Coombs, Brucellacapt, and ELISA, which can stay positive for years, e.g., 2–3 years. Persistence of residual positive titers in cured patients has doubtful meaning [2, 12, 15, 24]. Relapse has also been diagnosed by a detection of a resurgence in *Brucella*-specific IgA and IgG antibodies, not IgM [12, 15, 24, 27]. Markers for differentiating active disease from an inactive one are being sought. For example, anti-Brucella cytoplasmic or periplasmic protein antibodies increased only in patients with active brucellosis, as determined by ELISA, and were a better predictor of cure compared to anti-lipopolysaccharide antibodies [13, 16]. Also, some interleukins show a decrease post-therapy [23].

Several other challenges remain to be addressed, especially those pertaining to finding relevant diagnostic and prognostic markers associated with the different stages/categories of brucellosis [2].

Conclusion

Consequently, a combination of two agglutination tests (SAT and Brucellacapt, SAT and indirect Coombs test), or ELISA for IgM and IgG should be used when investigating patients with brucellosis. In this way, one would be able to determine antibodies in any stage of the disease, since in the acute stage any test can be positive, while in chronic, complicated, or focal disease (e.g., neurobrucellosis) cases, the SAT may be negative, while the Coombs test, ELISA using IgG, and Brucellacapt may be positive. Again, one should keep in mind that any serologic test findings need to be evaluated taking into account the patient's medical history [2, 30].

References

1. Al Dahouk S, Sprague LD, Neubauer H (2013) New developments in the diagnostic procedures for zoonotic brucellosis in humans. Rev Sci Tech Off Int Epiz 32:177–188
2. Araj GF (2010) Update on laboratory diagnosis of human brucellosis. Int J Antimicrob Agents 36:12–17
3. Araj GF (1997) Enzyme linked immunosorbent assay, not agglutination test is the test of choice for the diagnosis of neurobrucellosis (letter). Clin Infect Dis 25:1481
4. Araj GF, Lulu AR, Mustafa MY, Khateeb MI (1986) Evaluation of ELISA in the diagnosis of acute and chronic brucellosis in human beings. J Hyg (Lond) 97:457–469
5. Araj GF, Lulu AR, Saadah MA, Mousa AM, Strannegard I-L, Shakir RA (1986) Rapid diagnosis of central nervous system brucellosis by ELISA. J Neuroimmunol 12:73–82
6. Araj GF, Lulu AR, Khateeb MI, Saadah MA, Shakir RA (1988) ELISA versus routine tests in the diagnosis of patients with systemic and neurobrucellosis. Acta Pathol Microbiol Scand 96:171–176
7. Araj GF (1988) Profiles of Brucella-specific immunoglobulin G subclass in serum of patients with acute and chronic brucellosis. Serodiag Immun Other Infect Dis 2:401–410
8. Araj GF, Kaufman AF (1989) Determination by enzyme-linked immunosorbent assay of immunoglobulin G (IgG), IgM, and IgA to Brucella melitensis major outer membrane proteins and whole-cell heat-killed antigens in sera of patients with brucellosis. J Clin Microbiol 27:1909–1912
9. Araj GF, Kattar MM (2003) Rapid diagnosis of human brucellosis using Bact/Alert continuous culture monitoring system. Abstract of the 103rd annual meeting of the American Society for Microbiology, Washington, DC, 18–22 May, Abstract C-002
10. Araj G, Kattar M, Fattouh LG, Bajakian OK, Kobeissi SA (2005) Evaluation of the PANBIO Brucella immunoglobulin G (IgG) and IgM enzyme-linked immunosorbent assays for diagnosis of human brucellosis. Clin Diagn Lab Immunol 12:1334–1335
11. Araj GF, Lulu AR, Khateeb MI, Haj MM (1990) Specific IgE response in patients with brucellosis. Epidemiol Infect 105:571–577
12. Ariza J, Corredoira J, Pallares R, Vilarich PF, Rufi G, Pujol M, Gudiol F (1995) Characteristics of and risk factors for relapse of brucellosis in humans. Clin Infect Dis 20:1241–1249
13. Baldi PC, Miguel SE, Fossati CA, Wallach JC (1996) Serologic follow-up of human brucellosis by measuring IgG antibodies to lipopolysaccharide and cytoplasmic proteins of Brucella species. Clin Infect Dis 22:446–455
14. Dean AS, Crump L, Greter H, Schelling E, Zinsstag J (2012) Global burden of human brucellosis: a systematic review of disease frequency. PLoS Negl Trop Dis 6, e1865
15. Gazapo E, Gonzalez Lahoz J, Subiza JL, Banquero M, Jil J, de la Concha EG (1989) Changes in IgM and IgG antibody concentration in brucellosis over time: importance for diagnosis and follow-up. J Infect Dis 159:219–225
16. Goldbaum FA, Rubbi CP, Wallach JC, Miguel SE, Baladi PC, Fossati CA (1992) Differentiation between active and inactive human brucellosis by measuring antiprotein humoral immune responses. J Clin Microbiol 30:604–607
17. Gul HC, Erdem H, Bek S (2009) Overview of neurobrucellosis: a pooled analysis of 187 cases. Int J Infect Dis 13(e):339–343
18. Guven T, Ugurlu K, Ergonul O, Celikbas AK, Gok SE, Comoglu S, Baykam N, Dokuzoguz B (2013) Neurobrucellosis: clinical and diagnostic features. Clin Infect Dis 56:1407–1412
19. Karger A, Melzer F, Timke M, Bettin B, Kostrzewa M, Nöckler K, Hohmann A, Tomaso H, Neubauer H, Al Dahouk S (2013) Interlaboratory comparison of intact-cell matrix-assisted laser desorption ionization-time of flight mass spectrometry results for identification and differentiation of Brucella spp. J Clin Microbiol 51:3123–3126
20. Kattar MM, Zallou PA, Araj GF, Samaha-Kfoury J, Shbaklo H, Kanj SK, Khalife S, Deeb M (2007) Development and evaluation of real-time polymerase chain reaction assays on whole blood and paraffin-embedded tissues for rapid diagnosis of human brucellosis. Diagn Microbiol Infect Dis 59:23–32
21. Lubani MM, Doudin KI, Araj GF, Manandhar DS, Rashid FY (1989) Neurobrucellosis in children. Pediatr Infect Dis J 8:79–82
22. Lulu AR, Araj GF, Khateeb MI, Mustafa MY, Yusuf AR, Fenech FF (1988) Human brucellosis in Kuwait: a prospective study of 400 cases. Q J Med 66:39–54
23. Makis AC, Galanakis E, Hatzimichael EC, Papadopoulou ZL, Siamopoulou A, Bourantas KL (2005) Serum levels of soluble interleukin-2 receptor alpha (sIL-2Alpha) as a predictor of outcome in brucellosis. J Infect 51:206–210
24. Pellicer T, Ariza J, Fox Z, Pallares R, Gudiol F (1988) Specific antibodies during relapse of human brucellosis. J Infect Dis 157:918–924
25. Shakir RA, Al-Din ASN, Araj GF, Lulu AR, Mousa AR, Saadah MA (1987) Clinical categories of neurobrucellosis: a report on 19 cases. Brain 110:213–223

26. Sohrabi M, Mohabati MA, Khoramalbadi N, Hosseini DR, Behmanesh M (2014) Efficient diagnosis and treatment follow-up of human Brucellosis by a novel quantitative TaqMan real-time PCR assay: a human clinical survey. J Clin Microbiol 52:4239–4243
27. Solera J, Martinez-Alfaro E, Espinosa A, Castillejos ML, Geijo P, Rodriguez-Zapata M (1998) Multivariate model for predicting relapse in human brucellosis. J Infect 36:85–92
28. Wang Y, Wang Z, Zhang Y, Bai L, Zhao Y, Liu C, Ma A, Hui Yu H (2014) Polymerase chain reaction–based assays for the diagnosis of human brucellosis. Ann Clin Microbiol Antimicrob 13:31
29. Yagupsky P (1999) Detection of Brucellae in blood cultures. J Clin Microbiol 37:3437–3442
30. Young EJ (2010) Brucella species. In: Mandell GL, Bennet JE, Dolin R (eds) Principles and practice of infectious diseases. Churchill Livingstone, Philadelphia, pp 2921–2925
31. Yu WL, Nielsen K (2010) Review of detection of Brucella spp. by polymerase chain reaction. Croat Med J 51:306–313

Part VI

Therapy of Neuro-Brucellosis

Medical Therapy of Neurobrucellosis

20

Ana Cerván, Miguel Hirschfeld, Miguel Rodriguez, and Enrique Guerado

Contents

A. Cerván, MD • M. Hirschfeld, MD •
M. Rodriguez, MD • E. Guerado, MD, PhD, MSc (✉)
Department of Orthopedic Surgery and Traumatology, Hospital Universitario Costa del Sol., University of Malaga, Marbella (Málaga), Spain
e-mail: anacervan@me.com; miguelhirschfeld@gmail.com; miguelrodriguezsolera@hotmail.com; eguerado@hcs.es

Abstract

Antibiotics are the mainstay of brucellosis treatment; several dual or triple antibiotic combinations for spinal brucellosis have been compared in different studies. In uncomplicated brucellosis, the rifampicin plus doxycycline regimen is the most accepted treatment, but the scientific community is also in favor of streptomycin plus doxycycline, possibly because of its lower price and ease of administration. However there is still no consensus on the best treatment regimens and its duration. The treatment with the combination of ceftriaxone or trimethoprim/sulfamethoxazole, doxycycline, and rifampicin is effective in neurobrucellosis cases that affect the central nervous system and should be prolonged for no less than 3 months. Surgery usually is unnecessary for brucellosis spondylodiscitis. The surgical intervention is reserved for biopsy, severe neurological impairment, or spinal stabilization.

Keywords

Antibiotics • Central nervous system • Medical therapy • Neurobrucellosis • Treatment

M. Turgut et al. (eds.), *Neurobrucellosis: Clinical, Diagnostic and Therapeutic Features*,
DOI 10.1007/978-3-319-24639-0_20

Abbreviations

CNS	Central nervous system
CSF	Cerebrospinal fluid
TMP/SMZ	Trimethoprim/sulfamethoxazole
WHO	World Health Organization

20.1 Introduction

The main treatment for brucellosis is antibiotics. There are issues regarding medical treatment of neurobrucellosis. The difficulty in treatment is due to: the intracellular localization of the microorganism, the requirement for a sufficient antibiotic dose level in the cerebrospinal fluid (CSF), and the need for prolonged treatment to prevent relapse. Nowadays there is no consensus on regimens and duration of treatment being that it is not easy to choose the best treatment option [6, 22]. Some authors believe that long-term observation after the cessation of chemotherapy is essential to prevent relapses [48, 49].

20.2 Medical Treatment Options

Antibiotics are the mainstay of brucellosis treatment, with combinations recommended to prevent the high relapse rates reported with monotherapy. Several dual or triple antibiotic combinations for spinal brucellosis have been compared in different studies [10, 21, 51, 52].

The essential element in the treatment of all forms of human brucellosis is the administration of effective antibiotics for an adequate length of time [16]. There are some limitations in choosing the best regimen: the best choice of antibiotics that act intracellularly is limited, and prolonged treatment needed to prevent relapse may increase the occurrence of adverse reactions and may reduce adherence to the treatment [2].

The most frequently proposed and used combinations include streptomycin. Despite the known side effects of streptomycin, favorable results were reported in brucellosis with bone and joint involvement. In some studies ototoxicity and dizziness were the most prominent side effects of the drugs among their patients [50]. Clinicians may particularly hesitate to treat the disease with streptomycin in the elderly because they are more prone to side effects. The restricted use of a parenterally administered drug in clinical practice is another disadvantage of the treatment.

It is found that treatment with streptomycin in combination with doxycycline was reported to have a superior efficacy and lower relapse rates [2, 51]. Uncomplicated acute brucellosis almost invariably responds well to appropriate antibiotic treatment. Patients and their families should be reassured that full clinical and bacteriological recovery is usual in human brucellosis.

Regimens that combine two or more antibiotics are now recommended by most experts due to the high relapse rate with monotherapy [1, 38]. In addition, since the majority of brucellosis cases are in low socioeconomic areas of developing countries, where tuberculosis also is an endemic health problem, the overlap between treatment regimens of two diseases has raised concerns over the potential increase in resistance to tuberculosis drugs due to their prolonged use in brucellosis treatment [2]. The World Health Organization (WHO) issued recommendations for the treatment of human brucellosis in 1986 [24], suggesting the use of doxycycline, 100 mg twice daily for 6 weeks combined with either rifampicin, 600–900 mg daily for 6 weeks, or streptomycin, 1 g daily for 2–3 weeks. During the following years, a number of clinical studies assessed the efficacy of different regimens. Furthermore, reports from various regions of the world revealed that the WHO-recommended regimens have not been universally applied in clinical practice.

The significant health consequences of multiple drug-resistant tuberculosis have resulted in calls for new drug regimens and shorter brucellosis drug treatment regimens [53]. Solera et al. [46] performed a meta-analysis evaluating the efficacy of the two WHO-recommended regimens and concluded that the efficacy of the doxycycline-streptomycin regimen was superior to the doxycycline-rifampicin regimen. Pappas et al. [39] showed in his study that the doxycycline-rifampicin regimen is preferred by patients.

20.3 Drugs

20.3.1 Tetracyclines

Tetracycline (500 mg every 6 h orally) administered for at least 6 weeks has long been the standard treatment of human brucellosis. Doxycycline (a long-acting tetracycline analog) is now the preferred drug because it can be given once or twice daily and is associated with fewer gastrointestinal side effects than tetracycline.

20.3.2 Aminoglycosides

Streptomycin (1 g/day intramuscularly) administered for 2–3 weeks has long been the aminoglycoside of choice when used in combination with tetracycline or doxycycline. Although synergy between the two drugs is difficult to prove using routine in vitro assays, bacterial killing studies have shown that *Brucella* species undergo a more rapid rate of killing by the combination than by either drug alone. Gentamicin is more active in vitro against *Brucella* species than streptomycin and, when administered as a single daily dose, is associated with fewer adverse side effects.

20.3.3 Rifampicin

Rifampicin is active in vitro against *Brucella* species, is remarkably lipid soluble, and accumulates within eukaryotic cells.

20.3.4 Fluoroquinolones

Fluoroquinolone antibiotics have greater activity in vitro against *Brucella* species than the parent drug nalidixic acid. In addition, they are well absorbed after oral administration, and they achieve high concentrations within phagocytic cells. Although the minimum bactericidal concentration of quinolones is reported to be approximately four times the minimum inhibitory concentration, a lack of bactericidal activity was found at pH levels comparable to those found within cells. In addition, when quinolones were used as monotherapy in experimental animals and humans infected with *Brucella*, the rates of relapse were unacceptably high.

20.3.5 Trimethoprim/Sulfamethoxazole

Trimethoprim/sulfamethoxazole (TMP/SMZ, co-trimoxazole) in a fixed ratio of 1:5 (80 mg TMP/400 mg SMZ) is more active in vitro against *Brucella* species than either drug alone. Although initial studies with TMP/SMZ (co-trimoxazole) reported good results, prospective, controlled, comparative trials demonstrated that the drug was associated with an unacceptably high rate of relapse.

20.4 Regimens in Uncomplicated Brucellosis

Since 1971, when the WHO suggested a 21-day regimen of tetracycline plus streptomycin as the treatment of choice for human brucellosis, regimens for treatment of brucellosis have been changing for different reasons [23]. Although this regimen was successful in reducing the early symptoms, it failed to treat the disease completely, and immediate relapse was observed in some patients [3].

In 1986, the Joint Food and Agriculture Organization of the United Nations/WHO Expert Committee on Brucellosis proposed two new regimens: rifampicin (600–900 mg/day orally) plus doxycycline (200 mg/day orally) for 6 weeks and doxycycline (200 mg/day orally) for 45 days plus streptomycin (1 g/day intramuscularly) for 2–3 weeks [24].

However, later studies showed a treatable but high rate of relapse for the mentioned regimens.

The rifampicin plus doxycycline regimen is the most popular treatment and favorable to the more effective regimen of streptomycin plus doxycycline, possibly because of its lower price and ease of administration [34, 38], while streptomycin requires parenteral administration in a hospital setting or in an appropriately set-up primary care network, both of which are restricted to lower income countries [40].

The abovementioned treatment regimens were replicated in the 2006 WHO recommendations [11].

20.4.1 Monotherapy

It has been considered inadequate due to the high relapse rates. Many studies demonstrated disappointing results with different monotherapy antibiotic treatments (ceftriaxone, rifampicin, TMP/SMZ or co-trimoxazole, etc.) [12, 17, 18, 27, 31, 32].

20.4.2 Doxycycline-Gentamicin Regimen

Solera et al. [44] considered this combination an adequate regimen for the treatment of human brucellosis. Likewise, Hatala et al. [19] support the feasibility of once-daily dosing of aminoglycoside. Different studies show interventions with gentamicin-encapsulated microspheres, a useful future option of treatment [20, 28–30, 33, 41, 42].

20.4.3 Fluoroquinolone-Containing Regimens

Regimens of treatment that include combinations with fluoroquinolones can be acceptable, but not as a first option [15, 36]. There are no data on the efficacy of the fluoroquinolone in the treatment of brucellosis. More properly designed prospective clinical trials using this option will be necessary.

20.4.4 Trimethoprim/Sulfamethoxazole-Containing Regimens

It has been used in some countries, due to its lower cost. It makes it the most cost-effective drug against brucellosis. The important issue regarding the use of TMP/SMZ (co-trimoxazole) in brucellosis treatment is the development of resistance in *Brucella melitensis* [26].

20.4.5 Other Tetracyclines

Minocycline can be used instead of doxycycline in the treatment of brucellosis, used as monotherapy or in combination with rifampicin. It has been reported to carry a very low relapse rate [7]. Another option is the use of tigecycline, the first glycylcycline antibiotic. This new drug has specific efflux pump acquisition and ribosomal protection and is active against many gram-positive and gram-negative organisms [43]. But it has two problems: the high cost and the need to be administrated parenterally.

20.5 Regimens in Special Situations

20.5.1 Adults and Children 8 Years of Age and Older

The streptomycin plus doxycycline regimen was stated as the gold standard for the treatment of brucellosis by the recommendations [2]. Streptomycin plus doxycycline was considered superior to the doxycycline plus rifampicin regimen by the Ioannina expert panel, because of its higher effectiveness, some supporting evidence of pharmacokinetics, and its lack of overlap with tuberculosis treatments. However, the expert panel suggested the need for further studies on the potential side effects of aminoglycoside-containing regimens.

20.5.2 Children Less than 8 Years of Age

The optimal treatment for brucellosis in neonates and children less than 8 years of age has not been definitively determined. Tetracyclines are contraindicated because of the potential for permanent staining of deciduous teeth and inhibition of bone growth. Doxycycline binds less to calcium than other tetracyclines and may pose less of a risk; however, there are no studies to confirm this with certainty. Consequently, aminoglycosides, TMP/SMZ (co-trimoxazole), and rifampicin are the drugs generally recommended. TMP/SMZ (co-trimoxazole) and rifampicin are not recommended by the manufacturers for use in young children, and the rates of relapse are high when either agent is used alone. Satisfactory results have been reported with TMP/SMZ (co-trimoxazole) (8/40 mg/kg/day twice daily orally) administered for 6 weeks plus streptomycin (30 mg/kg/day once daily intramuscularly) administered for 3 weeks or gentamicin (5 mg/kg/day once daily intravenously or intramuscularly) administered for 7–10 days. Alternatives include TMP/SMZ (co-trimoxazole) plus rifampicin (15 mg/kg/day orally) each administered for 6 weeks or rifampicin plus an aminoglycoside. Until additional experience is obtained with these regimens, it is not possible to define the therapy of choice.

20.5.3 During Pregnancy

If promptly diagnosed, antimicrobial therapy of pregnant women with brucellosis can be lifesaving for the fetus. Pregnant women and nursing mothers pose special problems with regard to the selection of appropriate drugs. All drugs cross the placenta in varying degrees, thus exposing the fetus to potential adverse drug effects. Tetracyclines are contraindicated in pregnancy owing to the potential for permanent staining of fetal dentition and the susceptibility of pregnant women to drug-induced fatty necrosis of the liver and pancreatitis. The teratogenic potential of many drugs, such as the fluoroquinolones, rifampicin, and TMP/SMZ (co-trimoxazole), is simply unknown. Fetal toxicity has been reported in pregnant women treated with streptomycin; however, there are no reports of toxicity with gentamicin.

Consequently, the optimal therapy for brucellosis during pregnancy has not been determined with certainty. TMP/SMZ (co-trimoxazole) has been used in individual cases with reported success. Another alternative is rifampicin therapy for at least 45 days depending on the clinical outcome.

20.6 Regimens in Spinal Brucellosis

Early recognition of complicated cases is critical in preventing devastating complications. Selection of an appropriate antibiotic combination should be made on the basis of the patient and the population: age, side effects, and ease of application [50]. In case series including patients with paraspinal abscess, it was reported that patients were treated for a longer duration depending on the clinical and radiological response [45], and a magnetic resonance imaging of the spine should always be performed, if there is a suspicion of spinal involvement (Figs. 20.1, 20.2, and 20.3). Antimicrobial treatment should be prolonged in complicated spinal forms of brucellosis. A meta-analysis of the existing data concluded that the matter for the outcome is the duration of treatment, and not the specific (recommended) regimen used [37].

The treatment should last not less than 3 months [9, 37]. Solera et al. [44] believe that aminoglycoside-containing regimens may be better than rifampicin-containing ones and suggest that the outcome of spondylitis may potentially be improved when such a streptomycin-containing regimen is used.

There is no recommendation for the use of oral antibiotics for the treatment of acute central nervous system (CNS) infections [13, 47]. The use of the oral antibiotic combination including rifampicin, doxycycline, and TMP/SMZ (co-trimoxazole)

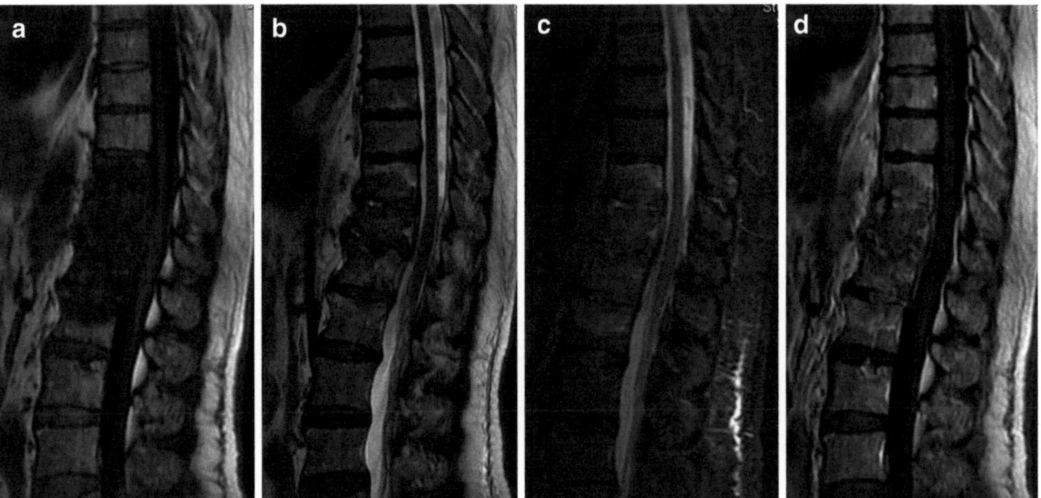

Fig. 20.1 Sagittal MRIs from a 62-year-old man with brucellar spondylodiscitis. (**a**) T1-weighted image showing irregularity and destruction of vertebral end plates and hypointensity at T11 to L2. (**b**) T2-weighted image showing increased signal intensity of the disk and loss of intervertebral disk height. (**c**) Sagittal STIR image shows hyperintense lesions vertebral contiguous. (**d**) Contrast-enhanced T1-weighted sagittal MRI shows involvement of intervertebral disk space between T11–L2 vertebral levels, vertebral bodies, and vertebral end plate

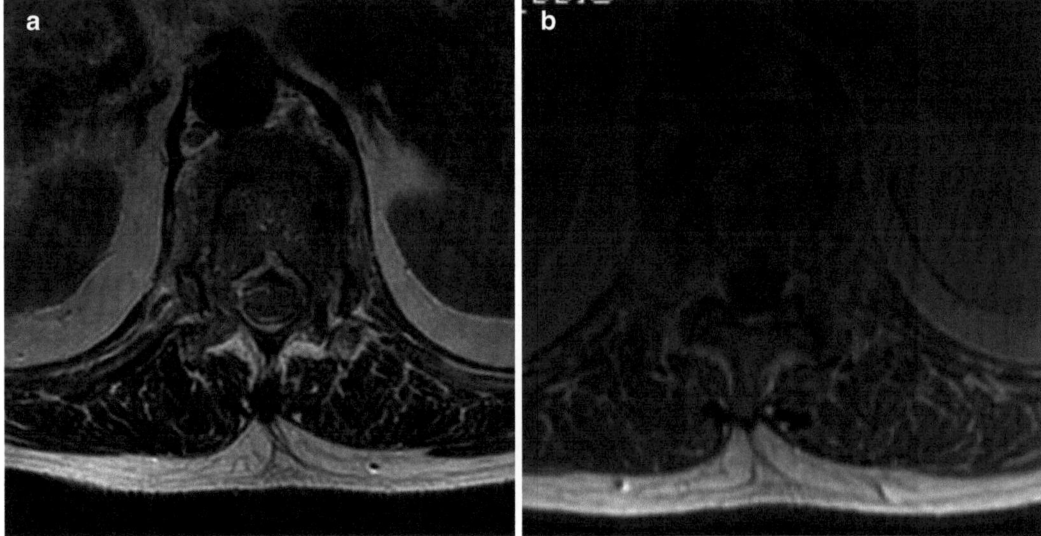

Fig. 20.2 (**a**) Axial T2-weighted MRI reveals a paravertebral abscess. (**b**) Contrast-enhanced T1-weighted axial image shows enhancement in affected vertebra and paravertebral soft tissue

can be considered in poor countries. The use of streptomycin is not recommended for its doubtful ability to penetrate into the CSF and its potential neurotoxicity that can confuse the clinical presentation of the illness [35].

Erdem et al. [14] concluded in their study (multicenter retrospective study) in favor of 1 month of parenteral ceftriaxone in combination with doxycycline and rifampicin for the treatment of neurobrucellosis.

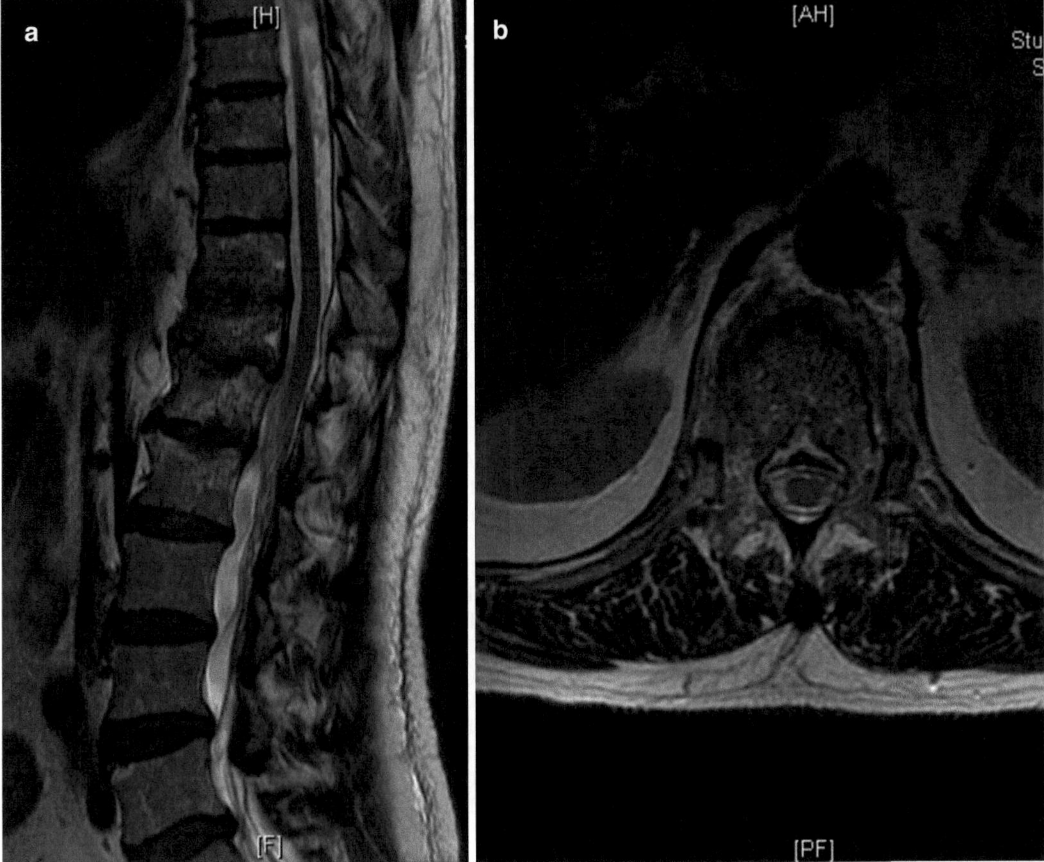

Fig. 20.3 (a) Sagittal and (b) axial MRIs after 1 year of diagnosis and treatment

Conclusion

Neurobrucellosis should always be considered in the differential diagnosis of neurological and psychiatric cases in endemic areas of brucellosis. Patients with spondylitis or meningoencephalitis may need to be treated for a longer period of time [4, 5, 9, 37]. The treatment with the combination of ceftriaxone or TMP/SMZ (co-trimoxazole), doxycycline, and rifampicin is effective in neurobrucellosis cases that affect the CNS [8, 25]. Complications need long treatment courses and possibly surgical treatment [5].

References

1. Agalar C, Usubutun S, Turkyilmaz R (1999) Ciprofloxacin and rifampicin versus doxycycline and rifampicin in the treatment of brucellosis. Eur J Clin Microbiol Infect Dis 18:535–538
2. Ariza J, Bosilkovski M, Cascio A, Colmenero JD, Corbel MJ, Falagas ME, Memish ZA, Roushan MR, Rubinstein E, Sipsas NV, Solera J, Young EJ, Pappas G (2007) Perspectives for the treatment of brucellosis in the 21st century: the Ioannina recommendations. PLoS Med 4, e317
3. Ariza J, Gudiol F, Valverde J, Pallarés R, Fernández-Viladrich P, Rufí G, Espadaler L, Fernández-Nogues F (1985) Comparative trial of rifampin-doxycycline

versus tetracycline-streptomycin in the therapy of human brucellosis. Antimicrob Agents Chemother 28:548–551
4. Bordur H, Erbay A, Akinci E, Colpan A, Cevik MA, Balaban N (2003) Neurobrucellosis in an endemic area of brucellosis. Scand J Infect Dis 5:94–97
5. Bossi P, Tegnell A, Baka A, Van Loock F, Hendriks J, Werner A, Maidhof H, Gouvras G, Task Force on Biological and Chemical Agent Threats, Public Health Directorate, European Commission, Luxembourg (2004) Bichat guidelines for the clinical management of brucellosis and bioterrorism-related brucellosis. Euro Surveill 9:1–5
6. Bouza E, García de la Torre M, Parras F, Guerrero A, Rodríguez-Créixems M, Gobernado J (1987) Brucellar menengitis. Rev Infect Dis 4:810–822
7. Cascio A, Scarlata F, Giordano S, Antinori S, Colomba C, Titone L (2003) Treatment of human brucellosis with rifampin plus minocycline. J Chemother 15:248–252
8. Ceran N, Turkoglu R, Erdem I, Inan A, Engin D, Tireli H, Goktas P (2011) Neurobrucellosis: clinical, diagnostic, therapeutic features and outcome. Unusual clinical presentations in an endemic region. Braz J Infect Dis 15:52–59
9. Colmenero JD, Reguera JM, Fernández-Nebro A, Cabrera-Franquelo F (1991) Osteoarticular complications of brucellosis. Ann Rheum Dis 50:23–26
10. Colmenero JD, Ruiz-Mesa JD, Plata A, Bermúdez P, Martín-Rico P, Queipo-Ortuño MI, Reguero JM (2008) Clinical findings, therapeutic approach, and outcome of brucellar vertebral osteomyelitis. Clin Infect Dis 46:426–433
11. Corbel MJ (2006) Brucellosis in humans and animals [WHO/CDS/ EPR/2006.7]. World Health Organization, Geneva, pp 36–41
12. Doğanay M, Aygen B (1992) Use of ciprofloxacin in the treatment of brucellosis. Eur J Clin Microbiol Infect Dis 11:74–75
13. Erdem H, Kilic S, Coskun O, Ersoy Y, Cagatay A, Onguru P, Alp S (2010) Community-acquired acute bacterial meningitis in the elderly in Turkey. Clin Microbiol Infect 16:1223–1229
14. Erdem H, Ulu-Kilic A, Kilic S, Karahocagil M, Shehata G, Eren-Tulek N, Yetkin F, Kemal M, Ceran N, Cem Gul H, Mert G, Tekin-Koruk S, Dizbay M, Seza Inal A, Nayman-Alpat S, Bosilkovski M, Inan D, Saltoglu N, Abdel-Baky L, Adeva-Bartolomé MT, Ceylan B, Sacar S, Turhan V, Yilmaz E, Elaldi N, Kocak-Tufan Z, Ugurlu K, Dokuzoguz B, Yilmaz H, Gundes S, Guner R, Ozgunes N, Ulcay A, Unal S, Dayan S, Gorenek L, Karakas A, Tasova Y, Usluer G, Bayindir Y, Kurtaran B, Resat O, Leblebicioglu H (2012) Efficacy and tolerability of antibiotic combinations in neurobrucellosis: results of the Istanbul study. Antimicrob Agents Chemother 56:1523–1528
15. Falagas ME, Bliziotis IA (2006) Quinolones for treatment of human brucellosis: critical review of the evidence from microbiological and clinical studies. Antimicrob Agents Chemother 50:22–33
16. Franco MP, Mulder M, Gilman RH, Smits HL (2007) Human brucellosis. Lancet Infect Dis 7:775–786
17. Hall WH (1990) Modern chemotherapy for brucellosis in humans. Rev Infect Dis 12:1060–1099
18. Hasanjani Roushan MR, Mohraz M, Hajiahmadi M, Ramzani A, Valayati AA (2006) Efficacy of gentamicin plus doxycycline versus streptomycin plus doxycycline in the treatment of brucellosis in humans. Clin Infect Dis 42:1075–1080
19. Hatala R, Dinh T, Cook DJ (1996) Once-daily aminoglycoside dosing in immunocompetent adults: a meta-analysis. Ann Intern Med 124:717–725
20. Imbuluzqueta E, Gamazo C, Lana H, Campanero MÁ, Salas D, Gil AG, Elizondo E, Ventosa N, Veciana J, Blanco-Prieto MJ (2013) Hydrophobic gentamicin-loaded nanoparticles are effective against Brucella melitensis infection in mice. Antimicrob Agents Chemother 57:3326–3333
21. Ioannou S, Karadima D, Pneumaticos S, Athanasiou H, Pontikis J, Zormpala A, Sipsas NV (2011) Efficacy of prolonged antimicrobial chemotherapy for brucellas spondylodiscitis. Clin Microbiol Infect 17:756–762
22. Izadi S (2001) Neurobrucellosis. SEMJ 2:1–7
23. Joint FAO/WHO Expert Committee on Brucellosis (1971) Joint FAO/WHO Expert Committee on Brucellosis [meeting held in Geneva, 29 June – 6 July 1970]: fifth report. WHO Technical Report Series No. 464/FAO Agricultural Series No. 85. World Health Organization, Geneva, pp 41–43
24. Joint FAO/WHO expert committee on brucellosis (1986) World Health Organ Tech Rep Ser. 740:1–132
25. Karsen H, Koruk ST, Duygu F, Yapici K, Kati M (2012) Review of 17 cases of neurobrucellosis: clinical manifestations, diagnosis and management. Arch Iran Med 15:491–494
26. Kinsara A, Al-Mowallad A, Osoba AO (1999) Increasing resistance of Brucellae to co-trimoxazole. Antimicrob Agents Chemother 43:1531
27. Lang R, Dagan R, Potasman I, Einhorn M, Raz R (1992) Failure of ceftriaxone in the treatment of acute brucellosis. Clin Infect Dis 14:506–509
28. Lecaroz C, Blanco-Prieto MJ, Burrell MA, Gamazo CJ (2006) Intracellular killing of Brucella melitensis in human macrophages with microsphere-encapsulated gentamicin. J Antimicrob Chemother 58:549–556
29. Lecaroz C, Gamazo C, Blanco-Prieto MJ (2006) Nanocarriers with gentamicin to treat intracellular pathogens. J Nanosci Nanotechnol 6:3296–3302
30. Lecaroz MC, Blanco-Prieto MJ, Campanero MA, Salman H, Gamazo C (2007) Poly (D, L-lactide-coglycolide) particles containing gentamicin: pharmacokinetics and pharmacodynamics in Brucella melitensis-infected mice. Antimicrob Agents Chemother 51:1185–1190
31. Lulu AR, Araj GF, Khateeb MI, Mustafa MY, Yusuf AR, Fenech FF (1988) Human brucellosis in Kuwait: a prospective study of 400 cases. Q J Med 66:39–54

32. Montejo JM, Alberola I, Glez-Zarate P, Alvarez A, Alonso J, Canovas A, Aguirre C (1993) Open, randomized therapeutic trial of six antimicrobial regimens in the treatment of human brucellosis. Clin Infect Dis 16:671–676
33. Mundargi RC, Babu VR, Rangaswamy V, Patel P, Aminabhavi TM (2008) Nano/micro technologies for delivering macromolecular therapeutics using poly (D, L-lactide-co-glycolide) and its derivatives. J Control Release 125:193–209
34. Pappas G, Akritidis N, Bosilkovski M, Tsianos E (2005) Brucellosis. N Engl J Med 352:2325–2336
35. Pappas G, Akritidis N, Christou L (2007) Treatment of neurobrucellosis: what is known and what remains to be answered. Expert Rev Anti Infect Ther 5:983–990
36. Pappas G, Christou L, Akritidis N, Tsianos EV (2006) Quinolones for brucellosis: treating old diseases with new drugs. Clin Microbiol Infect 12:823–825
37. Pappas G, Seitaridis S, Akritidis N, Tsianos E (2004) Treatment of brucella spondylitis: lessons from an impossible meta-analysis and initial report of efficacy of a fluoroquinolone-containing regimen. Int J Antimicrob Agents 24:502–507
38. Pappas G, Siozopoulou V, Akritidis N, Falagas ME (2007) Doxycycline-rifampicin: physicians' inferior choice in brucellosis or how convenience reigns over science. J Infect 54:459–462
39. Pappas G, Siozopoulou V, Saplaoura K, Vasiliou A, Christou L, Akritidis N, Tsianos EV (2007) Health literacy in the field of infectious diseases: the paradigm of brucellosis. J Infect 54:40–45
40. Pappas G, Solera J, Akritidis N, Tsianos E (2005) New approaches to the antibiotic treatment of brucellosis. Int J Antimicrob Agents 26:101–105
41. Prior S, Gander B, Blarer N, Merkle HP, Subirá ML, Irache JM, Gamazo C (2002) In vitro phagocytosis and monocyte-macrophage activation with poly(lactide) and poly(lactide-co-glycolide) microspheres. Eur J Pharm Sci 15:197–207
42. Prior S, Gander B, Lecároz C, Irache JM, Gamazo C (2004) Gentamicin-loaded microspheres for reducing the intracellular Brucella abortus load in infected monocytes. J Antimicrob Chemother 53:981–988
43. Rubinstein E, Vaughan D (2005) Tigecycline: a novel glycylcycline. Drugs 65:1317–1336
44. Solera J, Espinosa A, Martinez-Alfaro E, Sanchez L, Geijo P, Navarro E, Escribano J, Fernández JA (1997) Treatment of human brucellosis with doxycycline and gentamicin. Antimicrob Agents Chemother 41:80–84
45. Solera J, Lozano E, Martinez-Alfaro E, Espinosa A, Castillejos ML, Abad L (1999) Brucellar spondylitis: review of 35 cases and literature survey. Clin Infect Dis 29:1440–1449
46. Solera J, Martinez-Alfaro E, Saez L (1994) Meta-analysis of the efficacy of the combination of rifampicin and doxycycline in the treatment of human brucellosis. Med Clin (Barc) 102:731–738
47. Tunkel AR, Hartman BJ, Kaplan SL, Kaufman BA, Roos KL, Scheld WM, Whitley RJ (2004) Practice guidelines for the management of bacterial meningitis. Clin Infect Dis 39:1267–1284
48. Turgut M, Sendur OF, Gurel M (2003) Brucellar spondylodiscitis in the lumbar region-case report. Neurol Med Chir (Tokyo) 43:210–212
49. Turgut M, Cullu E, Sendur OF, Gurer G (2004) Brucellar spine infection. Four case reports. Neurol Med Chir (Tokyo) 44:562–567
50. Ulu-Kilic A, Karakas A, Erdem H, Turker T, Inai AS, Ak O, Turan H, Kazak E, Inan A, Duygu F, Demirasian H, Kader C, Sener A, Dayan S, Deveci O, Tekin R, Saltoglu N, Aydin M, Horasan ES, Gul HC, Ceylan B, Kadanal A, Karabay O, Karagoz G, Kayabas U, Turhan V, Engin D, Gulsun S, Elaldi N, Alabay S (2014) Update on treatment options for spinal brucellosis. Clin Microbiol Infect 20:O75–O82
51. Ulu-Kilic A, Sayar MS, Tutuncu E, Sezen F, Sencan I (2013) Complicated brucellar spondylodiscitis: experience from an endemic area. Rheumatol Int 33:2909–2912
52. Yilmaz E, Parlak M, Akalin H, Heper Y, Ozakin C, Mistik R, Oral B, Helvaci S, Töre O (2004) Brucellar spondylitis: review of 25 cases. J Clin Rheumatol 10:300–307
53. Yousefi-Nooraie R, Mortaz-Hejri S, MehraniM, Sadeghipour P (2012) Antibiotics for treating human brucellosis. Cochrane Database Syst Rev (10):CD007179

Surgical Therapy of Neurobrucellosis

21

Xenophon Sinopidis, Mehmet Turgut, Stylianos Roupakias, Ahmet Tuncay Turgut, and Oreste de Divitiis

Contents

Abstract

The presentation of the role of surgery in the treatment of neurobrucellosis is the scope of this chapter. As laboratory and imaging diagnostic methods and antibacterial drug regimens continuously evolve, the same occurs to operative equipment and methods. Surgical involvement in life-threatening conditions such as brain and spinal abscess is thoroughly presented. In this chapter, special issues such as cerebrovascular involvement or intraparenchymal lesions are addressed. Intervention in structures with high morbidity like the cervical spine is exposed. Minimal invasive techniques, stenting, grafts, and instrumentation are presented in a friendly way for anyone who is involved in the treatment of neurobrucellosis.

X. Sinopidis, MD, PhD (✉) • S. Roupakias, MD
Department of Pediatric Surgery, University of Patras, Patras, Greece
e-mail: xsinopid@upatras.gr; stylroup@yahoo.gr

M. Turgut, MD, PhD
Department of Neurosurgery, Adnan Menderes University School of Medicine, Aydın, Turkey
e-mail: drmturgut@yahoo.com

A.T. Turgut, MD
Department of Radiology, Hacettepe University School of Medicine, Ankara, Turkey
e-mail: ahmettuncayturgut@yahoo.com

O. de Divitiis, MD
Department of Neurosciences, Reproduction and Odontostomatological Sciences, School of Medicine and Surgery, University of Naples Federico II, Naples, Italy
e-mail: oreste.dedivitiis@unina.it

M. Turgut et al. (eds.), *Neurobrucellosis: Clinical, Diagnostic and Therapeutic Features*,
DOI 10.1007/978-3-319-24639-0_21

Keywords
Aspiration • Brain abscess • Craniotomy • Drainage • Neurobrucellosis • Spine stabilization • Stereotactic surgery • Treatment • Ventriculostomy

Abbreviations

ACA	Anterior cerebral artery
CSF	Cerebrospinal fluid
CT	Computed tomography
IICP	Increased intracranial pressure
IVD	Intervertebral disk herniation
MCA	Middle cerebral artery
MRI	Magnetic resonance imaging
SAH	Subarachnoid hemorrhage
US	Ultrasound

21.1 Introduction

Neurobrucellosis response to conservative therapy is satisfactory as a rule. However, in many patients diagnosis remains under question, or antibiotic regimens are not effective, and serious complications needing surgical intervention occur. The indications and performance of surgery for different forms of neurobrucellosis are presented in this chapter. It deals thoroughly with the modern techniques implicated in the surgical treatment of brain abscess and the cerebrovascular and the intraparenchymal lesions of the brain, all conditions with high morbidity and mortality. A part of the chapter is devoted to the indications and techniques of surgical treatment of spinal cord neurobrucellosis, giving special attention to contemporary procedures, grafting, and instrumentation. At the end of the chapter, there is a thorough presentation of the current relevant literature.

21.2 Surgical Therapy of Brain Abscess Due to Brucellosis

Outcome and quality of life in brain abscess patients still remain a continuous challenge, despite the modern surgical strategies and techniques [4, 89, 132]. There are no absolute guidelines for the treatment of brain abscess, and a multidisciplinary team approach on an individualized patient basis is paramount to the successful management [4, 89]. Advances in neuroimaging and neuroanesthesia, microbiological isolation, anaerobic culture techniques, and new generation antibiotics have revolutionized modern surgical treatment. Nevertheless, a brain abscess can still be fatal [6, 69, 74, 89].

21.2.1 History

The first successful operative procedure on brain abscess was performed by the French surgeon Morand in 1752 [21]. In 1891, Topuzlu operated successfully the first case of brain abscess in the Ottoman Empire, one of the first cases of neurological surgery performed using contemporary anesthesiological and surgical techniques, which reveals the importance of neurological examination and cerebral localization techniques in the era before radiology [81, 86, 88]. In 1893, MacEwen published the results of a case series on 19 patients with brain abscess and described the draining of the pus using decalcified chicken bones, with only one death [32, 81].

King introduced marsupialization in 1924, and Dandy introduced aspiration in 1926 [81, 88]. In 1928, Sargent considered the procedure of enucleation of an encapsulated brain abscess, and Vincent practiced complete excision and proved its value in 1936 [88, 104]. In 1978, Rosenblum et al. [103] reported zero mortality in a series of 20 patients, after the introduction of antibiotics, organism isolation techniques, and computed tomography (CT).

In 1987, Maurice Williams presented the "open evacuation of pus," a technique that has combined the advantages of both aspiration and excision, involving open surgical drainage via limited craniectomy and/or craniotomy [79]. Today, in the era of frameless image-guided stereotactic surgery and minimally invasive techniques, aspiration of brain abscess has become the preferred method of drainage [93].

21.2.2 Surgical Indications

Brain abscesses usually require drainage in addition to appropriate antibiotic therapy, so early neurosurgical consultation is recommended [78]. The controversy of medical or surgical treatment has been a challenge on an individualized patient basis, and the choice is influenced by age, neurological status, location, number, size, and stage of abscess formation [4, 6, 110]. Clinical status of the patient and CT imaging help in treatment planning. CT detects exact localization; accurate characterization; determination of number, size, and staging of the abscess; hydrocephalus; increased intracranial pressure (IICP); edema; and associated infections like subdural empyema or ventriculitis [89, 110].

Nonoperative treatment has been proposed for a brain abscess less than 2 cm with chronic encapsulation, for multiple small abscesses, and for patients who are extremely poor surgical candidates [94]. As diagnosis based only on clinical and neuroradiological findings can be erroneous, nonsurgical therapeutic decisions should not be taken without positive pathological diagnosis [89].

Surgery is not only a therapeutic option but also allows confirmation of the diagnosis and the sampling of material for microbiological diagnosis and often reduces the duration of antibiotic treatment, the toxicity risk, the hospitalization rate, and the frequency of controls [6]. Thus, for almost any brain abscess, emergent drainage is indicated both therapeutically and for diagnosis [4].

In general, medical treatment alone should not be used when the diagnosis is in doubt [110]. In selective patients under conservative treatment (alert and clinically stable patients with small abscess in early phase of cerebritis, where the organism has been identified presumptively from any material culture, and in high-risk patients with bleeding diathesis in whom even minimally invasive neurosurgery is contraindicated), serial CT scans are critical [110]. If serial CT shows growth of abscess any time during treatment with antibiotics, or no decrease in size within 2–3 weeks, or failure to resolve after 3–4 weeks, a surgical procedure should be performed to confirm the diagnosis, to obtain a sample for culture, for identification of the specific pathogen and sensitivity to particular antibiotics, and to remove as much purulent material as possible [4, 89, 110].

When a trend toward nonsurgical management is followed, there is potential for delay in operative intervention and death from IICP or rupture of abscess into ventricle or subarachnoid space [110]. Urgent surgery should be performed in patients presenting with significant mass expansion effect, obstructive hydrocephalus, edema, IICP, Glasgow Coma Scale less than 12, progressive focal neurological deficit, or clinical deterioration during conservative management (Fig. 21.1a) [4, 6, 89, 110]. Cerebellar or brain stem abscesses often require urgent surgery due to the high risk of brain herniation, just as periventricular brain abscess gives the risk of intraventricular rupture [4].

The established guiding indications for surgical management are confirmation of microbiological diagnosis; antibiotic therapy modification from obtained pus; unresponsiveness to medical management; significant clinical deterioration; a walled off abscess larger than 3 cm in diameter; a capsular staged abscess larger than 2 cm in diameter; deep located capsular staged abscess larger than 3 cm in diameter; cerebellar, subdural, epidural, brain-stem, or paraventricular abscess; and finally the presence of multiple lesions [4, 89, 93, 94, 110].

21.2.3 Operative Procedures

Surgical therapy provides samples for accurate diagnosis, reduces the mass of the abscess, improves the efficacy of the drug used for treatment, and in some conditions allows intrathecal, intraventricular, and intracavitary administration of the antibiotic agent [53]. Currently, the

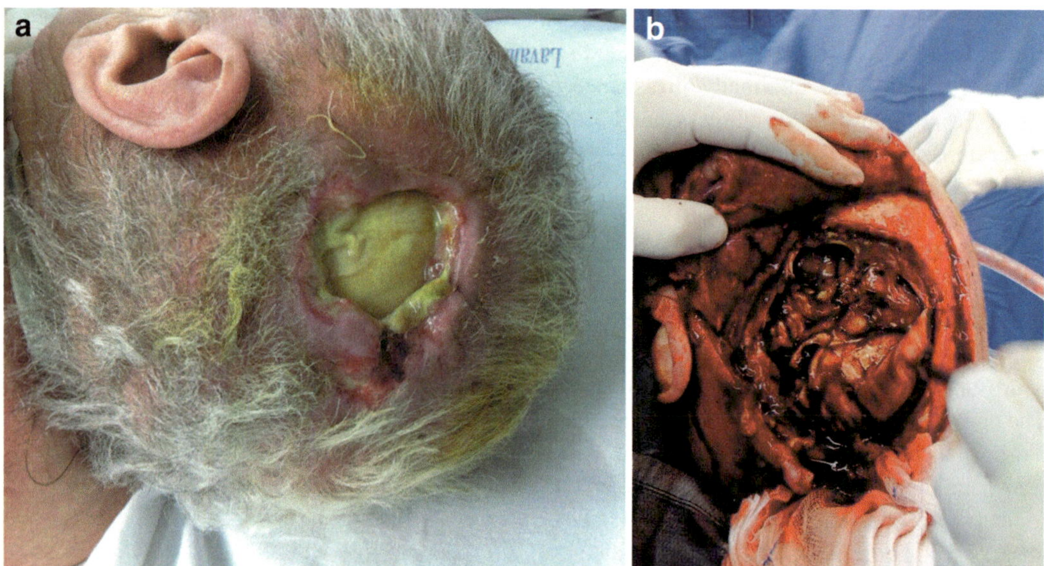

Fig. 21.1 An unusual presentation of unilateral brain, skull, and cutis abscess due to neurobrucellosis observed in a 64-year-old man, a country worker who gave no importance to the skin lesion, with a very low educational level and a history of fever, headache, vomiting, and seizures. When he arrived to the hospital, his abscess was initially misdiagnosed because he was comatose with a GCS score of 9 (**a**). During the operation the skull defect was enlarged with a wide craniotomy and curettage of the intracerebral portion of the abscess was performed, with a pathological diagnosis of brucellosis (**b**)

principal methods for surgical management involve freehand or endoscope-assisted aspiration of the pus with/without stereotactic CT guidance, drainage by craniotomy or craniectomy with/without intraoperative ultrasound (US) guidance, or excision of the abscess. The choice of procedure is a matter of debate, but the preference and the ability of the surgeon, as well as the ability of the patient to tolerate each procedure, should be taken into account [6, 88]. Craniotomy was advocated in the pre-CT era but is now rarely practiced as the first line of treatment [88]. Aspiration, repeated as necessary or combined with drainage, has widely replaced attempts at complete excision. Several reports have still advocated excision as the procedure of choice, because it is often followed by a lower incidence of recurrence and shorter hospitalization [88].

21.2.3.1 Aspiration

In most cases, aspiration of the purulent material is sufficient to initiate healing of the abscess [4]. Aspiration can be used in the cerebritis stage where biopsy gives positive culture and can discriminate abscess from other brain lesions (tuberculoma, metastasis, glioma, resolving hematoma) [106, 109]. Weekly or biweekly CT scans to monitor the size of the abscess are mandatory following aspiration or drainage in addition to parenteral antibiotic therapy for 6–8 weeks [82]. More than one aspiration may be needed for cure [109].

21.2.3.2 CT-Guided Stereotactic Procedure

Deep-seated abscess should be drained by a CT-guided stereotactic procedure [88]. Real-time US, particularly in infants with open fontanels, provides precise localization [110]. Multiloculated abscesses have been treated with stereotactic aspiration of all loculi in single or staged aspiration [109]. A question has been raised as to whether aspiration combined with immediate washout, with or without antibiotics, and drainage for several days could lead to even better results, with this point seeming to be more important for the treatment of subdural empyemas [102]. Sometimes though, the penetration of a thick abscess wall with the blunt-tipped stereotactic probes can be difficult, and one may fail to enter the abscess [83]. Impedance monitoring can avoid the false-negative result [101]. The ability to monitor the progress of the aspiration in real time and to detect intraoperative complications makes the use of the open magnetic resonance imaging (MRI) within the operating room attractive, although its availability is still extremely limited [64, 102]. Stranjalis [121] applied a stereotactic aspiration in a patient with a cerebral abscess due to *Brucella*. In general, aspiration is a rapid and safe procedure especially with the use of stereotactic US or CT-guided techniques, which can be done even under local anesthesia, on bedside, in seriously ill high-risk patients [110]. Often, the initial approach is to drain the abscess through a twist-drill craniostomy [88].

21.2.3.3 Burr Hole Drainage

If the pus is thick or inadequate drainage of abscess is suspected, the next procedure would be therapeutic burr hole evacuation with or without intraoperative radiography and neuronavigation [88]. The residual pus can be evacuated if the patient does not exhibit significant improvement, or serial CT reveals moderate to large residue [88].

21.2.3.4 Neuroendoscopic Stereotactic Evacuation

Neuroendoscopic stereotactic evacuation with rigid or flexible scope has shown encouraging results and additional advantages of more complete drainage and lavage [42, 55, 59, 73]. Deep-seated (thalamic, basal ganglia, brain stem) and hemispheric eloquent area abscess can be managed by frame-based stereotactic or neuronavigation-guided aspiration [83, 88].

21.2.3.5 Drainage by Craniotomy, Craniectomy, or Excision

Drainage by craniotomy, craniectomy, or excision is used more often in superficial abscesses and those found in the posterior cranial fossa (Fig. 21.1b) [6]. Surgical excision becomes mandatory if the pus is thick, if a peripherally placed abscess fails to respond to aspiration, and in multiloculated abscesses [4]. However, excision is inappropriate in the cerebritis stage; small, deep-seated abscesses in eloquent areas; and multiple abscesses [4, 110].

Open craniotomy for excision of brain abscess allows complete removal of purulent material and the surrounding abscess capsule, providing definitive treatment, like in a reported case of refractory epilepsy caused by a chronic abscess in brucellosis [22, 44]. The capsule often has anchor extensions into the surrounding white matter, and the surgical procedure may cause unplanned extensive damage to the adjacent viable cerebral tissue [54]. The ideal excision of the abscess in one piece, necessary to prevent the spillage of pus in the operative field and the reinfection of the traumatized brain tissue, contradicts the general neurosurgical tenet that removal of debulked lesions causes significantly less parenchymal and vascular brain damage [102].

21.2.3.6 Balloon Catheter-Assisted Excision

A balloon catheter-assisted excision averts spillage and allows the decompressed abscess to be pulled gently toward the surface while the cleavage plane from the brain is developed step by step [102]. In cases where complete excision is not feasible (wall of the abscess appeared too thin on US) during operation, open aspiration via craniotomy allows thorough irrigation of the abscess cavity and verification of complete evacuation of abscess contents using US [44].

Multiple abscesses are best treated by aspiration of the most superficial or the largest one for diagnosis and the others if they are causing mass effect or producing neurological deficit [4, 110]. Treating the remaining lesions with antibiotics and biweekly CT imaging is advocated [110].

21.2.3.7 Serial or Staged Stereotactic Aspiration

Serial or staged stereotactic aspiration can be performed in abscesses greater than 3 cm in diameter, deeply located in the brain stem or close to the ventricular wall, recollecting or enlarging, and failing to decrease or resolve

[109, 110]. When a peripherally placed abscess fails to respond to aspiration, consideration should be given to craniotomy and excision [4]. In multiple abscesses antibiotics are continued for 3 months [110]. Calik et al. [20] described a case of multiple brain abscesses and hydrocephalus in a 4-month-old infant, due to *Brucella melitensis* after isolation from cerebrospinal fluid (CSF), which was treated only with ventriculoperitoneal shunt and long-term antibiotic administration, but no abscess surgical drainage.

21.2.3.8 Craniotomy

A craniotomy should be performed for an epidural abscess, with a large osteoplastic craniotomy to be preferred in comparison with a free flap because of its better vascularity and its increased resistance to infection [102].

21.2.3.9 Ventriculostomy

Urgent evacuation of abscess is required for subdural empyema and cerebellar abscess, and a ventriculostomy is indicated for significantly IICP [88]. Tabatabai et al. [122] drained a delayed postsurgical subdural empyema in brucellosis via a burr hole-applied technique. Shoshan et al. [111] reported a surgical drained chronic subdural empyema during craniotomy in an 8-year-old girl, with the characteristic MRI appearance of diploic widening together with the thick capsule and meningeal-pial enhancement. Subdural empyema in infants may reoccur after repeated drainage and can be successfully resolved by craniectomy and juxtaposition of the temporal muscle [26]. Cerebellar abscess due to brucellosis has been reported [11]. Cerebellar or brain stem abscess is often an indication for posterior fossa craniotomy [4].

21.2.3.10 Cerebrospinal Fluid Diversion

Associated supra- or infratentorial abscess or empyema may be present with cerebellar abscess, but the latter one needs to be regarded differently from supratentorial abscess because of its ability to cause sudden total occlusion of CSF pathways early in the course of disease [88, 110]. Immediate CSF diversion with an external ventricular drain is mandatory in presence of overt or incipient hydrocephalus [95]. Persistent hydrocephalus is treated with a shunting procedure [88]. Presence of periventricular lucency is an absolute indication for immediate ventricular drainage regardless of level of consciousness [88].

Regardless of the suggestion that cerebellar abscess should be managed by primary excision, in recent years burr hole aspiration has emerged as a satisfactory method [19]. Drainage via a twist-drill craniostomy is as effective as burr hole drainage but is best avoided except in life-threatening situations or as a salvage procedure [88]. Cerebellar abscess should be completely excised through a suboccipital craniectomy or a craniotomy [88]. Solaroglu et al. [114] reported a case of surgical cyst aspiration with wide capsule resection via a bilateral suboccipital craniectomy and C_1 laminectomy after an ineffective operative spinal needle aspiration, in a patient with one solitary extra-axial posterior fossa abscess due to brucellosis. They were unable to remove completely the capsule of the abscess as the anterior part was firmly adhered to the brain stem [114]. Gündcş ct al. [50] evacuated a left cerebellar hemisphere brucellar abscess via an occipital (supratentorial) craniotomy. In cases of intraventricular rupture of brain abscesses, in addition to a combination of intrathecal and intravenous antimicrobial treatment, rapid evacuation and debridement of the abscess cavity via urgent craniotomy, lavage of the ventricles, intraventricular drainage, and intraventricular administration of antibiotics are recommended [72].

21.2.4 Complications and Outcome

The two most feared complications of cerebral abscess are herniation secondary to mass and abscess rupture into the ventricle and/or subarachnoid space [46]. In some rare cases, uncoagulated old hematoma-like fluid such as chronic subdural hematoma fills the drained or excised cavity, as a result of the significant revascularization with inflammatory cells in the remaining abscess capsule or cavity [102]. After aspiration and drainage of brain abscess, delayed minor bleeding from the capsule can be detected by MRI [131]. Late recurrent abscess is more common after aspiration alone than after excision [46].

About 30–50 % of survivors are found to have neurological sequelae, which fall into three major categories: focal neurological deficits, cognitive and learning impairment, and seizures [46, 110]. Epilepsy may occur during long-term follow-up; therefore, all patients with subdural empyema should be placed on anticonvulsants for at least several months after surgery [102].

Although the use of steroid treatment in brain abscess is controversial, corticosteroids may be beneficial in patients with IICP, significant cerebral edema with mass effect, compromised mental or neurological status, and potentially life-threatening complications such as impending cerebral herniation, despite maximal surgical treatment [39, 57]. Some feel that steroid therapy can reduce antibiotic penetration into the abscess or increase the risk of intraventricular rupture [44].

At present, major centers report a mortality rate of less than 10 % [71]. Many poor prognostic indicators have been described, which include neonates, infants, and elderly patients; delayed diagnosis and institution of treatment; rapidly progressing disease; sensory deterioration at presentation; coma; multiple and deep-seated lesions; intraventricular rupture and posterior fossa location; associated meningitis, ependymitis, or empyema; large size; and presence of hydrocephalus [4, 110]. Early aspiration, together with the absence of initial seizures, sterile CSF, and normal ventricles on CT scan, appeared to be a factor leading to a better prognosis in terms of epilepsy and mental sequelae [6].

Primary excision of brain abscess carries the risk of serious damage to the surrounding brain tissue with increased potential for neurological sequelae and epilepsy [4, 93]. Today, aspiration of brain abscess has become the preferred method of surgical drainage, with main disadvantages of the repeat procedures (because incomplete evacuation of thick purulent material), the hemorrhage into the abscess capsule and the possibility of iatrogenic puncture of ventricle, and subarachnoid or subdural leakage of pus leading to meningitis, or empyema, or ventriculitis [41, 54, 94].

Stereotactic aspiration avoids the so-called leukotomy effect that can occur with a freehand aspiration technique [83]. The incidence of residual neural deficits, such as hemiparesis, and cognitive and learning deficits in children is less with aspiration than excision [110]. Excision has been better than aspiration in regard to postoperative duration of antibiotics use, earlier improvement in neurological function and radiological clearance, rate of reoperative surgery, length of hospital stay, and overall cost of treatment [4, 87, 105, 106, 123].

21.3 Surgical Therapy of Neurobrucellosis with Cerebrovascular Involvement

Meningovascular complications of neurobrucellosis are reported in the medical literature, and some of them may lead to clinical presentations that necessitate urgent intervention [49]. Subarachnoid hemorrhage (SAH), subdural hematomas, mycotic aneurysms with or without rupture, ischemic attacks, and venous thrombosis are vascular involvement of neurobrucellosis [1, 3, 14, 15, 49].

Altekin et al. [3] described a case of intraparenchymal hematoma caused by rupture of a mycotic aneurysm of the right posterior cerebral artery in a patient with aortic valve endocarditis caused by *Brucella melitensis*. Because of high complication risk and low success rate of endovascular treatment without infection control and the patient's neurological stability, intervention for the aneurysm was planned after infection control and aortic valve surgery [3]. Although mycotic aneurysms are fragile, hemorrhage is an uncommon event, supporting more the conservative approach with prolonged courses of antibiotics and serial follow-up angiography to detect the dynamic or stable nature of aneurysm [91].

In a dynamic aneurysm, the aim of aggressive surgical therapy is to eliminate the mycotic aneurysm from circulation, prevent the ischemic events from arterial circulation, and evacuate any associated hematoma [28, 91]. Endovascular treatment of mycotic aneurysm due to neurobrucellosis can be achieved safely after the infection and vascular inflammation are taken under control [3]. Delayed surgery may reduce the risk of perioperative rupture and allow the aneurysm to mature from a friable acute lesion to a more fibrotic chronic lesion [28]. Erdoğan et al. [38] described a case of ruptured aneurysm of the distal anterior cerebral artery (ACA) associated with brucellosis, who presented with the symptoms of SAH. A right frontal interhemispheric approach was used, and a tiny aneurysm that had not been detected on angiography was found arising from the left distal ACA [39]. The ruptured fusiform aneurysm at the right callosomarginal artery was successfully clipped, and then the silent aneurysm was covered with muscle [39].

21.3.1 Endovascular and Surgical Techniques

21.3.1.1 Intracranial Stents

Intracranial stents provide the unique ability to simultaneously preserve parent vessel integrity while obliterating the aneurysmal sac, but their use for the treatment of mycotic intracranial aneurysms has only been reported in a few instances [34].

Ay presented a patient with brucellosis and a frontoparietotemporal infarct in the right cortical area, supplied by the middle cerebral artery (MCA) and a prominent stenotic segment distal to the right MCA. Reperfusion was achieved with a stent placed into the right MCA [10]. Although evidence regarding the efficacy of endovascular treatment in acute stroke has been equivocal, the recent publication of a large multicenter randomized controlled trial indicates benefit of intra-arterial stent retriever reperfusion in patients selected by appropriate imaging and treated early by experienced operators [8].

21.3.1.2 Endovascular Embolization or Trapping

Selective endovascular embolization or trapping with soft and ultrasoft detachable coils is an effective technique that should be considered for management of dynamic unruptured mycotic aneurysms, whereas conventional surgical intervention should be restricted to ruptured mycotic aneurysms with associated intracerebral hematoma and IICP [91]. Amiri et al. [5] reported a case of a small intracerebral and intraventricular hemorrhage accompanied with mild hydrocephalus occurring in a patient with three *Brucella-related* mycotic aneurysms treated with delayed surgery, resection, and excision after a left posterior temporoparietal craniotomy.

21.3.1.3 Sinus Thrombectomy, Bypass, Thrombolysis, and Clot Disruption

Zaidan and Al Tahan [134] described a case of complete sagittal sinus thrombosis in a patient with meningitis due to *Brucella melitensis* and a pseudotumor-like picture. The value of neurosurgical intervention in dural sinus thrombosis remains unproved [62]. Decompressive craniotomy or craniectomy has been used in patients with coma and significantly IICP, although benefit is unproved and outcomes are commonly poor [27, 90].

Surgical revascularization procedure such as sinus thrombectomy and bypass has been reported, when peripherally infused anticoagulant or thrombolytic agents fail [112]. Also, local thrombolysis via a frontal burr hole has been described [107]. Endovascular local intrasinus thrombolysis is an increasingly applied intervention, but this modality carries an increased risk of hemorrhage [27]. A reasonable indication for endovascular therapy would seem to include thrombus propagation and clinical deterioration despite adequate anticoagulation and reduction in consciousness followed by seizures and hemiparesis [84]. The endovascular approach allows local sinus thrombolysis directly targeted into the thrombus and for mechanical disruption or aspiration of thrombus, both of which contribute to recanalization [84]. The most widely applied endovascular technique in combination with local thrombolysis is clot disruption, performed with angioplasty balloons, microwires, snares, or microcatheters [16, 24, 100, 115, 119]. Revascularization of the occluded sinuses by stent placement was also described [40, 58].

Several recent studies report on the successful use of the Angiojet rheolytic endovascular device, that works by creating a vacuum to fragment and aspirate the thrombus [27, 82, 136]. The use of the MERCI clot retrieval device was also applied for clot disruption in combination with thrombolysis [96]. The penumbra thrombectomy system is an alternative aspiration-debulking device [68]. Due to the relative rarity of the disease, more studies are required to establish the full role of invasive endovascular therapy in this patient population [68, 84].

21.4 Surgical Therapy of Neurobrucellosis with Intraparenchymal Cerebral Lesions

Intraparenchymal mass lesions mimicking a cerebral tumor, as a *B. melitensis* infection-associated syndrome, have been documented radiographically [37, 77, 80, 113]. In these cases, MRI revealed an enhanced lesion with vasogenic edema associated or not with midline shift and mass effect, interpreted as a cerebral tumor [37, 80, 113]. The patients were misdiagnosed as a brain tumor and underwent a surgical biopsy, with/without total excision of the lesions, or partial lobectomy [37, 39, 113]. The diagnosis of granulomatous or non-granulomatous encephalitis was made after the mass biopsy, but histopathologic studies did not reveal the organism in tissue sections [37, 39, 113]. Only in one case the definitive diagnosis of neurobrucellosis was made via bacterial isolation of *Brucella* in postoperative brain tissue specimen culture [113]. Residual areas of brain atrophy and focal neurological deficits are possible long-term complications [37, 39, 113].

Neurobrucellosis must be considered in the differential diagnosis of cerebral tumors, particularly in endemic areas, especially if the patient has a history of previous brucellosis. Patients having these lesions, with either granulomatous or non-granulomatous encephalitis, should be studied for brucellosis with blood and CSF cultures and serological tests [37].

21.5 Surgical Therapy of Spinal Neurobrucellosis

The intimate anatomical association of the spinal cord and the spinal nerve routes with the vertebral column renders spinal neurobrucellosis in a direct relationship with the various forms of vertebral brucellosis. Spinal involvement of brucellosis was first described in 1932 [92]. Spondylitis and spondylodiscitis are the most common forms of osteoarticular brucellosis with a reported incidence from 10 % up to 60 % in different studies [12, 30, 31, 36, 63, 98, 126, 127]. Other spinal clinical types are arthritis, osteomyelitis, and paravertebral and epidural abscess [33].

The most frequent area of involvement in spinal brucellosis is the lumbosacral region, followed by the thoracic and cervical segments [30, 31, 116, 126]. In rare occasions the disease may affect simultaneously different vertebral segments [137]. Spondylodiscitis is a very serious form of *Brucella* osteoarticular involvement [128]. *Brucella* reaches the spinal central nervous divisions via either hematogenous route or by direct extension from spondylitis [92]. It may spread up to the cervical spine via the CSF route [92]. Epidural abscess or granuloma, radiculoneuritis, myelitis, and demyelinating neuropathy are the most critical causes of morbidity [7, 17, 30, 128].

Significant progress has been made on the guidelines of conservative and surgical therapy, thanks to the evolution of accurate diagnostic tools such as MRI and fine operative techniques and the invention of sophisticated operative spine stabilization devices. Though spinal neurobrucellosis is not as fatal as in other conditions such as brain abscess, it is a serious factor of morbidity, chronic disability, and medical care cost.

Before outlining the indications of surgical treatment of spinal neurobrucellosis, there are some points regarding the disease which affect the timing and the outcome of surgery, and they must be kept in mind. The point of surgical intervention in spinal neurobrucellosis has been under debate [128]. Brucellosis has a slowly progressive course with unspecific symptoms [12].

Spinal neurobrucellosis usually responds well to combined antibiotic therapy even in cases with serious and progressive neurological symptoms, such as spastic paraparesis, and sphincter abnormalities in bowel and bladder functions [45, 60]. The extent of conservative treatment usually may vary from 8 weeks to 2 years [130]. This duration combined with the efficacy of modern conservative treatment is a factor which renders the timing of surgical intervention in question [12, 117].

A serious factor that has to be considered is that the therapeutic decisions are based on evidenced data which originate from a relatively small number of cases in the relevant literature. For example, 52 % of publications on spinal brucellosis out of a total number of 64 articles regarding 452 cases from 34 secondary or tertiary referral centers in Turkey were merely case reports [128]. It should also be noted that treatment recommendations for all types of bacteria causing spinal epidural abscess (which is one of the most aggressive complications of brucellar spondylodiscitis) are based on retrospective studies, case series, and expert opinions [108].

Laboratory information (55 % of blood cultures and 30–50 % of cultural tests of specimens from drained abscesses) may not be diagnostic for a long period of time [13, 48]. In many occasions there is a differential diagnostic dilemma from vertebral or intervertebral disk herniation (IVD), malignant tumors, and other infectious diseases such as spinal tuberculosis [13, 48, 133]. History of raw dairy product consumption, occupation dealing with livestock, and the geographical distribution of brucellosis are often the critical factors that guide the diagnostic investigation [13, 48, 128, 132]. All these factors set hurdles on the final decision of the surgical team that confronts with the neurobrucellosis patient in terms of diagnosis and choice of treatment.

MRI is the gold standard diagnostic method for the accurate assessment of the anatomy and topography of the lesions in spinal neurobrucellosis [128]. The characteristic radiological features of each lesion have been coded, whereas experience is increasing [128].

Some authors suggest immediate and aggressive surgical intervention, especially in epidural spine abscesses, in cases with severe neurological deficits (spinal instability, cord compression, radiculopathy, cauda equina syndrome, severe muscle weakness, progressive crumple), fearing a significant risk of sudden neurological deterioration and vertebral collapse during the period of treatment with antibiotics [2, 30, 31, 117, 135]. The authors of this mentality also support that prompt surgical therapy can prevent and decrease severity, that the combination of medical and surgical treatment is necessary to alleviate the disease and shorten the time of therapy, and that they leave conservative treatment with close observation in selected cases, particularly the elderly [31, 51, 133].

There are more roles of surgery in the confrontation with spinal neurobrucellosis. One of them is the palliation and reduction of the mass effect on the neighboring neural elements; as the lesions from *Brucella* microorganisms are slow growing, encapsulated, elastic in nature, moderately vascular, and firmly adhered to neural structures, the dissection is challenging, with a serious possibility of severe complication of CSF perioperative leakage [31]. There are also authors who suggested percutaneous drainage or aspiration of epidural and paravertebral abscesses instead of surgery [124].

As shown in the algorithm, the location of surgical intervention in the multidisciplinary and time-consuming effort of treatment is actually in the last raw of the relevant algorithm [128]. Nevertheless, surgeons are familiar with this position of their role as it is obvious from the last pages reserved for the surgical therapy in any major medical textbook (Fig. 21.2).

There are three main indications of surgical intervention: diagnosis through tissue and pus harvesting (culture, histology), decompression of the affected important neural structures by abscess and granuloma debridement, and stabilization of the spine. Detailed and rationalized presentation of the indications can be seen at the end of the section.

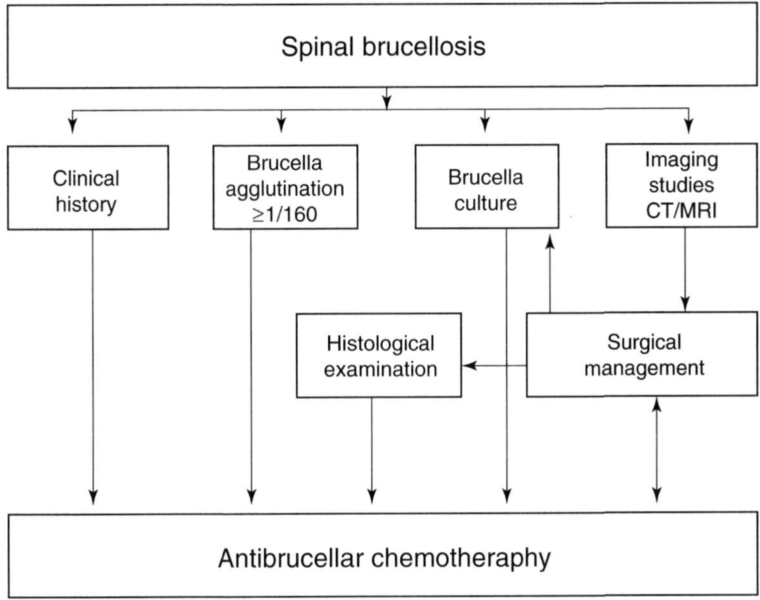

Fig. 21.2 Algorithm depicting the diagnosis, imaging, and treatment management pathway for spinal brucellosis (From Turgut et al. [128])

21.5.1 Different Forms of Spinal Brucellosis

21.5.1.1 Spondylodiscitis

Spinal cord compression is a complication of spondylodiscitis [125]. Involvement of the intervening IVD in addition to adjacent vertebral bodies is generally observed in MRI (Fig. 21.3) [12, 127]. Conservative treatment with a combination of antibiotics has been suggested as a sufficient option in many cases [12, 18, 70, 127]. However, there are conditions where surgical therapy has been considered mandatory. Incapacitating pain and severe neurological deficit often demand surgical intervention [61]. Lumbar laminectomy, drainage decompression, removal of epidural granulation tissue, and plate system stabilization are performed in cases of paraparesis, lumbar pain, and urinary incontinence [36]. There are various degrees of vertebral deterioration from mildly affected vertebral end plates to complete catastrophic destruction due to collapse of the affected vertebrae [30, 117, 135]. In the cases of acute spinal syndrome which may result, surgical intervention is mandatory to confront spinal instability, persistence or progression of neurological defect, and vertebral collapse. Debridement, cage screw construction, and stabilization have been reported [30, 117, 135].

21.5.1.2 Epidural Abscess

The epidural space is the most common area of abscess formation in spinal brucellosis, secondary to spondylodiscitis [9, 18, 129]. As in spinal epidural abscess caused by any microorganism, the management is multidisciplinary, involving spinal surgeons, radiologists, and infectious disease specialists, with drainage of the abscess and eradication of the microorganism considered the ultimate practice [108]. Laminectomy, hemilaminectomy, inferior laminectomy, and interlaminar fenestration are the preferred therapeutic surgical procedures for the drainage and decompression of lumbar epidural abscesses [31, 108, 120, 133]. Laminotomy has been proposed as an alternative operative technique for epidural abscesses in children [120]. Discectomy may be combined with laminectomy, which alternatively may be performed today with the use of microsurgery [92]. In the thoracic spine, as stability is maintained mostly by the rib cage, except the posterior approach with decompression and

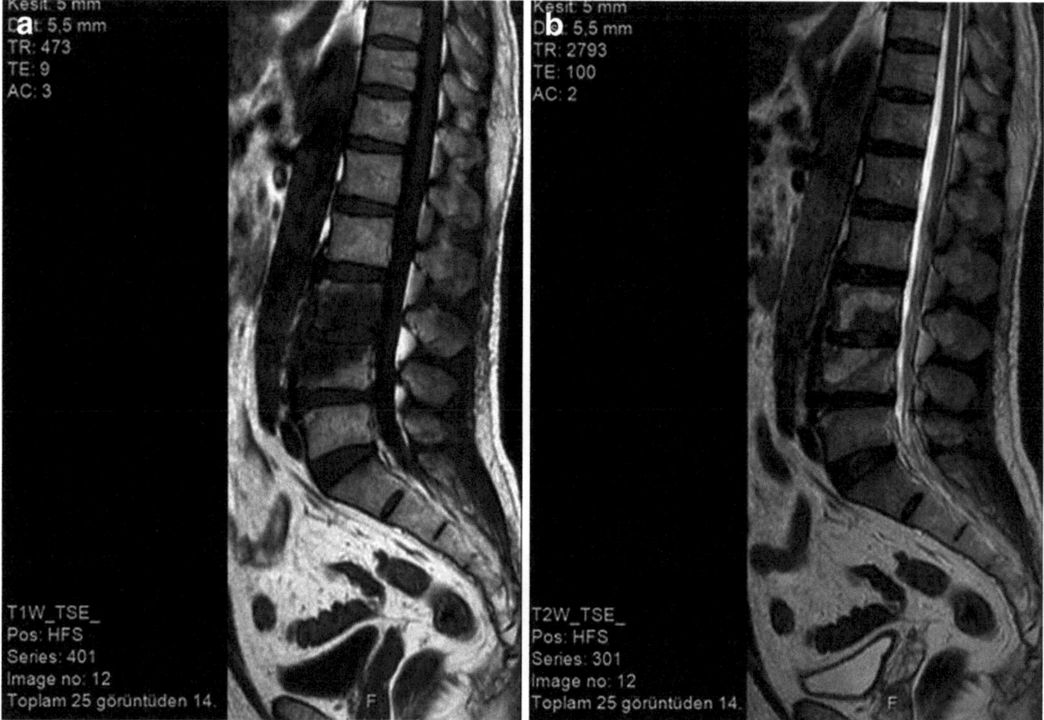

Fig. 21.3 Sagittal T1- (**a**) and T2- (**b**)weighted MRIs demonstrate brucellar involvement at the anterior surfaces of the L3 and L4 vertebrae. Note the presence of inflammatory reaction extended from L3 body through the disk space to L4 body (Courtesy of Y. Ozsunar, M.D.)

instrumentation, a purely anterior approach for decompression and fusion (transthoracic, posterolateral, or thoracoscopy) may be used for monosegmental lesions without involvement of posterior elements [35].

21.5.1.3 Paravertebral Abscess

Paravertebral abscess is a clinical presentation with potential neurological deterioration [23, 48, 76, 99]. A paravertebral *Brucella* abscess with spondylolysis and spondylolisthesis, initiated as discitis of the lumbosacral region, may be misdiagnosed and treated with peridural infiltration as lumbar sciatica (Fig. 21.4) [48]. Delayed pus draining surgery from the territory of the iliopsoas muscle was performed in such a case [48].

21.5.1.4 Intramedullary Abscess

Intramedullary abscess formation is a very rare condition. There are authors who performed conservative treatment with success. Bingol et al. [15] treated with antibiotics an intramedullary granuloma with surrounding edema with complete resolution of the disease, and Novati et al. [97] described the successful medical treatment of a focal abscess of 15 mm in diameter within the dorsal tract of the spinal cord. Early intervention is proposed for the prevention of neurological disability and achievement of improved functional outcome [130]. Multilevel T_{11}-L_2 laminectomy with limited myelotomy, purulent fluid drainage during abscess evacuation, and dura closure are reported in a case with lower limb disability and urinary incontinence [130]. An intramedullary dermoid in a boy was infected with *B. abortus*. At surgery multiple cavitary abscesses containing hair were drained. The patient responded well to surgical drainage and medical treatment [29]. A patient with a well-circumscribed intramedullary mass at T_{11} and T_{12} levels was drained and biopsied with considerable recovery after combined therapy with antibiotics [56].

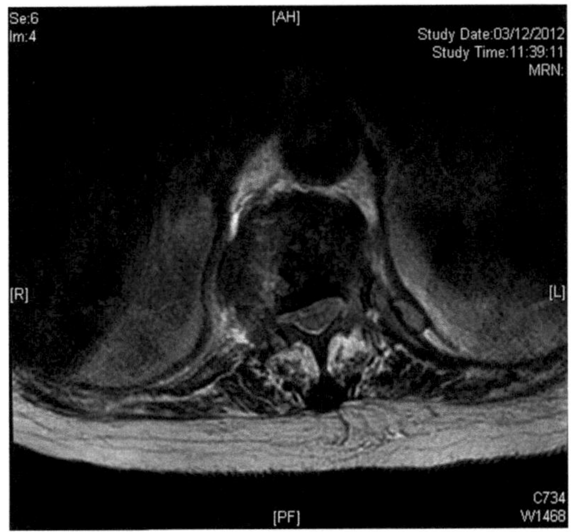

Fig. 21.4 Axial T2-weighted MRI shows paravertebral and muscle abscesses. Note the presence of medullary compression by T12 right pedicle (Courtesy of A. Cervan, M.D.)

21.5.1.5 Cervical Brucellosis

Cervical neurobrucellosis, though less frequent than lumbar and thoracic involvement, is accompanied by more severe manifestations, as a result of frequent inflammatory epidural masses with spinal cord compression and serious neurological disabilities [33, 47, 51, 67, 118]. A brucellar epidural abscess of cervical location is associated with a high incidence of devastating neurological complications [33].

Microscopic access to the anterior cervical spine by anterior approach, removal of a portion of the anterior longitudinal ligament and the involved IVDs, debridement of spinal infection, drainage of epidural abscess, and reconstruction are the methods preferred today for the cervical brucellosis [33]. Duarte added eventual corpectomy and fusion with bone graft and anterior plate [35]. He also suggested posterior cervical approach and posterior instrumentation for the cases of multilevel intervention and for those where involvement is mainly epidural with no severe destruction of the vertebral body [35]. Anterior cervical fusion is performed with an autogenous iliac strut bone graft and application of a halo vest for stabilization and prevention of autograft dislodgment [25, 33].

21.5.2 Minimal Invasive Surgery

Minimal invasive surgery is a modern and useful option [25]. Experience in video-assisted thoracoscopic surgery in other diseases has been proposed as an alternative therapeutic option in spinal infections, though debridement and instrumentation are technically demanding, with the use of special instruments with seldom use in other routine spine operations [52, 85, 92].

21.5.3 Grafting and Instrumentation

A consensus needed to be obtained is regarding the use of grafting and instrumentation in one- or two-stage surgery, in the cases of active infection. In the past surgeons preferred drainage and decompression in one stage and grafting and instrumentation in a second, because of the perceived risk of the residual bacterium contamination of the implants and persistence of the disease [25, 43]. Today, more and more authors adopt single-staged operation supporting the advantages of lower complication rate, shorter hospital stay, and earlier mobilization [25, 65, 66]. A classic bone graft with tricortical iliac autograft is recognized as a safe procedure, with excellent outcome [35]. Structural bone allograft can be used alternatively, avoiding donor site morbidity and reducing operative time [35, 75].

Conclusion

- The main treatment of brain abscess in neurobrucellosis is surgical, although medical therapy can be used for selected cases.
- The principal methods for surgical management involve freehand or endoscope-assisted aspiration of the pus with or without stereotactic guidance, drainage by craniotomy or craniectomy with or without intraoperative US guidance, or excision of the abscess.
- Today, aspiration of brain abscess has become the preferred method of surgical drainage.

- Aspiration is a rapid and safe procedure especially with the use of stereotactic CT guidance techniques.
- Surgical excision becomes mandatory if a peripherally placed abscess fails to respond to aspiration.
- Cerebellar abscesses are often an indication for posterior fossa craniotomy.
- Brain abscess due to brucellosis can still be fatal.
- Spinal brucellosis treatment is mainly conservative. Surgery is indicated for the drainage of paravertebral abscess, in anticipation of major anatomical deterioration and neurological deterioration.
- Surgery is also indicated when major neurological defects are present (spinal instability, cord compression, radiculopathy).
- Incapacitating pain and failure of conservative treatment in minimizing clinical symptoms may render surgical intervention necessary.
- If antibiotic treatment is chosen as initial therapy, the possibility of sudden neurological deterioration must be taken into account.
- The most important prognostic factor in recovery is the preoperative neurological status.
- Special attention should be given to the cervical neurobrucellosis, as morbidity is more serious than the other regions of the spine, and fine anterior access with microscopy is preferred instead of posterior access preferred elsewhere.
- Contrary to the high morbidity and mortality rates reported in the pyogenic or tuberculosis spondylodiscitis, the prognosis of *Brucella* spondylodiscitis is generally good with early diagnosis and adequate management.
- Finally, as stated in the section of the chapter on brucellar brain abscess, surgery is not only a therapeutic option but also allows confirmation of the diagnosis and the sampling of material for microbiological diagnosis and often reduces the duration of antibiotic treatment, the toxicity risk, the hospitalization rate, and the frequency of controls.

References

1. Adaletli I, Albayram S, Gurses B, Ozer H, Yilmaz MH, Gulsen F, Sirikci A (2006) Vasculopathic changes in the cerebral arterial system with neurobrucellosis. AJNR Am J Neuroradiol 27:384–386
2. Alp E, Doganay M (2008) Current therapeutic strategy in spinal brucellosis. Int J Infect Dis 12:573–577
3. Altekin RE, Karakas SM, Yanikoglou A, Ozbek SC, Akdemir B, Demitras H, Demirtas H, Deger N, Cekirge IS (2011) Aortic valve endocarditis and cerebral mycotic aneurysm due to brucellosis. J Cardiol Cases 4:e179–e182
4. Alvis Miranda H, Castellar Leones SM, Elzain MA, Moscote Salazar LR (2013) Brain abscess: current management. J Neurosci Rural Pract 4:S67–S81
5. Amiri RS, Hanif H, Ahmadi A, Amirjamshidi A (2014) Brucella-related multiple cerebral aneurysms: report of a case and review of the literature. Surg Neurol Int 21:152
6. Arlotti M, Grossi P, Pea F, Tomei G, Vullo V, De Rosa FG, Di Perri G, Nicastri E, Lauria FN, Carosi G, Moroni M, Ippolito G, GISIG (Gruppo Italiano di Studio sulle Infezioni Gravi) Working Group on Brain Abscesses (2010) Consensus document on controversial issues for the treatment of infections of the central nervous system: bacterial brain abscesses. Int J Infect Dis 14:S79–S92
7. Arslantas A, Kerimoglu A, Durmaz R, Cosan E, Atasoy M, Tel E (2002) Epidemiology and treatment of spinal infections. Annual meeting of Turkish Neurosurgical Society, Istanbul; Congress Book, PS 43, 03–08 June
8. Asadi H, Dowling R, Yan B, Wong S, Mitchell P (2015) Advances in endovascular treatment of acute ischemic stroke. Intern Med J 45:798–805. doi:10.1111/imj.12652
9. Ates O, Cayli SR, Kocak A, Kutlu R, Onal RE, Tekiner A (2005) Spinal epidural abscess caused by brucellosis. Neurol Med Chir 45:66–70
10. Ay S, Tur BS, Kutlay S (2010) Cerebral infarct due to meningovascular neurobrucellosis: a case report. Int J Infect Dis 14:e202–e204
11. Ayala-Gaytan JJ, Ortegon-Baqueiro H, de la Maza M (1989) Brucella melitensis cerebellar abscess. J Infect Dis 160:730–732
12. Aydin G, Tosun A, Keles I, Ayaslioglu E, Tosun O, Orkun S (2006) Brucellar spondylodiscitis: a case report. Int J Clin Pract 60:1502–1505
13. Aygen B, Doganay M, Sümerkan B, Yildiz O, Kayabas U (2002) Clinical manifestations, complications and treatment of brucellosis: a retrospective evaluation of 480 patients. Med Mal Infect 32:485–493
14. Bingöl A, Togay-Işikay C (2006) Neurobrucellosis as an exceptional cause of transient ischemic attacks. Eur J Neurol 13:544–548
15. Bingol A, Yucemen N, Meco O (1999) Medically treated intraspinal "Brucella" granuloma. Surg Neurol 52:570–576

16. Bishop FS, Finn MA, Samuelson M, Schmidt RH (2009) Endovascular balloon angioplasty for treatment of posttraumatic venous sinus thrombosis. Case report. J Neurosurg 111:17–21
17. Bodur H, Erbay A, Colpan A, Akinci E (2004) Brucellar spondylitis. Rheumatol Int 24:221–226
18. Boyaci A, Boyaci N, Tutoglu A, Dokumaci DS (2013) Spinal epidural abscess in brucellosis. BMJ Case Rep. pii: bcr2013200946. doi: 10.1136/bcr-2013-200946
19. Brydon HL, Hardwidge C (1994) The management of cerebellar abscess since introduction of CT scanning. Br J Neurosurg 8:447–455
20. Calik M, Iscan A, Gul M, Derme T, Cece H, Torun MF (2012) Severe neurobrucellosis in a young infant. Clin Neurol Neurosurg 114:1046–1048
21. Canale DJ (1996) William MacEwen and the treatment of brain abscesses: revisited after one hundred years. J Neurosurg 84:133–142
22. Carrasco-Moro R, García-Navarrete E, Pedrosa-Sánchez M, Pascual-Garvi JM, Minervini-Marín M, Sola RG (2006) Refractory epilepsy as the presenting symptom of a brucellar brain abscess. Rev Neurol 43:729–732
23. Cesur S, Ciftci A, Sōzen TH, Tekeli E (2003) A case of epididymo-orchitis and paravertebral abscess due to brucellosis. J Infect 46:251–253
24. Chaloupka JC, Mangla S, Huddle DC (1999) Use of mechanical thrombolysis via microballoon percutaneous transluminal angioplasty for the treatment of acute dural sinus thrombosis: case presentation and technical report. Neurosurgery 45:650–656
25. Chen WH, Jiang LS, Dai LY (2007) Surgical treatment of pyogenic vertebral osteomyelitis with spinal instrumentation. Eur Spine J 16:1307–1326
26. Choi CY, Datta NN (2000) Juxtapositioning of the temporalis muscle for intractable subdural empyema in infants. Surg Neurol 54:316–319
27. Chow K, Gobin YP, Saver J, Kidwell C, Dong P, Viñuela F (2000) Endovascular treatment of dural sinus thrombosis with rheolytic thrombectomy and intra-arterial thrombolysis. Stroke 31:1420–1425
28. Chun JY, Smith W, Halbach VV, Higashida RT, Wilson CB, Lawton MT (2001) Current multimodality management of infectious intracranial aneurysms. Neurosurgery 48:1203–1214
29. Çokça F, Meco O, Arasil E, Unlu A (1994) An intramedullary dermoid cyst abscess due to Brucella abortus biotype 3 at T11-L2 spinal levels. Case report. Infection 22:359–360
30. Colmenero JD, Reguera JM, Martos F, Sanchez-De-Mora D, Delgado M, Causse M, Martin-Farfân A, Juarez C (1996) Complications associated with Brucella melitensis infection: a study of 530 cases. Medicine (Baltimore) 75:195–211
31. Daglioglu E, Bayazit N, Okay O, Dalgic A, Hatipoglu HG, Ergungor F (2009) Lumbar epidural abscess caused by brucella species: report of two cases. Neurocirugia (Astur) 20:159–162
32. De Divitiis O, de Divitiis E (2012) Brain abscess: past and present. World Neurosurg 78:607–609
33. De Divitiis O, Elefante A (2012) Cervical spinal brucellosis. World Neurosurg 78:257–259
34. Ding D, Raper DM, Carswell AJ, Liu KC (2014) Endovascular stenting for treatment of mycotic intracranial aneurysms. J Clin Neurosci 21: 1163–1168
35. Duarte RM, Vaccaro AR (2013) Spinal infection: state of the art and management algorithm. Eur Spine J 22:2787–2799
36. El Mostarchid B, Okacha N, Akhddar A, Gazzaz M, Boucetta M (2008) Spinal cord compression caused by brucellar spondylitis. Pan Arab J Neurosurg 12:102–104
37. Erdem M, Namiduru M, Karaoglan I, Kecik VB, Aydin A, Tanriverdi M (2012) Unusual presentation of neurobrucellosis: a solitary intracranial mass lesion mimicking a cerebral tumor: a case of encephalitis caused by Brucella melitensis. J Infect Chemother 18:767–770
38. Erdogan B, Sener L, Ozsahin K, Savas L, Caner H (2005) An unusual case of ruptured distal anterior cerebral artery aneurysm associated with brucellosis. J Infect 51:e79–e82
39. Erdoğan E, Cansever T (2008) Pyogenic brain abscess. Neurosurg Focus 24, E2
40. Formaglio M, Catenoix H, Tahon F, Mauguière F, Vighetto A, Turjman F (2010) Stenting of a cerebral venous thrombosis. J Neuroradiol 37:182–184
41. Frazier JL, Ahn ES, Jallo GI (2008) Management of brain abscesses in children. Neurosurg Focus 24, E8
42. Fritsch M, Manwaring KH (1997) Endoscopic treatment of brain abscess in children. Minim Invasive Neurosurg 40:103–106
43. Fukuta S, Miyamoto K, Masuda T, Hosoe H, Kodama H, Nishimoto H, Sakaeda H, Shimizu K (2003) Two-stage (posterior and anterior) surgical treatment using posterior spinal instrumentation for pyogenic and tuberculotic spondylitis. Spine 28:E302–E308
44. Gadgil N, Patel AJ, Gopinath SP (2013) Open craniotomy for brain abscess: a forgotten experience? Surg Neurol Int 4:34
45. Gangi SMS, Roushan MRH, Janmohammadi N, Mehraeen R, Amiri MJS, Khalilian E (2012) Outcomes of treatment in 50 cases with spinal brucellosis in Babol, Northern Iran. J Infect Dev Ctries 6:654–659
46. Gorgan M, Neacsu A, Bucur N, Pruna V, Lipan C, Sandu AM, Cristescu CF (2012) Brain abscesses: management and outcome analysis in a series of 84 patients during 12 year period. Romanian Neurosurg 3:175–182
47. Gōrgulu A, Albayrak BS, Gorgulu E, Tural O, Karaaslan T, Oyar O, Yilmaz M (2006) Spinal epidural abscess due to Brucella. Surg Neurol 66:141–147
48. Guglielmino A, Sorbello M, Murabito O, Naimo J, Palumbo A, Lo Giudice E, Giuffrida S, Fazzio S, Parisi G, Mangiameli S (2007) A case of lumbar sciatica in a patient with spondylolysis and

spondylolysthesis and underlying misdiagnosed brucellar discitis. Minerva Anestesiol 73:307–312
49. Gul HC, Erdem H, Bek S (2009) Overview of neurobrucellosis: a pooled analysis of 187 cases. Int J Infect Dis 13:e339–e343
50. Gündeş S, Meriç M, Willke A, Erdenliğ S, Koç K (2004) A case of intracranial abscess due to Brucella melitensis. Int J Infect Dis 8:379–381
51. Guzey FK, Emel E, Sel B, Bas NS, Ozkan N, Karabulut C, Solak O, Esenyel M (2007) Cervical spinal brucellosis causing epidural and prevertebral abscesses and spinal cord compression: a case report. Spine J 7:240–244
52. Hadjipavlou AG, Katonis PK, Gaitanis IN, Muffoletto AJ, Tzermiadianos MN, Crow W (2004) Percutaneous transpendicular discectomy and drainage in pyogenic spondylodiscitis. Eur Spine J 13:707–713
53. Hakan T (2008) Management of bacterial brain abscesses. Neurosurg Focus 24, E4
54. Hall WA, Truwit CL (2008) The surgical management of infections involving the cerebrum. Neurosurgery 62:519–530
55. Hellwig D, Benes L, Bertalanfy H, Bauer BL (1997) Endoscopic stereotaxy-an eight years' experience. Stereotact Funct Neurosurg 68:90–97
56. Helvaci M, Kaslgra E, Çetin N, Yaprak I (2002) Intramedullary spinal cord abscess suspected of Brucella infection. Pediatr Int 44:446–448
57. Helweg-Larsen J, Astradsson A, Richhall H, Erdal J, Laursen A, Brennum J (2012) Pyogenic brain abscess, a 15 year survey. BMC Infect Dis 12:332
58. Hunt MG, Lee AG, Kardon K, Lesley WS, Chaloupka JC (2001) Improvement in papilledema and visual loss after endovascular stent placement in dural sinus thrombosis. Neuroophthalmology 26:85–92
59. Kamikawa S, Inui A, Miyake S, Kobayashi N, Kasuga M, Yamadori T, Tamaki N (1997) Neuroendoscopic surgery for brain abscess. Eur J Paediatr Neurol 1:121–122
60. Karaca S, Demiroglu YZ, Karatas M, Tan M (2007) Acquired progressive spastic paraparesis due to neurobrucellosis: a case report. Acta Neurol Belg 107:118–121
61. Katonis P, Tzermiadianos M, Gikas A, Papagelopoulos P, Hadjipavlou A (2006) Surgical treatment of spinal brucellosis. Clin Orthop Relat Res 444:66–72
62. Kimber J (2002) Cerebral venous sinus thrombosis. QJM 95:137–142
63. Kōkes F, Aciduman A, Günaydin A, Kinikli S (2007) A rare cause of "foot drop": spinal epidural Brucella granuloma. Turk Neurosurg 17:255–259
64. Kollias SS, Bernays RL (2001) Interactive magnetic resonance imaging-guided management of intracranial cystic lesions by using an open magnetic resonance imaging system. J Neurosurg 95:15–23
65. Korovessis P, Petsinis G, Koureas G, Iliopoulos P, Zacharatos S (2006) One stage combined surgery with mesh cages for treatment of septic spondylitis. Clin Orthop 444:51–59
66. Korovessis P, Sidiropoulos P, Piperos G, Karagiannis A (1993) Spinal epidural abscess complicated closed vertebral fracture: a case report and review of literature. Spine 18:671–674
67. Kose S, Senger SS, Çavdar G, Yavas S (2011) Case report on the development of a brucellosis-related epidural abscess. J Infect Dev Ctries 5:403–405
68. Kulcsár Z, Marosfõi M, Berentei Z, Szikora I (2010) Continuous thrombolysis and repeated thrombectomy with the Penumbra System in a child with hemorrhagic sinus thrombosis: technical note. Acta Neurochir (Wien) 152:911–916
69. Kumar A, Saeed H, Alamri A, Crocker M, Dave J (2011) Twenty years of intracranial abscesses: prognostic indicators and treatment review. J Infect 63:491–492
70. Lampropoulos C, Kamposos P, Papaioannou I, Niarou V (2012) Cervical epidural abscess caused by brucellosis. BMJ Case Rep 2012. pii: bcr2012007070. doi:10.1136/bcr-2012-007070
71. Landriel F, Ajler P, Hem S, Bendersky D, Goldschmidt E, Garategui L, Vecchi E, Konsol O, Carrizo A (2012) Supratentorial and infratentorial brain abscesses: surgical treatment, complications and outcomes-a 10-year single-center study. Acta Neurochir (Wien) 154:903–911
72. Lee TH, Chang WN, Su TM, Chang HW, Lui CC, Ho JT, Wang HC, Lu CH (2007) Clinical features and predictive factors of intraventricular rupture in patients who have bacterial brain abscesses. J Neurol Neurosurg Psychiatry 78:303–309
73. Longatti P, Perin A, Ettorre F, Fiorindi A, Baratto V (2006) Endoscopic treatment of brain abscesses. Childs Nerv Syst 22:1447–1450
74. Lu CH, Chang WN, Lui CC (2006) Strategies for the management of bacterial brain abscess. J Clin Neurosci 13:979–985
75. Lu DC, Wang V, Chou D (2009) The use of allograft or autograft and expandable titanium cages for the treatment of vertebral osteomyelitis. Neurosurgery 64:122–129
76. Malavolta N, Frigato M, Zanardi M, Mule R, Lisi L, Gnudi S, Fini M (2002) Brucella spondylitis with paravertebral abscess due to Brucella melitensis infection: a case report. Drugs Exp Clin Res 28:95–98
77. Martinez-Chamorro E, Muñoz EJ, Muñoz Giangaspro E (2002) Focal cerebral involvement by neurobrucellosis: pathological and MRI findings. Eur J Radiol 43:28–30
78. Mathisen GE, Johnson JP (1997) Brain abscess. Clin Infect Dis 25:763–779
79. Maurice-Williams RS (1987) Experience with 'open evacuation of pus' in the treatment of intracerebral abscess. Br J Neurosurg 1:343–351
80. Miguel PS, Fernández G, Vasallo FJ, Hortas M, Lorenzo JR, Rodriguez I, Ortiz-Rey JA, Anton I (2006) Neurobrucellosis mimicking cerebral tumor:

case report and literature review. Clin Neurol Neurosurg 108:404–406
81. Misra BK (2011) Management of brain abscess. World Neurosurg 75:612–613
82. Modi K, Misra V, Reddy P (2008) Rheolytic thrombectomy for dural venous sinus thrombosis. J Neuroimaging 19:366–369
83. Moorthy RK, Rajshekhar V (2008) Management of brain abscess: an overview. Neurosurg Focus 24, E3
84. Mortimer AM, Bradley MD, O'Leary S, Renowden SA (2013) Endovascular treatment of children with cerebral venous sinus thrombosis: a case series. Pediatr Neurol 49:305–312
85. Mückley T, Schütz T, Schmidt MH, Potulski M, Buhren V, Beisse R (2004) The role of thoracoscopic spinal surgery in the management of pyogenic vertebral osteomyelitis. Spine 29:E227–E233
86. Mut M, Dinç G, Naderi S (2007) On the report of the first successful surgical treatment of brain abscess in the Ottoman Empire by Dr. Cemil Topuzlu in 1891. Neurosurgery 61:869–872
87. Mut M, Hazer B, Narin F, Akalan N, Ozgen T (2009) Aspiration or capsule excision? Analysis of treatment results for brain abscesses at single institute. Turk Neurosurg 19:36–41
88. Muzumdar D (2011) Central nervous system infections and the neurosurgeon: a perspective. Int J Surg 9:113–116
89. Muzumdar D, Jhawar S, Goel A (2011) Brain abscess: an overview. Int J Surg 9:136–144
90. Nagpal RD (1983) Dural sinus and cerebral venous thrombosis. Neurosurg Rev 6:155–160
91. Nakahara I, Taha MM, Higashi T, Iwamuro Y, Iwaasa M, Watanabe Y, Tsunetoshi K, Munemitsu T (2006) Different modalities of treatment of intracranial mycotic aneurysms: report of 4 cases. Surg Neurol 66:405–409
92. Nas K, Güre A, Kemaloglu MS, Geyik MF, Cevik R, Büke Y, Ceviz A, Sarac AJ, Aksa Y (2001) Management of spinal brucellosis and outcome of rehabilitation. Spinal Cord 39:223–227
93. Nathoo N, Nadvi SS, Narotam PK, van Dellen JR (2011) Brain abscess: management and outcome analysis of a computed tomography era experience with 973 patients. World Neurosurg 75:716–726
94. Nathoo N, Narotam PK, Nadvi S, van Dellen JR (2012) Taming an old enemy: a profile of intracranial suppuration. World Neurosurg 77:484–490
95. Navdi SS, Parboosing R, Van Dellen JR (1997) Cerebellar abscess: the significance of cerebrospinal fluid diversion. Neurosurgery 41:61–67
96. Newman CB, Pakbaz RS, Nguyen AD, Kerber CW (2009) Endovascular treatment of extensive cerebral sinus thrombosis. J Neurosurg 110:442–445
97. Novati R, Vigano MG, De Bona A, Nocita B, Finazzi R, Lazzarin A (2002) Neurobrucellosis with spinal cord abscess of the dorsal tract: a case report. Int J Infect Dis 6:149–150
98. Ozgocmen S, Ardicoglu A, Kocakoc E, Kiris A, Ardicoglu O (2001) Paravertebral abscess formation due to brucellosis in a patient with ankylosing spondylitis. Joint Bone Spine 68:521–524
99. Papaioannides D, Giotis C, Korantzopoulos P, Akritidis N (2003) Brucellar spinal epidural abscess. Am Fam Physician 67:2071–2072
100. Philips MF, Bagley LJ, Sinson GP, Raps EC, Galetta SL, Zager EL, Hurst RW (1999) Endovascular thrombolysis for symptomatic cerebral venous thrombosis. J Neurosurg 90:65–71
101. Rajshekhar V (1992) Continuous impedance monitoring during CT-guided stereotactic surgery: relative value in cystic and solid lesions. Br J Neurosurg 6:439–444
102. Rappaport ZH, Vajda J (2002) Intracranial abscess: current concepts in management. Neurosurg Quart 12:238–250
103. Rosenblum ML, Hoff JT, Norman D, Weinstein PR, Pitts L (1978) Decreased mortality from brain abscesses since advent of computerized tomography. J Neurosurg 49:658–668
104. Sargent P (1928) Remarks on drainage of brain abscess. Br Med J 2:971–972
105. Sarmast AH, Showkat HI, Bhat AR, Kirmani AR, Kachroo MY, Mir SF, Lone YA, Khan AA (2012) Analysis and management of brain abscess; a ten year hospital based study. Turk Neurosurg 22:682–689
106. Sarmast AH, Showkat HI, Kirmani AR, Bhat AR, Patloo AM, Ahmad SR, Khan OM (2012) Aspiration versus excision: a single center experience of forty-seven patients with brain abscess over 10 years. Neurol Med Chir (Tokyo) 52:724–730
107. Scott JA, Pascuzzi RM, Hall PV, Becker GJ (1988) Treatment of dural sinus thrombosis with local urokinase infusion. Case report. J Neurosurg 68:284–287
108. Sendi P, Bregenzer T, Zimmerli W (2008) Spinal epidural abscess in clinical practice. Q J Med 101:1–12
109. Sharma BS, Gupta SK, Khosla VK (2000) Current concepts in the management of pyogenic brain abscess. Neurol India 48:105–111
110. Sharma BS, Khosla VK, Kak VK, Gupta VK, Tewari MK, Mathuriya SN, Pathak A (1995) Multiple pyogenic brain abscess. Acta Neurochir (Wien) 133:36–43
111. Shoshan Y, Maayan S, Gomori MJ, Israel Z (1996) Chronic subdural empyema: a new presentation of neurobrucellosis. Clin Infect Dis 23:400–401
112. Sindou M, Mercier P, Bokor J, Brunon J (1980) Bilateral thrombosis of the transverse sinuses: microsurgical revascularization with venous bypass. Surg Neurol 13:215–220
113. Sohn AH, Probert WS, Glaser CA, Gupta N, Bollen AW, Wong JD, Grace EM, McDonald WC (2003) Human neurobrucellosis with intracerebral granuloma caused by amarine mammal Brucella spp. Emerg Infect Dis 9:485–488
114. Solaroglu I, Kaptanoglu E, Okutan O, Beskonakli E (2003) Solitary extra-axial posterior fossa abscess

due to neurobrucellosis. J Clin Neurosci 10: 710–712
115. Soleau SW, Schmidt R, Stevens S, Osborn A, MacDonald JD (2003) Extensive experience with dural sinus thrombosis. Neurosurgery 52:534–544
116. Solera J, Lozano E, Martinez-Alfaro E, Espinosa A, Castilejos ML (1999) Brucellar spondylitis: review of 35 cases and literature survey. Clin Infect Dis 29:1440–1449
117. Solera J, Martinez-Alfaro E, Espinosa A (1997) Recognition and optimum treatment of brucellosis. Drugs 53:245–256
118. Song KJ, Yoon SJ, Lee KB (2012) Cervical spinal brucellosis with epidural abscess causing neurologic deficit with negative serologic tests. World Neurosurg 78(375):375e15–375e19
119. Stam J, Majoie CBLM, van Delden OM, van Lienden KP, Reekers JA (2008) Endovascular thrombectomy and thrombolysis for severe cerebral sinus thrombosis: a prospective study. Stroke 39:1487–1490
120. Starakis I, Solomou K, Konstantinou D, Karatza C (2009) Brucellosis presenting as spinal epidural abscess in a 41-year-old farmer: a case report. Cases J 2:7614
121. Stranjalis G, Singounas E, Boutsikakis I, Saroglou G (2000) Chronic intracerebral Brucella abscess. J Neurosurg 92:189
122. Tabatabai SA, Saberi H, Mehrazin M (2000) Intracranial suppuration following neurosurgical procedures due to brucella species. Med J Islamic Republic Iran 14:97–100
123. Tan WM, Adnan JS, Mohamad Haspani MS (2010) Treatment outcome of superficial cerebral abscess: an analysis of two surgical methods. Malays J Med Sci 17:23–29
124. Tekkok IH, Berker M, Ozcan OE, Ozgen T, Akalin E (1993) Brucellosis of the spine. Neurosurgery 33:838–844
125. Tur SB, Suldur N, Ataman S, Ozturk EA, Bingol A, Atay MB (2004) Brucellar spondylitis: a rare case of spinal cord compression. A case report. Spinal Cord 42:321–324
126. Turgut M, Çullu E, Sendur OF, Gulcan G (2004) Brucellar spine infection. Neurol Med Chir 44:562–567
127. Turgut M, Sendur OF, Gurel M (2003) Brucellar spondylodiscitis in the lumbar region. Case report. Neurol Med Chir 43:210–212
128. Turgut M, Turgut AT, Kosar U (2006) Spinal brucellosis: Turkish experience based on 452 cases published during the last century. Acta Neurochir 148:1033–1044
129. Ugarizza LF, Porras LF, Lorenzana LM, Rodriguez-Sanchez JA, Garcia-Yague LM, Cabezudo JM (2005) Brucellar spinal epidural abscesses. Analysis of eleven of cases. Br J Neurosurg 19:235–240
130. Vajramani GV, Nagmoti MB, Patil CS (2005) Neurobrucellosis presenting as an intra-medullary spinal cord abscess. Ann Clin Microbiol Antimicrob 4:14
131. Wakamoto H, Tomita H, Tabuse M, Miyazaki H, Ishiyama N (2001) Aspiration and drainage for a gas-producing brain abscess causing delayed bleeding from the abscess capsule. A case report. No Shinkei Geka 29:445–449
132. Yetkin MA, Bulut C, Erdinc FS, Oral B, Tulek N (2006) Evaluation of the clinical presentations in neurobrucellosis. Int J Infect Dis 10:446–452
133. Yuksel KZ, Senoglu M, Yuksel M, Gul M (2006) Brucellar spondylodiscitis with rapidly progressive spinal epidural abscess presenting with sciatica. Spinal Cord 44:805–808
134. Zaidan R, Al Tahan AR (1999) Cerebral venous thrombosis: a new manifestation of neurobrucellosis. Clin Infect Dis 28:399–400
135. Zakaria AH, Al-share B, Al-Yacoub MA (2014) Acute spinal syndrome due to thoracic vertebral brucellosis: a case report. J Neuroinfect Dis 5:2
136. Zhang A, Collinson RL, Hurst RW, Weigele JB (2008) Rheolytic thrombectomy for cerebral sinus thrombosis. Neurocrit Care 9:17–26
137. Zormpala A, Skopelitis E, Thanos L, Artinopoulos C, Kordossis T, Sipsas NV (2000) An unusual case of brucellar spondylitis involving both the cervical and lumbar spine. Clin Imaging 24:273–275

Conclusion

Brucellosis represents a rare zoonotic disease due to *Brucella* species, whose incidence rate is actually declining worldwide; still, it is endemic in several areas along the Mediterranean basin, South Asia, and South America. As a matter of fact, it involves both the central and peripheral nervous systems in its most severe form, i.e., neurobrucellosis causing a conspicuous number of patients to develop neurological disabilities, especially when not diagnosed and treated on time.

Owing to that, the aim of this book is to provide the reader with a backbone of symptoms and signs of this entity in an attempt to reveal and identify neurobrucellosis at the earliest stage and thus prevent late effects on different parts of the central and peripheral nervous systems. Indeed, this protean disease may involve the nervous system at different levels and severity, although seldomly the brain and/or the spinal cord is involved if the disease has already spread elsewhere.

As a general rule, the diagnosis of neurobrucellosis should be suspected in cases with neurological deficits, especially in endemic countries. Cogent medical treatment should be administered as soon as possible, while surgery should be reserved for those cases which are not prone to medical therapy and/or in those cases with neurobrucellosis that seriously impairs neurological functions and/or represents a clinical emergency or is life threatening.

M. Turgut et al. (eds.), *Neurobrucellosis: Clinical, Diagnostic and Therapeutic Features*,
DOI 10.1007/978-3-319-24639-0

Index

M. Turgut et al. (eds.), *Neurobrucellosis: Clinical, Diagnostic and Therapeutic Features*,
DOI 10.1007/978-3-319-24639-0

9783319246376